THE WAR
ON PAIN

THE WAR ON PAIN

S COTT F ISHMAN , M.D.

with L ISA B ERGER

Quill

An Imprint of HarperCollins*Publishers*

A hardcover edition of this book was published in 2000 by HarperCollins Publishers.

THE WAR ON PAIN. Copyright © 2000 by Scott Fishman, M.D., with Lisa Berger. All rights reserved. Printed in the United States of America. No part of this book may be used or reproduced in any manner whatsoever without written permission except in the case of brief quotations embodied in critical articles and reviews. For information address HarperCollins Publishers Inc., 10 East 53rd Street, New York, NY 10022.

HarperCollins books may be purchased for educational, business, or sales promotional use. For information please write: Special Markets Department, HarperCollins Publishers Inc., 10 East 53rd Street, New York, NY 10022.

First Quill edition published 2001.

Designed by Jessica Shatan

The Library of Congress has catalogued the hardcover edition as follows:

Fishman, Scott.
    The war on pain: how breakthroughs in the new field of pain medicine are turning the tide against suffering/Scott Fishman, with Lisa Berger—1st ed.
        p.cm.
    "A Living planet book."
    Includes index.
    ISBN 0-06-019297-6
     1. Pain—Popular works. 2. Chronic pain—Popular works. 3. Holistic medicine.
    4. Analgesia. 5. Pain—Alternative treatment. 6. Mind and body therapies. I. Berger, Lisa.
    II.Title.

RB127 .F57 2000
616'.0472—dc21   99-042965

ISBN 0-06-093078-0 (pbk.)

01 02 03 04 05 ❖/RRD 10 9 8 7 6 5 4 3 2 1

CONTENTS

FOREWORD
by Thomas Moore

Let me say from the start that if my child, my wife, or my friend were in pain, I would do almost anything to lessen their suffering. It is the noblest gift of human life to feel compassion for another and in a way, all of human activity comes down to this one issue: responding to the suffering of others. The Buddha focused the heart of his wisdom, the Four Noble Truths, around the theme of suffering. Jesus demonstrated his spiritual teaching by healing the physical and emotional suffering he encountered on his path. And in this useful book, Dr. Scott Fishman brings his experience, his expertise in many medical areas, and his compassion to bear on understanding pain and treating chronic suffering.

I come to suffering not as a physician, but, to use language favored in the Renaissance, as a doctor of the soul, and I would like to speak for the soul as it is present in pain and in healing. For human beings there is no such thing as a plain fact. Each person in pain experiences that pain in a particular way that to him has a special meaning. This meaning may not be fully conscious, but it is present. It tends to be experienced as narrative, a fragment of a story or an image. Usually, with a little encouragement, a person in pain will be willing to tell the story of his experience. As a soul doctor, I am interested in these stories, for they tell how the person is experiencing the pain, not just sensing it.

Whenever I have to think about medicine and healing, I turn to a doctor from the sixteenth century, Paracelsus, who has remarkable things to say about illness and treatment, things that we have forgotten in our technological age. For example, Paracelsus says that all illnesses can be cured, without exception. But, he says, to effect these cures we must get to the essence of our pain and not just the symptoms. We have to treat not just the mortal body, but the eternal body as well. I'm sure this challenging statement could be read in many ways, including highly spiritual ones. But I take it to mean that we human beings are never only hunks of physical flesh. Certainly the body considered physically is wondrously complex and miraculous in its workings, but a human being is more than this physical body. We are persons with constant thoughts, memories, associations, anxieties, and hopes. We are connected people, with families, friends, and neighbors. When we lie in pain, we are still concerned about beauty, justice, and love.

A physician, too, is filled with images as he goes about his work of dealing with pain. He lives in a specific culture, comes with a particular family story, and has a complex personality as well. Although we healers may go about our work as though the imagination were not present, it is, and it may hold the key to our success in curing every illness and alleviating every pain. As the pages of this book reveal, the humanity, imagination, and creativity which Dr. Fishman brings to his healing is critical to his success.

Modern medicine currently appears to be pushing the envelope of our materialistic view of the human body. We are relatively free in our use of so-called "alternative medicines," and we are beginning to see the importance of lifestyle in relation to health. But although we have far surpassed Paracelsus in the physical science and technology of health and treatment, we have a long way to go towards seeing our suffering in a larger context.

What is the essence of our illness? Perhaps ultimately we suffer from the way we picture life. We don't complain about the poisons around us and in us. We don't respond seriously to suffering children. And yet we expect modern medicine to do a constantly better job of ridding us of pain. Perhaps it is time to open our minds to the essence of our illness as a society. When I allow my imagination to soar and move beyond the confines of current approaches to health, I foresee hospitals designed not for treating the material body but for responding to whole, complicated, imagining persons. From Dr. Fishman's descriptions of the frontiers of Pain Medicine, I expect medicine one day to become as sophisticated about the interplay of emotion and physical symptoms as we are today about imaging and surgery.

For now, I am pleased to say a word in praise of Dr. Fishman's dedication to the alleviation of pain. He applies both highly technical skill, within the mythology of our time, along with a flexible and caring vision. I have seen him firsthand as he gently tries to stretch the mind of modern medicine in highly technical contexts, and I feel rare confidence as I read his advice for I sense that he is moving in the direction of my Paracelsian ideal. Pacifist that I am, seeped in the unbelligerent imagery of Taoism, I admit that I worry some about his root metaphor of conducting a war on pain. Yet Paracelsus himself refers to pain as the enemy, and there is a long, valuable tradition in the religions of the world about the spiritual warrior. Perhaps a physician has to have the spirit of the war-gods and goddesses in him as well as the strong but peaceable Christ-healer. As I know from my own experience as a psychotherapist, if you don't have a warrior spirit, you will be overcome, and certainly working with pain does require courage and forcefulness.

We are all called to be healers, whether it is bandaging a child's injured finger or suggesting medication for a spouse's migraine. Our doctors help us to heal each other, and ourselves. Dr. Fishman's book is one I want to keep at hand to help me deal with pain wherever I encounter it. I hope his excellent drawing together of effective responses to pain will inspire the reader to be a healer. We can all renew our compassion and take more seriously our call to work caringly on behalf of those who are suffering. We can also be more radical about our way of life, educating ourselves in those things that contribute to pain and changing our lifestyle where needed. The Hindu scriptures say, "At least do not contribute to the unconsciousness of the time." If we were to be creative individuals, taking full responsibility for making a world in which pain is mitigated, we would enjoy at least the internal rewards of a compassionate life.

The ultimate war on pain is the toughest of them all—shifting out of the self-destructive mind-set of our consumerist, self-focused culture, and recovering a profound sense of mutuality and community. Our pain is a signal asking us to change the way we live as a society. In Dr. Scott Fishman we have a model of compassion in a technological setting. We could all help alleviate pain by allowing our compassion to come first and our personal comforts second. Pain is a language. It says that something is wrong. If we are to be healers, we have to heed the pain around us and dare to respond with a strong caring style—and yes, a militant attitude.

INTRODUCTION

Pain is something we all know about. Our first lessons begin at birth, and we quickly learn enough about pain to steer clear of it. Ordinarily, pain is something that looms in the background but doesn't interfere with our lives. But for people in chronic pain, life is a very different place. On any given day in my pain management clinic, I see chronic pain debilitate and isolate its victims while it devastates families, relationships, and careers. A staggering number of people suffer chronic pain—by conservative estimates, it afflicts well over 10 percent of the population, leaving tens of millions disabled. The economic cost to society is immense, but the cost in suffering is immeasurable.

Understanding pain—and translating that knowledge into strategies for overcoming and coping with it—has been my continuing challenge, and is the subject of this book. As a physician who specializes in pain medicine, I see the many faces of pain every day. I may be called on to treat a child with burns, someone recovering from surgery or a car accident, an eighty-year-old with terminal cancer, or a person afflicted with chronic pain, often of unknown cause. The common denominator for these people is suffering. By the time patients arrive at my office, they have frequently sought help from multiple doctors at numerous hospitals and clinics and been shunted from one specialist to another. Despite batteries of tests and an exhausting stream of medications, suffering continues while they clash with a new adversary: a medical culture that is largely ill prepared to cope with chronic pain. Too often they understandably feel that the medical system has failed them.

In contrast to the suffering it brings, pain offers a rare perspective on one of the most important features of being human: the connection between body and mind. Pain is a consummate mind-body event where sensation and emotion become inextricably intertwined; it is impossible to say where the realm of physical pain ends and psychic suffering begins. While this makes pain difficult to combat, it is also what makes it one of the most fascinating aspects of the human condition.

Throughout history, mankind has struggled to defeat pain. But no different than our ancestors, we continue to live in a world where pain is possible at any moment. In every culture and in every era throughout time, shamans, doctors, and theologians have experimented with almost every conceivable therapy for pain, from herbal remedies to faith healing. Because it renders us powerless, often robbing us of our happiness, our identity, our very humanity, pain has remained our most feared and, until recently, unassailable enemy.

Dramatic breakthroughs in neuroscience in the past few years have revolutionized our understanding of the way our brains process sensation and emotion. In just the past decade, pain medicine has developed into an exciting and fast-moving medical specialty; interdisciplinary pain centers have sprung up around the country and around the world; pharmaceutical companies and research centers are racing to develop new classes of painkillers at an unprecedented rate. But despite this progress, there is much we still don't know about pain. Such mysteries make pain a tantalizing phenomenon. It beckons with mysteries and myths, and with the possibility of riches and rewards, should it be mastered.

As a physician who routinely treats the most difficult pain cases in my medical community, I try to cultivate an inclusive, open-minded, and pragmatic approach to treating pain. Everything that's safe and works is in play—and an astounding range of techniques *do* work, from acupuncture to surgical nerve blocks, from common analgesics to opioids, from psychiatric drugs to cognitive behavioral therapies. We still don't know why some of these agents work. But for the patients I treat, whose quality of life has become intolerable, results are what matter, first and foremost.

In choosing to specialize in this new field, I understood that I would be grappling with pain's physical devastation and, equally important, helping to ease patients' suffering. To prepare, I studied internal medicine and trained in psychiatry as well as pain management through anesthesiology. The battle with pain would demand that I bring together often disparate treatments and incorporate the most effective tools of physical and psychiatric medicine, surgical and anesthetic interventions, and a range of cognitive and alternative therapies. But despite my diverse medical background, on many days I still don't feel broadly enough trained for every nuance of my job. As I have immersed myself in pain medicine, I have learned that while it is a distinct specialty, it requires the breadth and versatility of an old-fashioned family physician who's ready to treat the widest variety of problems at any given time.

The War on Pain offers a view of the new collective artillery that we can use to counter the destructive effects of pain throughout the body and mind. It presents a hopeful appraisal of how far we've come and what we can expect to achieve in the near future. This approach combines the best of technology with the growing understanding of the whole person while remaining open to the many mysteries and possibilities of how we work and how we may help ourselves to heal. It respects the place of pain as an essential part of normal human life, a part we can't live without but to which we need not surrender.

Throughout this book, I'll take you behind the scenes at some of the country's leading pain centers to meet an array of health-care professionals who are fighting on the front lines of the war on pain. And I'll depict the many faces of pain by narrating the personal journeys of real patients. While many of the specific details of their lives have been changed to protect their individual identities, the essence of their genuine experiences is portrayed as a foundation for understanding why pain goes awry and how it can be subdued. Thus, the book is divided into two parts, initially describing the many problems pain can cause (Part I) and then the many solutions (Part II).

I hope that after reading *The War on Pain* you will feel armed with enough information—and perhaps inspiration—to enter any level of health care as your own best advocate against pain and suffering. This book is for the tens of millions of people afflicted by pain and for the many millions of healthy people who suffer along with a loved one in pain. It is for anyone curious about how our sum of molecules and cells is capable of feeling the world around us. It is for all of us in awe of how human beings can feel pain and then overcome it.

SCOTT FISHMAN, M.D.
Chief, Division of Pain Medicine
University of California, Davis

PART I

THE ANATOMY OF PAIN AND SUFFERING

Charting Its Pathways Through Mind and Body

Effectively confronting pain requires two distinct sets of information: an understanding of what pain is and knowing what to do about it. You may think that remedies are all you really need to know, but without an appreciation of the widespread causes of pain that span the mind-body continuum, you'll be operating under the same misconceptions that have so ill served mankind throughout the ages. Only recently have we understood enough about this enemy within us to take the upper hand. As the labyrinth of sensation and emotion becomes more and more visible to scientists, we've been able to develop increasingly effective strategies for penetrating to the sources of pain and suffering, and disarming them.

In his classic book, *The Art of War,* the ancient Chinese warrior Sun-tzu declared, "Know the enemy and know yourself; in a hundred battles, you will never be defeated." In that spirit, the first half of this book examines the anatomy of pain in all its forms and explores its pathways through the body and mind.

The first chapter shows how pain, an elementary part of being human, serves a vital evolutionary function. You'll read about the kind of pain that acts as an alarm, alerting you to bodily damage and dangers that could threaten your survival. Chapter 2 will uncover some of the secrets of acute pain—the variety that assaults all of us from time to time—and give a brief historical perspective on how previous generations have grappled with it, including the modern era's first big victory over pain, the discovery of anesthesia. Chapter 3 takes us deeper into enemy territory, focusing on chronic pain through the stories of people who have suffered from back pain. As its name suggests, chronic pain persists long after normal healing and treatment should have eradicated it. The type of chronic pain featured in chapter 4 is especially insidious because it attacks individual nerve fibers or entire nerve pathways. In chapter 5 you'll travel to the command center in charge of all pain sensation: the brain. The brain determines when, if, and how you feel pain, and defines the nature of your pain as well. This chapter helps explain why the brain and the mind are always involved in chronic pain. Chapter 6 shows how the body and brain are capable of controlling and defeating even the most excruciating sensations by manufacturing their own painkilling chemicals.

1

WHY PAIN HURTS
The Anatomy of Ouch

Illness is the doctor to whom we pay most heed. To kindness, to knowledge, we make promises only. Pain we obey.
—MARCEL PROUST

You know what acute pain feels like. The stubbed toe, the burned finger, the scraped knee. It's an inevitable and universal part of the
human experience, an unpleasant sensation that seizes your attention
and demands treatment. As Proust astutely observed, pain is a tyrant
whose commands everyone is impelled to obey. Yet much of what pain
commands is for your own good. While pain may seem like your
adversary, it's also your protector and ally of health. Most people know
from experience that you ignore pain at your own peril. You must pay
attention to it or risk further physical harm.

When I talk to patients about pain, I frequently compare it to a
sophisticated alarm system designed to protect you from impending
damage, as essential to your survival as eating and sleeping. Ordinary
pain, what doctors call *acute* pain, is a barometer of tissue health. Like
a warning system around the edge of a house, it raises an alarm when
it has been breached and you have been injured, alerting you to potential danger and the need for help.

Pain is a daily reminder that we are little more than a fragile collection of cells and fluids that can be easily pierced, burned, torn, or broken.
Unlike many of nature's other creatures, we have no armor, no rough

scales or thick hides to protect us from assault. All we have is our skin, a surface area of about twenty-one square feet composed of microscopically thin layers of cells that not only protect us from invasion by microorganisms but, more importantly, contain millions of sensory nerves specially designed to detect all sorts of sensations, including pain.

Paradoxically, this delicate epidermal perimeter *is* your body armor; your ability to feel pain enables you to avoid or survive life-threatening incursions on your body. Without pain, you would be in constant danger of fatally harming yourself and would not be aware of when you need medical attention. Acute pain is the reason most people seek out a doctor—after a sports injury, a car accident, a mishap in the home, a change in our health, after suffering fractures, sprains, strains, lacerations, wounds, contusions, and burns. According to government experts, Americans experience about sixty-four million such injuries a year. Most people experience acute pain about four times a year, usually lasting between one and five days.

If you have any doubts about pain's role as your protector and ally, consider what happens to people who don't feel pain. People suffering from a rare syndrome called congenital analgesia are born without innate pain sensors, leaving them senseless to any kind of physical assault. The story of Edward Gibson, who called himself "the Human Pincushion," is portrayed in the fascinating book *The Culture of Pain*. Gibson performed in vaudeville shows in the 1920s where twice a day he invited audiences to stick needles into him. Each day, they pushed in fifty or sixty pins up to their heads, yet Gibson felt nothing.

People like Gibson can tear tendons, twist ligaments, even break bones and feel close to nothing. They are constantly hurting themselves without knowing it. They burn their skin, suffer damage to internal organs, and live with dangerous infections completely unaware of the danger they are in. Not surprisingly, most of these people usually die by the time they reach their thirties, often from unfelt injuries. Unlike most of us, they don't have knee pain that says "lay off" or chest pain that might warn of a heart attack.

DECODING THE ANATOMY OF "OUCH!"

When I'm treating a patient, I often begin with the question "Where does it hurt?" But understanding a patient's pain really begins with another question: "What is pain?" There are many answers—all true, and all incomplete. Pain has many definitions because it's an intensely subjective experience that we filter through our emotions as well as our bodies. It's any sensation amplified to an uncomfortable level, and it's a constellation of negative emotions called "suffering." When you feel pain, there is much more going on than just nerves signaling the message "Ouch!" If you've lived with any sort of chronic pain, you know that "Ouch!" is a complicated phenomenon that quickly can turn a constant, unpleasant sensation into a life in pain.

Because pain is an intangible sensation, it challenges doctors and patients alike to describe and fathom it. It's usually a symptom, not a disease. I can't see it under a microscope or in a blood test. It's not an event, like a heart attack, that concentrates on a single organ or system in the body. And it's not solely an emotional or cognitive phenomenon, like a mental illness. Yet, pain is all these things, and more.

Compounding the riddle is the subjective nature of pain. There is no single accepted pain experience—no one feels it the same. Like the perception of beauty, it's very real, but only in the eye of the beholder. What hurts me may not hurt you. "Pain is what the patient says it is" is one of the few definitive, universal statements about pain. What is the difference between a patient who complains of the pain from losing a leg or the pain from losing a loved one? I hold emotional distress and physical torment to be equally painful experiences. I often see patients who claim a physical cause for their pain yet also tell me about great psychic pain, such as deep depression. Pain comprises a wide spectrum of feelings and is as individual as our fingerprint. Pain's inherently emotional quality is what makes it so difficult to define. Emotions like sadness, fear, anxiety, and anger, as well as childhood memories, all contribute to the landscape of pain.

TALKING ABOUT PAIN

If you've ever talked to a doctor about a persistent pain, you know how frustrating it can be. Talking about pain represents a huge challenge: What words can describe an experience that, for many people, is so intense that it defies language? One of the intriguing features of pain is that people all have a slightly different perspective on it, and these varying viewpoints are reflected in the language they use to describe these experiences. I frequently hear patients utter noises to convey what they are feeling. Or they resort to the tools of poetry like onomatopoeia, in which words sound like the experience they express, like "sizzle" or "zap." One of pain medicine's standard methods for assessing a child's pain involves not words but pictures of faces in various stages of pleasure or distress. Pain forces you to be imaginative and creative in the words you use to talk about it.

In recent years, doctors and nurses have begun to inquire more than ever into a patient's pain level as an indicator of general health. Understanding your pain means going beyond the purely physical. You may have encountered a doctor asking about your feeling of well-being and whether you are in any physical or mental distress. In short, are you suffering in any way? To quantify this feeling, a doctor might ask you to rate your pain or suffering on a one-to-ten scale (one being no pain and ten the most pain imaginable) and note this on a chart. As with the other vital signs, this gives the doctor a starting point or baseline for tracking any changes. What's most often helpful about this measurement is not necessarily the number you assign to your pain but whether it goes up or down over time. On its own, a pain rating of six might mean very noticeable pain or moderate, bearable pain, depending on the individual. Yet, if it quickly shifts to a nine, your doctor knows that your health has worsened.

Pain is so fundamental to your well-being, as both an alarm for protecting you and as a red flag signaling unseen damage, that it is sometimes called the "fifth vital sign." You've probably heard of vital signs, those four basic measures of a person's health: blood pressure, pulse rate, temperature, and respiration. If one of these vital signs is off, doctors surmise that something may be wrong with a patient's health. As an acknowledged vital sign, pain offers doctors valuable insight into a patient's general state of wellness or illness.

THINKING ABOUT PAIN

Most patients resort to using metaphors to describe how pain feels and how that feeling travels through their bodies and psyches. If you say that a headache feels like a sledgehammer, everyone knows exactly what you're feeling. Metaphor offers rich visual images of pain's power as well as insights into its illusive nature. Doctors also need metaphors to deal with pain. Let me give you a brief tour of the discoveries and resulting metaphors that have shaped doctors' evolving understanding of pain.

Pain Pathways: The Rope and Bell

One of the first modern notions of how pain moves through the body was the concept of nerve pathways. Until the mid-seventeenth century, doctors believed that all pain was felt in the heart. However, the philosopher and scientist René Descartes focused his studies on the anatomy and physiology of the senses. He is famous for having developed the idea of pain pathways. Descartes believed that pain was a unique sensation, separate from touch or other senses, that operated on its own sensory highway. He envisioned numerous threads or fibers forming nerves that ran between the skin and areas of the brain. Descartes' metaphor for how pain signals travel from the injury site to the brain is a rope pulling on a bell.

Considering that Descartes' methods of exploration were limited to crude microscopes and dissected cadavers, his concept of the sensory nervous system was wonderfully advanced. Pain *does* travel along pathways of nerves, although not along a single primary interstate, so to speak, but via two main routes: the central nervous system involving the brain and spinal cord and the peripheral nervous system involving everything else. These two main routes fan into many more pathways and numerous intersections, detours, and feedback and feed-forward loops. Imagine the most complex urban highway system and complicate it many times more. The pain system is more complex than science can fully comprehend at present.

Although science is still refining the pathways theory—and especially learning more about what happens at the central command station, the brain—the freeways-of-pain metaphor says much about the nature of pain. It illustrates that pain is not a static event but a process. It moves from point to point along any number of paths and is shaped and defined as it reaches certain nerve intersections. Lately, scientists have been even more surprised to find that pain can change the organization of nerve cells, having an impact on your health far beyond what they previously thought.

A Magnifying Glass on Sensation

A competing concept of pain at the time of Descartes was the intensive theory, which described pain as any sensation that had become magnified. Imagine the pleasant sensation of putting your hand in warm water. But as hot water is added, the heat and sensation are intensified to the point that you feel pain. The intensive theory was based on Aristotle's notion of pain as excessive sensitivity, mainly to heat and touch. Nineteenth-century scientists expanded the concept to all the senses. The idea of pain as a magnifying glass applied to any sensory experience persists today and provides yet another perspective on the mystery of pain.

If you think of pain as a magnifying glass that can distort any sensory experience, then you begin to understand why everyone feels it differently. Each individual has specially ground magnifying glasses that amplify some sensations and reduce others. The magnifying-glass metaphor explains not only the subjective nature of pain but also suggests that each person has a slightly different glass, or put another way, a slightly different pain tolerance. We're all aware of our different pain tolerances, not only from person to person but within ourselves. A tolerable pain one day can be intolerable the next. Patients frequently tell me that sometimes an injection really hurts, but a week later the same shot feels like a mere pinch. This is a great example of how your mind and body interact to influence how you feel pain. The mind-body collaboration can either magnify or demagnify your perception of pain. You can unconsciously amplify pain or consciously push it from the center of your consciousness. If you're in pain, this is heartening news. It means that you possess the ability, somewhere within the complex network of your mind-body connection, to transform pain into either less pain or no pain. Although I have found that patients often feel that treatments to harness the mind's ability to "demagnify" pain are somehow less than legitimate, these are powerful tools for pain management that I'll explain later.

The equation can be flipped, too. Too much sensation can magnify pain. The sensation may be a strong emotion, like anxiety, which can worsen physical pain. Think of how a simple hangover makes any loud noise less bearable, the stress of daily life harder to cope with, and any ache or pain seem less manageable. A bad mood can activate the same magnifying effect.

The Gateway and the Gatekeeper

The gateway, suggesting a neurological gate at the entrance to the brain and in the spinal cord, is a more recent metaphor for pain. The gate control theory, which was developed in the mid-1960s by Patrick Wall and Ronald Melzack, gave a big boost to pain medicine because it helped explain some of the more vexing puzzles of pain and became the basis for developing new drugs and treatments.

According to this theory, neurochemical signals open and close the gateway to the brain, regulating which pain signals get in, and when. Picture a gate that is controlled not by what's on the outside knocking to come in but by a command center on the inside, directing the gate to admit only certain sensations. By barring some sensations, the gate-keeper—your central nervous system, comprising the brain and spinal cord—enables you to filter out some types of pain while admitting others. The gate theory explains why your brain is not bombarded by a cacophony of sensations, emotions, and thoughts. While an individual painful signal might sound like a harsh drum, the composite of all the other incoming sounds is selectively channeled so that its result is a soothing melody.

While the nervous system is far more complicated than this simpli-fied model, the gate control theory still explains many mysteries of pain, including the marvel of "mind over matter." I'm sure you've heard of the injured athlete who ignores broken bones to continue playing or the accident victim who manages to escape the scene of the accident. These people have the same sensations that would overwhelm the aver-age person, but under their special circumstances they do not feel them as pain. Why does pain stimulus hurt at some times, but not at others? According to the gate control theory, the brain bars the entry of the pain sensation long enough for an injured person to escape. Sensory nerves and chemicals in the spinal cord act as "gatekeepers" by admit-ting or blocking pain signals to the brain. Depending on the circum-stances, this switching station may intensify, mute, or integrate differ-ent pain sensations.

Have you ever wondered why you instinctively rub an injured area of your body and why this helps soothe the pain? This is another example of how the gatekeeper moderates pain. When you bang your knee on a table, the pain sensation travels straight through the ner-vous system to the brain. The rubbing sensation then competes for the brain's attention. The gatekeeper brain listens to both sensations, allows the rubbing sensation to override the sharp uncomfortable sen-sation, and presto, less pain. The same dynamic is at work when you kiss a child's "owie" to make it better. The nurturing sensation of the kiss quickly overrides the pain of the child's scrape or bruise.

A Little Man with a Large Mouth

As you may have figured out by now, each of these pain theories not only adds to medicine's understanding of what you're feeling but better yet, adds to doctors' arsenal of resources for combating pain. Another of pain's mysteries is why an injury at one place in your body hurts more than at another place. In the mid-1980s, scientists discovered an intriguing feature of the brain—that sensory nerves in the most developed part of the brain, the cortex, are organized hierarchically according to various body parts. To illustrate this, scientists created a vivid metaphor of a Homunculus, or "Little Man" (the word is a diminutive of the Latin *homo,* meaning "human being").

A cross between E. T. and "It Came from the Swamp," the Homunculus has very full lips and mouth, a large, hairless head, huge hands, a shriveled torso, skinny legs, and modestly developed feet with oversized big toes. The Homunculus's proportions, which reflect the number of nerve connections between each body part and the brain, can tell you a lot about how you sense the world around you. For instance, it explains why a stubbed toe hurts more than a banged shoulder. The oversized representation of nerve connections for fingers and thumbs illustrates the heightened tactile sensitivity that equips you for fine motor tasks like sewing or slicing an onion, an evolutionary advance that separates man from the rest of the animal kingdom.

The Little Man is also a vivid depiction of how pain functions as man's evolutionary ally. Nature designed you to be especially sensitive to anything that might undermine your survival—namely, your ability to use your hands, to see, to breathe, to eat, and to speak (or yell for help). The Homunculus's enormous facial features explain why dental pain is so discomforting—your mouth is one of the most sensitive areas of the body. The sensory cortex of our brain has more nerve receptors for the mouth and face than any other part of the body—which is why even a small cut on the tongue can hurt as much as a serious injury elsewhere.

The Perimeter Alarm

One of the best metaphors for how pain works is a perimeter alarm system that not only registers pain but also activates the body's defenses. In simple terms, it works like this:

You encounter acute pain throughout the day as you cut yourself shaving, burn your hands with hot coffee cups, or bang a leg on an open drawer. When something unpleasant touches your skin or internal structures, special nerves called nociceptors flash a signal to regions of the brain that identify the pain's intensity and location. This kind of pain acts like a perimeter alarm, the equivalent of a red light telling you that the window in the back bedroom has been tampered with. That's why when you bump your elbow, you know the pain is at the elbow. You don't have to guess where the injury is or look for swollen or reddened skin.

At the moment of injury, pain emits two alarms—one is urgent and forces you to seek safety immediately, such as reflexively pulling your hand away from a flame, while the other ramps up more slowly and may signal to your cognitive functions that something truly serious has happened. (The message may then be passed to other areas of the brain, like the limbic system, where pain may acquire emotional characteristics.)

Your internal structures, as well as your skin, are laced with pain sensors. Just as some areas of your skin are more sensitive to pain than others, so too are your innards. Your muscles possess the richest supply of internal sensory nerves, followed in order of declining sensitivity by the fibrous sheets of tissue that wrap around muscles and organs, tendons, joints, ligaments, and the outer layer of bones. The hierarchy of pain nerve distribution explains why muscle aches are so common and why musculoskeletal pain is what often propels people to consult a doctor.

Pain moves from the damage site along many nerve pathways, each carrying distinctive pieces of information and operating at different speeds. While low-threshold nerve pathways constantly register fine tactile sensation, higher threshold pathways are reserved for pain sensation. (It's clearly not in the body's interest to have a hair-trigger pain threshold.) Certain pathways specialize in sharp, pointed feelings and transmit stinging pain very quickly—so fast it feels instantaneous. Other nerves move information along much more slowly and transmit dull, aching, or burning pain. So, when you cut your finger with a knife, you first feel the sharp sting and only later feel the aching or uncomfortable burning feeling.

Nerves are the highways that the pain signals travel along, and they're always open for traffic. The pain sensation makes a number of stops en route to the brain, then circulates to various regions of the brain, like the thalamus and hypothalamus. Depending on which part of the brain the pain arrives at first, the message may evoke a verbal "Ouch!" or it may be forwarded to motor nerves that command a physical flinch, or both. As sensory signals hustle along nerve routes carrying messages back and forth between injured tissue and the brain, other nerves are relaying information about the damage and instigating a response. Along the way, pain stimulates a chain reaction of neurochemicals that either intensify or dampen the sensation. Neurochemicals bearing messages about pain speed to various parts of the body and brain and account for a host of reactions, including swelling, inflammation, itching, muscle spasm, accelerated heart rate, even sweating.

At this point in the pain alarm system, your mind has registered some type of discomfort and your body is on the verge of reacting. You're at that instant when the needle has broken through your skin and you're about to flinch. One of the most dramatic responses comes from specialized nerves called the autonomic nervous system, which jump into action and rev up the stress response. This system makes your heart race when you run uphill, makes goose bumps break out when you are cold, and makes you blush when you're embarrassed. You have no control over this part of your nervous system, although you can influence it.

Like running from an attacker or bitter cold, extreme pain also activates the body's stress system, which blares out an alarm—"Battle stations, battle stations!" It activates the autonomic nerves and triggers the production of potent stress hormones. These nerves and hormones pump up the immune system, and they regulate heart rate and blood pressure to better handle the crisis. They also help the liver and muscles produce and absorb more glycogen (high-octane sugar), generating more energy to fight or flee harm.

This is when pain reveals its Jekyll-and-Hyde personality. While it's making you miserable, it's also spurring the release of chemicals that speed healing. For instance, while inflammation hurts, it also heals—by increasing blood flow, delivering nutrients to the injury site, and removing dead cells. An inflamed sunburn, for instance, is flooded with healing chemicals, though the pain arrives after the sun has done its damage. (Many of the most serious pain syndromes meander along a slow course, too late to warn us of danger. For instance, pain associated with cancer is notorious for surfacing long after irreparable damage has been done.)

One of the many powerful chemicals produced by your brain in pain are called prostaglandins, and they can have many different effects on nerves. Some prostaglandins dispatch a cascade of chemicals that make sensory nerves even more sensitive. At the same time, some of the nerve signals reach cells that produce several pain-suppressing hormones, known as endorphins. Endorphins are a group of naturally produced chemicals that work just like morphine—hence the name, from *endogenous* (meaning "in the body") and *morphine*. When endorphins are in the neighborhood, the reverberating loop of pain—leading to nerves and hormones stimulating even more pain—is broken.

WHEN PAIN KINDLES SUFFERING

The many metaphors of pain are useful models, though they are partial models because they describe only the physical aspect of the pain experience. As you may have suspected, pain does much more than disturb your body—it mingles with your emotions and generates an entirely new layer of discomfort. Recent advances in neuroscience have proven what scientists have long suspected, that pain is a tightly interwoven physiological *and* emotional event comprising both physical and psychic suffering. Everyone has a different idea of what it means to suffer, yet the suffering that pain may stir up has features common for all people even though everyone thinks his pain is unique. Pain and suffering—they go together like love and longing. Not the same thing, and not cause and effect, but so tightly woven that it's hard to imagine one without the other. Although suffering is usually associated with pain that goes on and on, it can surface with any blow to our physical well-being. Among my patients, the common denominator of their suffering frequently entails a sense of loss: loss of function, loss of daily routine, loss of good health, loss of a feeling of control, loss of autonomy, or the loss of feeling invulnerable—there are infinite varieties of loss.

Sometimes, I see patients suffering from what might be described as the spiritual dimension of their pain. People with strong religious beliefs may believe that their pain is a form of punishment for known or unknown sins. The English poet C. S. Lewis once referred to pain as

"God's megaphone," and indeed I have known patients who felt mental anguish because they believe that they somehow deserved what befell them.

The randomness and unfairness of an accident or violence that causes pain may also kindle suffering. Pain can seem so arbitrary, so unjustified, and make you feel as if you have little control over your world. Perhaps one of the most eloquent thinkers to delve into the nature of suffering is Viktor Frankl, a psychiatrist who survived a Nazi concentration camp and wrote about it in his seminal work, *Man's Search for Meaning*. Early in the book, he recounts his reaction to a guard beating him. "At such a moment, it is not the physical pain which hurts the most (and this applies to adults as much as to punished children), it is the mental agony caused by the injustice, the unreasonableness of it all." For many, this is the nexus of pain and suffering. Pain forces you to keep asking "Why me?" yet offers no answer.

Shame and isolation are other emotional by-products of pain.

Suffering is fertile ground for doubt, disbelief, and mistaken assumptions. How often have you heard someone question another's back pain and wonder if that person is trying to get out of work or escape some responsibility? Headaches can also raise doubts—while we've all heard the jokes about using headaches to avoid sex, there is contained in that joke a belief that headaches are one way to avoid personal interaction. Without a pain thermometer, as it were, people in pain must rely on their language skills to describe what they are feeling. Inevitably, their descriptions don't do justice to what they are going through, and so doctors, and others, may be skeptical of the severity of their pain. Doctors and loved ones may question a patient's pain and suspect some ulterior motive or even outright faking. People can be great cynics when it comes to others' misery, and I suspect this is one reason behind our culture of stoicism.

Patients learn that too many complaints raise eyebrows. They know from experience that even at a time of great need they may be unheard, helpless, and shunned. So rather than run the risk of being suspected of angling for sympathy, control, or power, people in pain may just grit their teeth and say nothing. Some people feel that admitting they are in pain is a sign of weakness. These feelings, and many more, become fodder for pain sufferers' internal turmoil and intensify the pain they feel.

FEAR, THE ULTIMATE PAIN MAGNIFIER

You may be wondering which feelings or experiences can make your pain worse. Although the formula is unique for everyone, an almost universal emotion that magnifies pain is fear. And one of the most common fears of pain involves visiting the dentist. The prospect of pain in your mouth epitomizes your vulnerability to what most people always try to avoid—unpleasant physical sensation. For many, the words "dental," "pain," and "fear" are synonymous.

A couple of months ago, I awoke in the middle of the night with a throbbing pain in my jaw. I instantly found a tooth that wanted nothing near it. The pain was so intense that it lifted me from a deep sleep. On top of being annoyed because I couldn't get back to sleep, I was also unsettled about the prospect of seeing the dentist and maybe needing a filling or, worse yet, a root canal. I tried to distract myself and stop thinking about it, but nothing helped. I gradually drifted back to sleep only to awaken trying to figure out if I had gum disease or just a cavity.

It was a few days before I could see the dentist, and I was constantly reminded of my damaged tooth. Drinking anything cold made me jump to the ceiling. I figured that I probably only had a cavity. A tooth is filled with dental pulp, a collection of blood vessels, nerves, and tissues. When pulp gets inflamed because of an invasion of bacteria, it aches. Too much bacteria produces toxins that eat away at the tooth and ultimately trigger the pain alarm.

Until I could get to the dentist, I brooded over my toothache. It made me irritable and brusque. I didn't feel like talking, because any air around it hurt, and feeling pressured at work, I resented the time it was going to take to fix it. The hypochondriac in me (a part that lurks in all of us) worried that it could be more than a cavity and require some gruesome form of dental surgery. I was anxious about the whole process, a feeling that made it even more difficult to cope. As a pain specialist, I marveled at how my mind and body colluded to make me miserable. Yet I did find a small comfort from friends and colleagues who sympathized with my distress. Everyone knows what dental pain feels like, so it's pretty easy to empathize. In my case, I could barely move my jaw to speak, so I didn't encounter the suspicions that often accompany pain that is less apparent or understandable.

For what turned out to be a cavity, I was treated with a shot of Novocain (local anesthetic) and a filling. I must reluctantly admit that like almost everyone else, I don't like shots. The dentist, knowing I'm a pain management specialist—and a scared pain management specialist at that—suggested trying "a little something to help with the experience." I was given a commonly used mixture of oxygen and nitrous oxide ("laughing gas") through a mask. Within seconds, the gas mixture dulled my attention to the dentist's drilling but allowed me to remain awake and alert and to cooperate with his requests. I became extremely relaxed, and although aware of the drilling and its somewhat unpleasant sensation, I was no longer clenching my hands around the armrests and somehow able to tolerate what I had expected would be a nightmare.

"Dental fear." It sounds like a horror movie. But it is very real, so real that it's being explored by the National Institute of Dental Research, where scientists are looking into how particular behaviors and attitudes can accentuate or diminish a person's fear. The reality of dental fear is personified by the unforgettable movie *The Marathon Man,* which plays on our most primitive fears about the vulnerability of our mouth and nerves beneath the teeth by pitting the helpless Dustin Hoffman against a Mengele-type Nazi dentist played by Laurence Olivier. Early in the movie, Hoffman, a marathon runner, declares, "I don't give in to pain," which is a setup for the scene when the sadistic Olivier uses his dental instruments to extract information.

It is no coincidence that before Olivier digs into Dustin Hoffman's tooth, he elaborately displays his instruments and forces Hoffman to watch him. Elaine Scarry, in her book *The Body in Pain,* notes that torture victims almost always are made to stare at the weapon that is going to be used against them. The mind is capable of intensifying almost any sensation, including fear. It is also capable of decreasing the intensity. Many people use this process to cope with disturbing feelings. Sometimes you can conjure up fear with nothing more than your imagination, in which case you may have some control over it. Other times, fears can be stirred up by circumstances beyond your control. When the source of the fear is out of your hands, the potential for discomfort is even greater.

You may know this intuitively. If you've sat in the dentist's chair with your mouth open and winced before the chrome probe even came near a tooth, you know how expectation can accentuate pain. There are sound physiological reasons for why fear of what's to come can make pain worse. Thinking about pain, waiting for pain—in short, mounting fear—produces many physical responses, including neurochemical changes. When you feel stress emotions such as fear and anxiety, your body releases hormones called catecholamines (such as adrenaline). They can make you feel nervous, jittery, and out of control, which may heighten your fear. In other circumstances, these chemicals can give you a jump start and boost your energy, clarity of thinking, and ability to perform tasks that might otherwise be impossible. Extra adrenaline circulating around sensory nerves makes them especially alert to incoming stimuli, which doctors think of as having become "sensitized." Although the stress response can release pain-dampening substances like endorphins, in some pain situations your body's stress reaction magnifies fear and pain instead of diminishing it.

PAIN THRESHOLDS

Fear is one of pain's most familiar emotional ingredients, but other emotions can join the fray. Emotions like depression or anger can increase pain's decibel level or lower it. Some sensations make a huge impact and others barely produce a beep, and likewise the pain alarm is louder in some people than in others. This is what is known as your pain tolerance, namely why a given injury produces an awful pain in me but feels mild to you.

Patients frequently wonder if what they're feeling is "normal," worrying that they're either being a hypochondriac or too stoical for their own good. I try to relieve their concerns by explaining the limits of a person's influence over pain, and the difference between pain threshold and pain tolerance. Here's a simple test that you can do to measure your personal pain threshold and pain tolerance. Fill a bowl with water and ice, plunge your hand into the bowl, and count the number of seconds before you feel the cold as painful. That's your pain threshold. Next, wait and see how much time passes before the pain of the cold forces you to withdraw your hand from the bowl. That's your pain tolerance level. Someone with a high tolerance for pain or high level of stoicism might be able to leave his hand in the bowl until he experiences frostbite. Another person, whose fear of cold acts as a magnifier, might have to withdraw his hand at the first flash of pain.

Your pain threshold is the point at which a sensation first becomes uncomfortable, and it is different from pain tolerance, which is how much discomfort you can endure until instinct or reason makes you pull away. Experiments with pain reveal that most people have the same sensation threshold: Everyone jumps when touched with a certain amount of electricity. Where people part ways is with pain tolerance.

While there's little you can do about your pain threshold—it's as much a part of you as the pigment of your skin—you can tinker with your pain tolerance. Learning to manage pain successfully often means adjusting pain tolerance. I'm not suggesting that you become a stoic, but instead that it is possible to control your level of discomfort so that what might have sidelined you last year is now only a minor annoyance.

But before you launch into some kind of toughening regimen, it may be helpful to know that how you feel pain is influenced by more than just your genes or determination. Culture and gender also color how you feel pain. For instance, people from warm, Mediterranean countries, like Italians, are thought to be more sensitive to heat than northern Europeans. Culture also plays a role when it comes to your pain tolerance. A study of women from different backgrounds—Irish, Italian, Jewish, and what experimenters called "Old American"— found that the white, Anglo-Saxon group had the highest tolerance, followed by Jewish, Irish, and Italian women, and that each group had its own attitudes and expectations about pain. While the "Old American" women tended to be matter-of-fact and more stoic, the Italian women at the other end of the spectrum focused on the immediate pain sensation and reacted strongly.

A recent study that surprised me looked at pain and cultural influence in the Baltic country of Lithuania. It suggests that people's reaction to pain may be influenced by whether the society compensates the pain sufferer. It was a study of whiplash and neck pain in which researchers looked at more than two hundred people who survived serious car accidents. Lithuania was investigated because at the time there was no legal system in place in which an individual could sue for damages resulting from a car accident. Only a third of these survivors reported headaches or neck pain, and most of those said that they had had the pain before the accident. In short, the study found that *there were no reported cases of whiplash*—a situation that would almost certainly have been dramatically different if the two hundred people had been Americans! The investigators concluded that expectations played a role in complaints of pain and injury. This doesn't mean that anyone with injuries from a car accident is faking pain for cash. I always tell my students, "Be suspicious but don't be overly judgmental." But be reminded that lots of factors may contribute to your pain and suffering, and social or cultural influences could be a vital piece of your pain puzzle.

GENDER AND PAIN

I have a hard time making generalizations about men, women, and pain. At times, it seems like all the men I treat are stoical and grin-and-bear-it types, then I meet a female patient who's a silent sufferer or a male patient who's exceedingly expressive and reacts to the slightest touch. So I keep my eye on what researchers are discovering about pain and gender, knowing that they're studying larger groups of people and coming up with conclusions that can shed light on patients' reactions to treatment.

Although it's clear that men and women differ in their experiences of pain, less certain is whether their complaints and symptoms are more influenced by culture, social convention, or physiology. Gender biology surely plays a role; men's and women's hormones wax and wane and probably contribute to different types of pain. For instance, headaches have long been considered largely a female domain, and there is some data to support this assertion. Recently, scientists at the University of Bergen in Sweden compiled an analysis of thirteen separate studies involving about seventy-five thousand people with non-migraine headaches, looking particularly at the gender split. They concluded: "Non-migraine headache is a woman's disease."

Yet as you read this, keep in mind the motto "Pain is what the patient says it is." It's possible that women appear to suffer from more headaches because they are better able and more likely than men to express their complaint. Put another way, men may be more culturally programmed to accept pain without complaint and "be a man" about it.

Researchers seem to believe that women tend to have lower pain thresholds and higher pain tolerance. In a controlled study at Graduate Hospital in Philadelphia, nine healthy men and ten healthy women allowed doctors to insert a balloon down their esophagus and reported how it felt. The women, researchers found, "had a significantly lower pain threshold." On the other hand, a study of arthritis conducted by doctors at Florida State University and Ohio University found that women handled discomfort much better than men. While the distress of arthritis tended to put men in a bad mood, women interpreted their pain as a call to action and took steps to relieve it. One possible conclusion is that women have a stronger initial reaction to pain but handle it better than men.

Unfortunately, women in pain are frequently treated differently than men who describe the same symptoms. For instance, studies confirm that men's pain is more often attributed to physiological causes and, as a result, men are more likely to receive a complete physical workup. Likewise, men are more likely to receive surgery in response to pain complaints, whereas women are more likely to receive medication to treat anxiety or depression. In short, women's pain is more often attributed to a mood problem and psychological disorder, while men's is likely to be attributed to organic causes.

Occasionally, gender can help pinpoint the exact cause of a pain. Doctors at the University Hospital in Kuopio, Finland, examined the records of 639 men and women who were admitted with some kind of abdominal pain. When they investigated the source of this pain, they found that by and large the underlying causes were different for men and women. Young men's stomach pain most likely came from appendicitis, and men of all ages were more likely to be suffering from alcoholic pancreatitis, gastritis, renal stones, and peptic ulcer. Young women, on the other hand, were more prone to what's called "nonspecific abdominal pain."

Recent studies also suggest that men and women respond differently to pain relievers. Following wisdom-tooth extraction, men and women revealed that a particular narcotic medication worked much better for women—perhaps because they also reported more pain before it was administered. The scientist leading the study, Dr. Jon Levine at the University of California at San Francisco, had searched the medical literature before the study and found that no one had asked the question, "Do women and men respond differently to drugs used in the treatment of pain?" Answering this question has become a topic of keen interest to researchers, and much more will likely be known in the months and years to come.

Other big influences on how you react to pain are the social expectations of how someone in pain should act and the possible meaning of the pain. For instance, the initiation rite of fraternity hazing often includes a steady stream of pain, from paddling to burning, but there are rarely any complaints from the boys. Group acceptance depends on their stoic endurance and their ability to block their bodies' reactions to pain. Tattooing among teens and young people is another painful experience that requires them to elevate their pain tolerance levels. Even though tattooing is rarely done with any anesthesia and requires hundreds of pinpricks, and sometimes superficial cutting, people frequently withstand it without much more than a grimace.

What pain "means" to a person—the context of the experience—can strongly influence how bad it feels. The extreme pain of childbirth is often easier to bear and quickly forgotten because the mother is focused on her child's well-being (and soon awash in postpartum hormones). A father who has injured his arm rescuing his daughter from danger may feel little pain at the time because of his urgent attention to the rescue. However, that doesn't mean that the experience is forgotten. The father may see his pain as a badge of courage but later recall the frightening experience with uneasy flashbacks, even to the point of anxiety. This anxiety can reach such a pitch that it's transformed into post-traumatic memory and becomes a new source of suffering.

BRIDGING THE MIND AND BODY

You first learn how to react to pain from your parents. As a child, you closely watch their response to your injuries: Do they seem to expect crying and lots of emotion? Do they dismiss what might hurt and sternly forbid outbursts with "Don't be a crybaby"? Or, do they sympathize with a smile and a hug, acknowledging the pain but discouraging you from letting it take charge? While no particular response is ever perfect or completely damaging, these formative experiences stay with you for a lifetime and may be more persuasive than any genetic predisposition to pain sensitivity.

Personal psychology and physiology—the mind and the body—mingle to shape the exact outline of a your experience of pain. Like personality, your pain tolerance is the product of personal biology as well as memories, experiences, behavior patterns, family history, and culture. The nature of your perceptions are equally diverse: There are infinite degrees of sensitivity to hot and cold, to sharp cuts and injections, to blows and traumas, to aching and burning—some painful and some not. I remember once asking my dentist about patients who could sit through crown work without so much as a whiff of Novocain and whether they had high thresholds for all sensation. He told me that often the same patients who may not feel drilling on their teeth may be hair-trigger sensitive to a metal instrument on their gums.

The psychological side of pain tolerance is a jumble of feelings that are conscious and unconscious. Your attitude toward pain, or more precisely, how much anxiety you experience around pain, is another part of the pain threshold. Extreme, persistent anxiety can set in motion a reverberating loop of anxiety and pain, which stirs up more anxiety, and more pain. Depression often lowers a person's pain threshold, making a person vulnerable to a wider range of uncomfortable feelings than he or she normally would be. Neuroscientists believe that depression has complex biological effects that may suppress the body's ability to tolerate pain and even reduce its pain-muting abilities.

TRIUMPH OVER ACUTE PAIN

I think one of the unheralded triumphs of medicine is how pain doctors have defeated acute pain. I see it every day. In fact, medicine's ability to contain the temporary pain that can come from an injury or after a medical procedure is so commonplace that anyone admitted to a modern hospital should expect that their acute pain will be controlled. If you're in the hospital recovering from surgery and getting good medical care, in most cases you should feel only minimal post-op acute pain. However, pain can only be treated successfully if it's treated. Even with modern technological wonders, too many patients feel more pain than necessary because it is either overlooked or not made a priority. Effective treatment starts with recognizing the need for treatment and taking action. Too many patients are afraid to complain. And, too, many doctors and nurses are either unaware of their patients' pain or disregard it. Medical practitioners are doing better with treating acute pain, but more needs to be done.

Medicine's ability to treat pain has been helped greatly by recently discovered links between mind and body that point toward a long-sought unified field theory of pain: *It's all in our heads.* This new paradigm doesn't mean that pain is imaginary; on the contrary, it's an inescapable and excruciating reality to pain sufferers. Pain can't occur without a brain and a mind. Cracking the code of pain lies in deciphering the brain's stew of neurochemicals. Understanding the mystery of pain lies in comprehending the complex mix of emotions and physical sensations that define the balance of pain and pleasure in your moment-to-moment consciousness—the interface of the mind and body.

But it's easy for well-meaning doctors to become so focused on the microscopic nerve cells transmitting electrical messages to the brain that they overlook the human emotions that can transform pain signals into nightmarish sensations. Patients in pain are also often suffering from fear, anxiety, loss of hope, frustration, and depression that can't be separated from the physical aspects of their condition. Add to this mix the other wounds of chronic pain—loss of income from disability, social stigma and isolation, dashed hopes for the future—and you have much more than a physical disease.

Nowhere is Hippocrates' directive to "Study the patient rather than the disease" more critical than in pain medicine, *because pain is a symptom of a patient's suffering.* Physical and emotional suffering are inseparable. To me, treating one without the other, particularly when pain becomes chronic, just doesn't make sense.

Discoveries about new treatments for pain are building on a growing body of knowledge not only about the connection between the mind and body but also about how your brain and nerve cells react to pain. While it may seem that the war on pain is a direct result of recent technological advances, pain remains man's oldest adversary and the battle against it is not new. Almost every month I read about a "revolutionary" new drug or new procedures for pain, only to learn later that this novel approach is really a refinement or improvement on pain remedies that have been around for many years. The history of pain management has a great deal to teach about combating this ancient enemy.

2

DISCONNECTING THE PAIN ALARM

The Dawn of Anesthesia and How It Revolutionized Pain Medicine

> Our craft has, once and for all, been robbed of its terrors.
> —DR. HENRY BIGELOW
> Surgeon, Harvard Medical School, 1846

Often in medical history, monumental discoveries spring not from earth-shattering events but from daily, mundane concerns. One of the most bothersome health problems and sources of pain in the nineteenth century was the toothache. Back then, everyone's teeth hurt—I think it was the equivalent of lower back pain today. The absence of oral hygiene, particularly brushing, and a diet light on calcium and heavy on sugar exposed people to a lifetime of tooth decay. Toothaches were ubiquitous, and dentistry was a flourishing profession whose chief skills were speed and strength for quick extraction. In fact, dentistry and surgery were considered a single profession. (In England, where barbers also performed dental work, the Barber-Surgeons Company later became the Royal College of Surgeons.) So, it is not a coincidence that the man credited with the discovery of anesthesia was a dentist.

CONQUERING PAIN IN THE ETHERDOME

When I was at Massachusetts General Hospital, I often walked by the Etherdome, the hospital's original operating theater. It's a large domed room housing one hundred steeply tiered wooden seats that tower in a semicircle above a stage and the scene of one of pain medicine's momentous events. On the morning of October 16, 1846, it was crammed with students and doctors curious about a surgery that was billed as a demonstration of a miraculous new technique for preventing pain. William Morton, a twenty-seven-year-old dentist, had cajoled the hospital's leading surgeon, John Collins Warren, into letting him administer a preparation he called Letheon to a patient about to undergo major surgery. Morton had fabricated the name from the Greek word "Lethe," a mythological river that brought on forgetfulness. Morton's preparation was largely ether, a gas made by heating alcohol with oil of vitriol, which is otherwise known as sulfuric acid. Doctors had been using ether, known as sweet vitriol, for centuries, but since Morton hoped to patent his application and make a fortune, he had to disguise its true nature and give it a catchy, yet vague-sounding name.

Despite many previous attempts to demonstrate his discovery, Morton had been snubbed by almost all of the top surgeons until Dr. Warren recognized its possible significance. Warren had too often witnessed the torture of surgery without pain control. He had known patients who had committed suicide rather than go under the dreaded knife. So Dr. Warren disregarded the skepticism of his colleagues and gave the dentist a chance to work a miracle.

On the operating couch lay twenty-year-old Gil Abbott, whose lower jaw pulsed from the pain of a tumor. Standing around him were Dr. Warren and six other doctors in black frock coats and starched white shirts. Against the wall stood an Egyptian mummy, placed there to make the place look more scientific. (The mummy is still there today.) It was fifteen minutes past the time Morton was supposed to arrive, and Warren, known for his impatience, was poised to begin cutting. Gil Abbott was growing visibly anxious at the prospect of deep cutting in his face (remember the Homunculus!) without any type of pain relief. At the last minute Morton rushed in, hurriedly explaining that his instrument maker had kept him waiting while he put the finishing touches on the special apparatus before them.

Warren curtly informed Morton that the patient was ready. Morton placed his apparatus—an inhaler consisting of a glass globe with a sponge inside and a wooden tube leading from it—beside Abbott and put the tube in his mouth. The sponge was soaked in sulfuric ether, although Morton had added aromatics, including oil of orange, to disguise the fact that his secret preparation was simple ether. The patient became tranquil and soon thereafter appeared to be asleep.

As Warren began his first incision, the entire operating theater fell silent. It was as if everyone was holding his breath, waiting for a cry of pain from the patient. But he was in a deep sleep, even as blood from severed arteries spurted out. Within minutes, Warren had removed the mass from the bloody jaw and Abbott was still unconscious. Dr. Warren's assistant sewed up and bandaged the incision, then waited for Abbott to regain consciousness.

Morton was probably most nervous at this juncture because in earlier surgeries with other types of anesthesia, some patients never woke up. I can imagine Morton's relief when a few minutes later, Abbott opened his eyes and, responding to Dr. Warren's question about how he felt, declared that he had felt no pain throughout the operation. At that point, Dr. Warren announced to the now astonished crowd, who had expected failure or at least some kind of parlor trick, "Gentlemen, this is no humbug." Another famous Harvard surgeon, W. J. Bigalow, then chimed in from his seat in the audience, "We have today witnessed something of the utmost importance to the art of surgery. Our craft has, once and for all, been robbed of its terrors."

THE WORLD'S MOST IMPORTANT MEDICAL DISCOVERY

The discovery of general anesthesia was hailed as "the world's most important medical discovery" and opened a surgical floodgate. People who dreaded the prospect of pain to the point of choosing death by infection or disease now agreed to undergo surgery. According to Dr. Warren's notes on how the news of ether's wondrous properties was received, within days "its use resorted to every considerable operation in the city of Boston." Bostonians still recognize "Ether Day." Although ether is no longer used in surgical operations, other similar but safer inhaled gases remain the mainstay of modern general anesthesia.

William Morton, the entrepreneurial young dentist, had to settle for fame and forgo fortune. In order to promote "the world's most important medical discovery," he had to reveal Letheon's not-so-novel active ingredient. Since ether was commonly available, Morton never got his patent, or his ticket to easy street. He spent the next twenty years in a bitter dispute with two other doctors who claimed to have been the real scientists behind the discovery of ether. After using his invention on thousands of Civil War soldiers undergoing amputation, Morton died in near poverty and still struggling for recognition as the father of anesthesia.

Before Morton's demonstration, doctors at Mass General had been performing surgery about once a week, often having to strap patients to tables in order to get them through the operation. Medical practitioners had no way to excise tumors, amputate infected limbs, or repair internal damage without inflicting horrendous pain. Unable to control the pain that accompanied treatment and surgery, medical practitioners were limited to superficial procedures or rushed operations. "The quicker the surgeon, the greater the surgeon" was the prevailing opinion of medical care. When major surgery was undertaken, patients were first given whisky. According to a history of the time, "Surgeons were known to enter the operating room with a bottle of whisky in each hand—one for the patient and the other for the doctor so that he could endure his patient's screams."

The enormous improvement in the quality of medical care that accompanied the advent of anesthesia rippled through the population's general health. Life expectancy rates gained by leaps and bounds. In the mid-nineteenth century, before anesthesia, the average life expectancy was an incredibly young thirty-five years. As use of general anesthesia swept through hospital operating rooms, life expectancy rates marched steadily upward and increased more than 25 percent. Anyone born around 1900 could expect to live to be over fifty years old.

The Etherdome where William Morton defeated pain is now a museum on the grounds of Massachusetts General Hospital. It is one of my favorite places, and whenever I had visitors or was interviewing doctors for recruiting into pain specialty training, I would take them up to the Etherdome to sit in the narrow wooden theater seats and imagine the day that changed medicine forever.

General anesthesia, by deactivating the body's alarms, revolutionized doctors' ability to make repairs, replace damaged or worn parts, or remove diseased tissue without causing further harm or pain. The marvel of general anesthesia is that it enables doctors to lower a patient's consciousness and metabolism to a point just before the entire system shuts down—to the brink of death—then restore the alarms and the basic life systems such as circulation and respiration, bringing the patient back in better shape than before. Many of today's procedures and surgeries are unthinkable without anesthesia, or its sibling, analgesia. Though people now take it for granted as a daily part of medical care, the development of anesthesia 150 years ago was a watershed event that opened the door for medical practitioners to explore, and heal, the human body.

ANESTHESIA IN ANCIENT TIMES

For hundreds of years prior to the Etherdome, pain science advanced only glacially. Stories of ancient pain remedies remind me of tales of alchemists trying to turn base metals into gold. Fantastic theories about bodily humors as the source of pain or ersatz medications containing such ingredients as snake venom or animal urine formed the basis of pain treatment for centuries. Until the nineteenth century, many of these pain remedies were refinements of opium and alcohol mixtures. The other leading methods for controlling pain were refrigeration and compression—freezing or squeezing around damaged tissue. Excavations in Egypt have reportedly uncovered tableaus from before Christ depicting an operation that included compressing nerves in a patient's arm, presumably to control pain. Napoleon's chief surgeon amputated hundreds of limbs by freezing them first. Some of these ideas, although crude, were on the right track and have led to present-day treatments.

The science of controlling pain before the modern era had always presented a daunting challenge: How can a doctor render a person senseless without inflicting more discomfort or without causing death? How far can medicine take senselessness? Ordinary pain can be controlled by shutting off the body's awareness of it, somehow making a patient insensible. While this sounds logical and simple, doing it effectively and in essence mastering unconsciousness have eluded medical wizards for centuries. Through the ages, doctors' only experience with unconsciousness was with sleep, which was virtually impossible to control. They experimented with a procedure known as garroting, in which pressure on a carotid artery leading to the brain produced unconsciousness. But they had no way of ensuring that the patient would remain unconscious throughout an operation or that the brain would not be injured from lack of oxygen.

Without a way to control pain, medical treatment was either limited or inflicted enormous physical suffering. Doctors had only crude tools, if any, to penetrate the perimeter alarm system of our skin, and usually tripped the pain sensors. The skin barrier not only prevented all types of surgery and internal repairs but also limited what could be learned about the human body. Medical knowledge about how the body responded to disease and injury was confined to what could be deciphered from cadavers. Thus, for centuries, imagination as much as science fueled ideas about the nervous system, musculature, and the functioning of organs like the heart and lungs.

Medicine men and philosophers concocted theories that had very little to do with biological reality. Early civilizations believed that pain came from the gods as punishment for misdeeds and evil. Around the time of Christ, Greeks considered pain to be caused by bodily fluids out of balance. Finally, in the seventeenth century, scientists began to home in on the causes of pain as they learned about human anatomy and constructed a new medical science—physiology, the study of how the human body functions.

SYNCHRONICITY AND SERENDIPITY IN SCIENCE

Scientific discoveries frequently occur in clusters. A mystery that has baffled scientists for decades, sometimes centuries, will suddenly be solved virtually simultaneously by many scientists working independently and unaware of each other's research. One of the wonderful quirks of science is how, after years of research, breakthroughs seem to happen by chance around the globe and more or less at the same time. You may recall a recent example of this with the numerous simultaneous announcements of successful animal cloning. A century ago—catalyzed by William Morton's breakthrough in the Etherdome—doctors in various countries were unraveling the secrets of anesthesia and devising a variety of practical applications.

Nitrous oxide, a common ingredient of anesthesia in contemporary operating rooms and dental offices, had first been discovered in the late 1700s by Joseph Priestley, who also first detected oxygen, ammonia, and sulfur dioxide. But it was used sparingly because scientists feared that even a small amount could kill someone. A hundred years later, Sir Humphrey Davy tried it himself and found that it cured his toothache, and also produced uncontrollable laughter. Only then did nitrous oxide begin to find its way as a pain reliever for medical procedures. Davy became a "laughing gas" addict and even wrote about its pain-relieving effects, but he never actually used it in surgery. Since it is not as potent an anesthetic as ether, nitrous oxide did not attract as much attention. Fears about it persisted, largely because if inhaled in high enough concentrations for prolonged periods of time, it can be deadly.

Another form of anesthesia, chloroform, was also gaining currency around this time. Like ether, it was inhaled after being dissolved in alcohol. After doctors found that it rendered animals unconscious, they wondered if it would work on people. One of its earliest investigators was a Scottish gynecologist named James Simpson, who, in 1847, gave it to a delivering mother whose previous labor had lasted three days. The operation was such a success that Simpson continued to use it daily, delivering thirty babies within the next six days. Probably his most famous patient was Queen Victoria, who gave birth to her seventh child while under chloroform.

Yet many doctors of the period questioned the safety of chloroform. As with nitrous oxide, a number of patients died of asphyxia when given too large a dose. So, ether became the first general anesthetic—the word *anesthesia* was coined by Oliver Wendell Holmes from the Greek *an,* meaning "without," and *aisthesis,* meaning "feeling" or "sensation"—and was often preferred to nitrous oxide or chloroform until doctors figured out how to deliver these gases without endangering patients' lives. A German surgeon eventually found the secret: premedication with morphine so that smaller doses of gas would be needed for a full operation. Patients given a preoperation shot of morphine (the newly invented hypodermic syringe and hollow needle had been simultaneously developed in the 1850s at two medical centers) did not need continuous, dangerous doses of pain-numbing gas. To this day, I routinely use one medicine to augment or limit the toxicity of another.

Even today, scientists continue to be baffled by exactly how ether, nitrous oxide, and chloroform quiet our brains and steal our consciousness. One theory suggests that they permeate cell membranes to halt the neurochemical communication between cells. But not understanding the underlying science of a wondrous discovery did not stop the nineteenth-century pioneers from using it, and I apply the same pragmatic philosophy. Many of my tools are directly descended from cruder instruments and principles no one fully understands. Take the marvelous common drug acetaminophen, what we all know as Tylenol. Medical science knows a lot about what it does but not exactly how it relieves pain and many other symptoms. I think Tylenol has wondrous properties yet to be discovered. There is much about pain medicine that's still a mystery, but as long as a pain reliever is safe and effective, it's welcome in my repertoire. If doctors had to know why treatments work before using them, Morton's discovery of general anesthesia would never have spread beyond the Etherdome.

THE MANY USES OF MORPHINE

It may surprise you to learn that even with the advances of biotechnology and chemical engineering, the gold standard of pain relief is still old-fashioned opiates. The medical profession has long had opiates to induce senselessness, and until the late nineteenth century there were few rivals in the realm of painkillers. Mankind has known about the power of opium and its offspring for thousands of years. Squeezed from bright blue-purple, white, or red poppies, opium's potent mind-bending properties over the ages have been applied to a procession of conditions—gallbladder pain, kidney stones, headaches, asthma, congestive heart failure, colic, insomnia, toothaches, and more. One of its first formulations as a medical compound was created in the sixteenth century by the famous chemist Paracelsus, who concocted a stew of opium, alcohol, and probably frog sperm and cinnamon as well, and labeled it "laudanum."

Over the centuries, opium's reputation grew, and by the 1800s it was used as a medical panacea. The popular, highly touted patent medicines of the period invariably contained opium. Amazingly, through the course of opium's long history, its addictive quality appears to have been ignored, and so it was given to one and all. During the American Civil War, doctors gave opiates liberally to soldiers, believing that if they were administered through the vein and did not reach the stomach, they would not cause hunger or addiction. Surgeons reportedly held out handfuls of morphine for soldiers on horseback as they rode past.

By the end of the war, more than 400,000 men suffered from what was called "soldier's disease." They were addicted, and some were treated with a potion packed with morphine that may have helped reduce their withdrawal. This is not dissimilar from the present-day practice of treating heroin addicts with methadone, a synthetic opioid with less chance of producing euphoric highs than heroin while preventing unpleasant withdrawal symptoms.

Morphine, opium's most potent ingredient, was extracted from the plant in 1803 by a German scientist. But it wasn't until doctors devised a way to get it into the human bloodstream, via the hollow syringe and hypodermic needle, that its use soared. Science wasn't altogether happy to leave morphine alone, and in 1875 chemists made a very subtle chemical change by adding two acetyl groups to morphine and created the first semisynthetic derivative. Twenty years later, a scientist at the Bayer Company named it "heroisch," for its strong, heroic qualities. Heroin was initially prescribed as a cure for morphine addiction and a treatment for coughs, although as we know, its use and abuse spread. (The acetyl groups allowed heroin to dissolve more quickly in brain fat and generate the notorious "rush" that makes it a choice for abuse over morphine.) Opiates, especially codeine, are still considered effective cough suppressants. They also can inhibit breathing to the point of death, which is what may happen during an overdose.

Since morphine was first extracted from opium, more than forty other alkaloids have been found in the plant, although fewer than half can be formed into active drugs. Later alterations and modifications of opium stimulated a host of painkilling variations, including codeine (one-sixth as strong as morphine), meperidine (now known as Demerol and distilled in 1939 as the first synthetic opioid), methadone (developed by the Germans during World War II as a substitute for hard-to-get morphine), hydromorphone (now known as Dilaudid, which is ten times stronger than morphine), and fentanyl (at present the only opioid that is given in a patch form and absorbed through the skin).

Opioids—"opium" is the plant extract, "opiate" is a drug made from opium, and an "opioid" is a drug, natural or synthetic, that acts like an opiate—work systemically and circulate throughout our bodies to latch onto specific receptors on the outside of cells in the brain and elsewhere. Think of a receptor as a lock on the door of the cell. Molecules, in the form of a naturally produced hormone or an opioid drug, act like a key that fits into a lock to open the door to the cell.

Once a cell door is "open," there are infinite possibilities for any variety of effects, depending on the cell, the receptor, the timing, and other reactions in other cells or parts of the body. In the case of morphine, once the opioid has unlocked the receptor, it may cause the nerve to fire more slowly or more quickly, and such change in cell action ultimately produces pain relief as well as other sensations. Opioid molecules function as if they are tailor-made because they perfectly fit the body's own opioid receptors. It is this precise fit that makes them so fast-acting and potent.

Scientists are rarely satisfied with simply making a discovery; they always want to know "Why?" Why does the body have its own opioid receptors? What use would we have for a lock system where the keys are substances like opium, heroin, or morphine? These questions led scientists to uncover some of the secrets of your ability to manage pain, which I'll tell you much more about later.

In the past fifteen years neurophysiologists have learned that the areas of the brain that receive incoming signals about pain are especially rich in opioid receptors. Yet opioids do not block all pain. Sharp, instantaneous pain that you feel from a cut or burn travels along a nerve path with scarce opioid receptors. While opioids may well be wonder drugs, they can't do it all.

CONQUERING PAIN AFTER SURGERY

The discovery of general anesthesia signaled the dawn of pain medicine. Anesthesia was able to temporarily disrupt consciousness so that patients could virtually sleep through otherwise painful interventions. But what about pain that lingers after you've woken up from surgery?

Over the next fifty years, scientists and doctors devised an assortment of devices and medications that combated pain without completely putting the patient to sleep. The spirit of stupendous discoveries continued with the revelation by the famous psychiatrist Sigmund Freud and a prominent ophthalmologist colleague of his that some drugs were wonderful numbing agents when applied to the skin. These drugs soon acquired the name "local anesthetics." The same doctors and dentists who had been experimenting with general anesthetics were also testing these chemicals for their impact on discrete parts of the body. For instance, a French physician dripped ether into an incision site, then blew cold air on it, hoping for numbness.

Sometimes ether was sprayed on an area that a doctor was about to repair. None of these worked as well as when ether was inhaled, but inhalation meant that doctors had to accept full unconsciousness and the mortal risks that came with it.

Local anesthetics offered doctors the chance to refine the impact of their painkillers, limiting the insensibility they delivered to a particular body part and avoiding the life-threatening risks of general anesthesia. They devised new gadgets, concocted new potions, experimented with exotic herbs. One such plant, the coca leaf, arrived in Europe from South America. Ancient Incans had used it as a source of energy for their exhaustive gold-mining labor, and ever since, natives had been chewing the deep green leaves and absorbing the juices into their bloodstream.

Four years after it was first introduced in Europe around 1859, coca was extracted into a wine called "Vin Mariani," after the chemist who formulated it. Vin Mariani quickly became Europe's most popular drink, renowned for raising spirits and even lifting them from deep depression. Twenty years later, a chemist in Georgia, John Pemberton, also used the plant to create a drink he called Coca-Cola, which he promoted as a cure for headaches and as a stimulant. (In 1906, coca was removed from Coca-Cola and replaced by caffeine.)

Scientists began experimenting with coca leaves to see what drugs they could extract. It was the German scientist Albert Niemann who in 1860 mixed a beaker of Peruvian coca leaves with water and other solvents to produce pure cocaine. Although he extracted other substances, cocaine was the only ingredient that affected people's minds. Cocaine was an intriguing chemical, able to lift spirits, energize, and alter thinking.

Its mind-bending qualities attracted the attention of young Sigmund Freud, whose specialty was neurology (psychiatry wasn't a science yet) and treating patients for "nervous exhaustion." Freud gave cocaine to patients as a tonic for all sorts of psychological troubles, particularly depression, and to treat morphine addiction. Like other scientists of the day, Freud experimented on himself and applied it to various parts of his body. As he wrote a few years later, he was especially impressed by its ability to desensitize the throat and tongue. "Cocaine and its salts have a marked anesthetizing effect when brought in contact with the skin and mucous membrane in concentrated solution," he wrote in 1884. "This property suggests its occasional use as a local anesthetic. . . ." Freud's proclivity for cocaine led to accounts of him being one of the most prominent cocaine addicts of the day. He went on to be acclaimed as one of the brilliant theorists of the mind, but he is rarely recognized for his significant contribution to anesthesia.

When Freud told an ophthalmologist, Carl Koller, about cocaine, he immediately decided to see whether this new numbing chemical would anesthetize the eye. After testing it on the eyes of a frog and guinea pig, he tried the drug on himself and found that his cornea could be made numb to prodding by a blunt instrument (remember, self-experimentation was prevalent during these times). Within a very short time, he was using it during eye surgery, freezing the eye so that it wouldn't move during the delicate procedure, while allowing the patient to remain awake and follow instructions.

Although Freud and Koller share the credit for discovering local anesthesia, a monumental advance that would have a profound impact on virtually every medical specialty, they used cocaine in limited cases. Only when an American doctor, William Halsted, used it to block nerve sensation all over the body did doctors begin to realize its potential. At Roosevelt Hospital in New York, Halsted—best known as the first surgeon to wear rubber gloves during surgery—came up with the idea of injecting cocaine into major nerve trunks as well as nerves around the eye and in the legs. Though the injections sometimes produced nausea and lightheadedness, the practice of injecting local anesthesia into sensitized nerves—particularly nerves in the skin where most pain is felt—became a mainstay of all medical procedures. Inspired by reports of injections of cocaine into spinal nerves, doctors began applying local or regional nerve blocks to all sorts of pain management, from treating hemorrhoids to removing bullets.

Medical science has a rough idea of how cocaine works, although much of its molecular activity continues to mystify researchers. Cocaine's ability to produce euphoria and suppress appetite may stem from its interaction with norephinephrine and dopamine, chemicals naturally generated by the body. When cocaine gets into the system, it stirs up these chemicals and causes more of them to circulate. Nerve cells designed to lock onto these chemicals and generate more chemical activity are especially rich in the brain's limbic system, the headquarters for your emotional responses. Cocaine's numbing action seems to come from its ability to block certain channels of nerve cells.

When applied to the eye or mucus membranes, cocaine makes its way into the bloodstream and to the brain, where it buoys thoughts and feelings. This is what made it so addictive (even Halsted was hooked for a while) and so troublesome as a local anesthetic. Cocaine would so flood a person's nervous system that it reached toxic levels. Early medical users reported many complications and at least a dozen deaths. But cocaine's amazing powers inspired laboratory chemists, and around 1905 they synthesized a chemical that acted like cocaine to numb skin and other tissues but didn't have its other effects on mood. Thus, the new agent was good at numbing but wasn't addictive. They labeled this chemical "procaine," which you know as Novocain—a member of a group of local anesthetics that I use all the time. Other synthesized siblings followed, such as benzocaine, bupivacine, lidocaine, and tetracaine. They, too, are superb locals.

FROM NARCOTICS TO OVER-THE-COUNTER DRUGS

The advent of local anesthesia in the nineteenth century totally altered general medicine and surgical procedures, but it rested in the hands of doctors and medical professionals. People still had to resort to home remedies or questionable compounds in order to treat run-of-the-mill aches and pain. Anesthesia did nothing for garden-variety, everyday pain like a headache. The folk remedies or over-the-counter medications of the day were mostly patent medicines and "soothing syrups," concoctions of opium, alcohol, and plants with names like Lydia Pinkham's Vegetable Compound and Kickapoo Indian Sagwa Blood Liver and Stomach Renovator. Patent medicines did not so much quiet specific aches and pains as stupefy a person so that little sensation was felt anywhere; or they put a person into a twilight sleep so he or she felt pain but just didn't care. I suspect that they just soused people!

Ancient folk remedies for pain and fever that had persisted through the ages were preparations made from the poplar tree or willow bark, or other leaves or fruits that contained forms of salicylate, a naturally occurring salt. Mixtures with vinegar were applied to ulcers, powdered forms or crushed leaves were used for diarrhea, and alcohol-based potions were recommended for a host of ailments. Scientists and doctors had been tinkering with variations of salicylate, mostly salicylic acid, for decades and had published papers describing how it reduced fevers. One such scientist was Fabrik von Heyden, whose company undertook the commercial production of sodium salicylate around 1880.

But the preparation had its drawbacks: It caused small blood vessels in the stomach to bleed, producing nausea, vomiting, and gastrointestinal distress. One of von Heyden's chemists, Felix Hoffman, had a father who suffered from crippling arthritis but couldn't tolerate the side effects of sodium salicylate. Young Hoffman scrounged through the company records of preparations that it had previously tested, looking for a pain reliever that might help his father. The most promising was a medication labeled "aspirin" ("a" for acetyl, part of its chemical composition, "spir" from a plant that contained salicin, and "in" because it was a popular medical suffix). Hoffman's father responded wonderfully, and within two years, Hoffman's employer, Friedrich Bayer and Company, was marketing aspirin. Just as Morton tried to disguise his common ether with the unique name of "Letheon," the Bayer company packaged its relatively simple substance under a patented trade name, Bayer Aspirin.

By 1899, Bayer Aspirin could be found in pharmacies throughout Europe, and it quickly became the leading remedy for arthritis, pain, and fever. At first, aspirin was sold as a powder, but within two years Bayer developed a water-soluble tablet, making it the first major drug to be offered in this convenient form. With a patented name, the Bayer company was able to control the production and sale of this common chemical substance until the beginning of World War I. It lost its monopoly when the U.S. Supreme Court ruled in a trademark infringement case that the company had advertised and marketed aspirin so heavily as to make the name a common term. Soon afterward, other companies began manufacturing and selling their brands of aspirin.

When aspirin went over the counter in 1915, the mass production of pain relievers for the general public was launched. But for many years aspirin had few competitors. Patent medicines had quickly disappeared because the U.S. government finally realized that narcotic-infused potions could be very harmful and needed to be controlled. The Harrison Act of 1914 put a stop to all the feel-good potions and required doctors and pharmacies to obtain and use a license number for writing prescriptions or selling medications. For people looking for something to treat their mild pain, this left them with nonprescription analgesics. For decades, aspirin reigned supreme. Its first real competition did not arrive until around 1960 when the FDA approved a new pain remedy available over the counter called acetaminophen, which you know by its brand name, Tylenol.

In fact, acetaminophen had been around since the late 1800s, but for fifty years it was ignored. Its original discovery was an accident— if it weren't for the sloppy work of a German pharmacist, we might have never heard of Tylenol. The doctors credited with recognizing that it helps relieve pain, Arnold Cahn and Paul Hepp, were treating patients for intestinal parasites and fever when the local pharmacy mistakenly supplied them with acetanilid instead of the drug they had been using. (The body metabolizes acetanilid into acetaminophen.) Then this drug seems to have fallen off the map, attracting virtually no scientific interest until 1951 when scientists at a Pennsylvania pharmaceutical company heard about it at a medical symposium.

McNeil Laboratories of Fort Washington, Pennsylvania, liked the looks of acetaminophen because it appeared to be as potent as aspirin without irritating the stomach and gastrointestinal tract. But acetaminophen had other shortcomings, especially its effect in large doses on the liver or when mixed with alcohol. The company launched full-scale testing and in 1955 introduced a liquid pain reliever for children called Tylenol. Because acetaminophen does not upset the stomach and can be suspended in a liquid, it was perfect as a child's medication. Five years later, McNeil brought to market the first adult variety.

THE MYSTERY OF ANTI-INFLAMMATORIES

If you think about it, even your mildest injury usually brings out redness and swelling, the telltale signs of inflammation. Inflammation and pain go hand-in-hand as much as dry mouth and thirst. It should come as no surprise to you that when pharmaceutical companies started hunting for new pain relievers, they focused on a compound's effect on inflamed tissue. In the race to develop new pharmaceuticals, Upjohn forged an alliance with a British pharmaceutical firm, Boots Pure Drug Company, in the 1960s to share research results. As it reviewed data and early tests from its English partner, Upjohn was particularly intrigued by a chemical compound called ibuprofen and began its own experiments. Despite some skepticism from executives who thought the drug was "just another aspirin," the American firm investigated the compound for five years and then began human tests in 1969. The first trials of ibuprofen, which Upjohn had given the name Motrin, were conducted on patients with arthritis.

In 1974 Upjohn applied for and received U.S. Food and Drug Administration approval for the marketing and sale of its new treatment for osteoarthritis and rheumatoid arthritis. It was such a hit that within two years the company had churned out 1.7 billion tablets of ibuprofen. As happens with many medications, there was considerable "off-label" use of the anti-inflammatory. People couldn't help but notice that it eased all sorts of aches and pains, from pulled muscles to sore throats. Five years later, the FDA approved Motrin as a drug to relieve a variety of pains.

Analgesics are a huge group of drugs—in essence, any drug that reduces pain. Over-the-counter or nonprescription analgesics are nonopioid medications that generally fall into two categories. There's the extended family of anti-inflammatories, which includes aspirin and ibuprofen (these are sometimes referred to as NSAIDs—nonsteroidal anti-inflammatory drugs) and there are drugs that contain acetaminophen, which are questionable anti-inflammatory agents but still are potent pain relievers.

It was only recently that scientists and doctors had a clear idea of how or why anti-inflammatories reduced fevers and eased pain. For seventy years, millions of people swallowed anti-inflammatory analgesics knowing only that they were remarkably effective. In 1971, an English doctor, John Vane, and two Swedish doctors, Bengt Samuelson and Sune Bergstrom, revealed the secret of the anti-inflammatories, and eleven years later, the Swedish Academy awarded them the Nobel Prize for Medicine.

When tissue is damaged—for instance when you're burned or cut— it releases a flood of chemicals including a peptide (a very small protein molecule) called bradykinin. Bradykinin swirls about, probably making your pain nerves more sensitive and creating tiny leaks in blood vessels in the neighborhood of the injury. The injury site is soon flooded with fluid and infection-fighting white blood cells—simply put, it becomes inflamed. The fight between fluids and infection draws another group of chemicals called prostaglandins into the fray. Prostaglandins kick off chemical activity and let your body know what's happening in its far-flung corners. Prostaglandins are produced by tissue throughout your body when there's some kind of trauma or damage. They help blood clot, regulate blood pressure, protect the stomach lining from injury and ulcers, and spur contractions during labor. Prostaglandins are also active in your immune system, and when a trauma prompts tissue to produce an excess of them, they join the fight with bradykinin and many other substances in helping fuel inflammation. While you know from experience that inflammation usually feels uncomfortable, it is probably necessary for healing because it sounds your perimeter pain alarm as well as activating the flow of healing hormones.

The prize-winning scientists studying these chemicals found that aspirin and other anti-inflammatories like ibuprofen decreased pain and swelling by curtailing the effects of an enzyme, cyclooxygenase (COX, for short), that is a key ingredient in the making of prostaglandins. What makes anti-inflammatories hard on your gut is that they lower COX production all over, including tissue in your gastrointestinal tract and kidneys, where these chemicals normally protect us. So by reducing inflammation in one type of tissue, where there's been damage, the pain relievers strip other tissue of their ability to protect. The result? Your gut aches. In the short run, you usually can get away with pain relief without too many side effects. If you take them for prolonged periods, however, side effects often set in and the cost of pain relief becomes too high.

Medicine's search for a better pain pill has recently found that there are two COX enzymes. The anti-inflammatories you've been taking for decades suppress activity of both of these. Now researchers have found that blocking only a particular one of these, called COX-2, may have the same or better effects right at the spots where blocking the enzyme for pain relief is necessary while avoiding the other places where its effects may be harmful. These highly selective drugs, only recently produced in high-tech, computerized labs, quiet inflamed tissue but leave the stomach and other organs alone. You'll be hearing much more about these selective "COX-2" inhibitors because they are now hitting the marketplace. They promise to offer the same pain relief with much fewer side effects. So unlike present drugs, they may be much more tolerable at high pain-relieving dosages over long periods of time.

THE RISE OF HYPNOTISM AND MIND-BODY MEDICINE

In reading about the wonders of nineteenth-century pain medicine, I am often captivated by stories about what was considered a highly questionable medical practice of the time, hypnotism. Accounts of hypnotic treatments offer clues about the power of the mind to manipulate pain. Hypnotism was a term coined by a British surgeon, James Braid, who followed in the path of the late-eighteenth-century Austrian doctor Franz Anton Mesmer. Although Mesmer is usually credited as the "father" of hypnosis, his experiments were more entertaining performances akin to the ether and the laughing-gas parties of the eighteenth century. It was Braid who translated mesmerism into hypnotism and put the entertaining practice on a scientific footing.

Mesmer's medicine reflected the thinking of the time, which mingled the scientific method of objective observation and experimentation with religious teachings and belief in "life forces." When he was a medical student at the University of Vienna, he theorized that people's health was strongly influenced by the gravitation of planets pulling on bodily fluids. He surmised that this force field was like electricity, or ocean tides that rise and fall. As a practicing doctor, he refined this idea into his theory of "Animal Magnetism" and attributed changes in a person's bodily fluids to magnetism rather than the planets. Disease or pain, Mesmer believed, was the result of blockages of an individual's fluids and could be cured by putting a person into a trance that would enable the body to restore its natural balance.

At first, Mesmer's ideas were greeted with skepticism and charges of fraud, so he moved from Vienna to Paris and set up a clinic-salon to treat mostly women for a variety of ailments, mainly "nervous" disorders. The centerpiece of his salon was a large tub filled with water and iron filings, with metal bars sticking out that served as handles. Mesmer's treatment consisted of asking a patient to stand beside the tub with her hands gripping its metal handles, and willing the magnetic energy inside the tub to enter the patient's body, placing her into a trance and reestablishing the "harmonious flow" of her fluids.

For a few years, Mesmer's parlor entertainment was quite popular, and he frequently treated groups of people using elaborate ceremony, which added to the party atmosphere of his treatments. His patrons frequently claimed that they had been cured, and the invention of electricity around this time seemed to buttress people's belief in unseen forces. Mesmer's popularity was short-lived. His lucrative practice, as well as his questionable therapeutics, drew criticism from other doctors. An investigation by a government commission composed of scientists and doctors concluded that there was no scientific evidence to support his claims, and mesmerism quickly faded from public view.

However, I don't think that Mesmer's "science" was completely bogus. Many of his theories sound similar to current explanations behind Chinese healing arts, especially the manipulation of a person's "chi" during acupuncture. (Like mesmerism, acupuncture is a medical technique that Western science has never completely understood or explained.) Much of the criticism surrounding Mesmer's treatments arose because they were not repeatable, which is one of the benchmarks for scientific credibility. Yet, reading accounts of his magnetic tub cures, I am struck by the psychological effect his trance-inducing ceremonies produced. His patients seemed to slip into an unconscious fog, like someone who is sleepwalking. And he was reputedly very successful in soothing mental illness or nervous states.

The fact that scientists of Mesmer's time could not duplicate the psychological impact that he produced does not necessarily mean all was fakery. The power of charismatic healers is well known today, and I suspect that much of Mesmer's magic had to do with therapeutic phenomena doctors continue to try to harness through relaxation, stress reduction, as well as the placebo effect. The story of what happened to Mesmer's techniques and how they were refined and reshaped into hypnotism, a very effective pain treatment for some people, has reinforced my conviction that thoughts and feelings can be as powerful as drugs when it comes to controlling pain.

Not all of Mesmer's ideas and unusual treatments were discarded. A few decades later, French physician Victor Burq modified Mesmer's animal magnetism theories into a treatment he called "metallotherapy," which he practiced at the famous Paris hospital, Salpetrière. Here, at one of the world's first psychiatric hospitals, which catered largely to women suffering from "hysteria" or other so-called nervous disorders, Burq used metal plates placed on women's bodies to restore lost sensation. Burq reputedly was very successful and claimed many cures, and so other doctors, most notably the famous neurologist Jean-Martin Charcot, adopted his methods. But while the French public and medical community loudly debated whether mesmerism was truly effective against mental disorders, James Braid was adapting the technique for use as an anesthetic.

Braid was a doctor in Manchester, England, who had attended demonstrations of mesmerism. While he thought much about it was hocus-pocus, he was impressed by how mesmerized patients' psychological states altered their physiological reactions, quickening their pulses and stiffening their muscles, then making them insensitive to pain or turning them pliable and hypersensitive. Braid could not explain how or why a person slipped into a trance, but he began experimenting with ways to put people into a trance and to attempt, through the power of suggestion, certain cures.

Determined to create a more scientific atmosphere, Braid eschewed Mesmer's elaborate ceremony and fanciful theory of metal affecting bodily fluids. He used the term "hypnotism," from the Greek *hypnos,* meaning "sleep," to separate the practice from the shaky science of its founder. He wanted to take hypnosis out of the realm of parlor game and into the medical laboratory, believing that rather than a metallurgic phenomenon, it was a kind of nervous sleep. He used any available shiny object, preferably a scalpel, to focus a patient's eyes and concentration and put them in a state of semiconsciousness in ten to fifteen seconds. During a trance, Braid suggested to the patient that pain was reduced if not gone. When Braid later wrote about his experiments, he reported successfully treating migraine headaches, tic douloureux (excruciating facial seizures known today as trigeminal neuralgia), "spinal irritations" (perhaps backache), and postsurgical pain.

Hypnosis both captivated and frightened people. It was constantly under suspicion and being challenged, yet it seemed to have amazing medicinal properties. There is even an account in the prestigious British medical journal *Lancet* from the mid-1800s of it being used as anesthesia for the amputation of a gangrenous limb. Even though the patient remained awake during the operation and said he was in no pain, the journal article claimed that he was not a genuine patient but really an actor trained not to show pain. (He certainly mastered an extraordinary form of acting.)

The possibility that hypnosis offered miraculous cures captured the public imagination, and as with mesmerism fifty years earlier, it became a popular, spellbinding entertainment. Street artists hypnotized "volunteers" and apparently cured the blind, deaf, and paralyzed. People believed that the power of hypnotic suggestion could make them commit crimes, even murder, when under its influence. A bestseller of the era, *Trilby,* by George Du Maurier, immortalized the notion of an evil, hypnotic seducer in the fictional character of Svengali. In the novel, Svengali is a music teacher who, through hypnosis, molds his young wife into a glorious singer who can perform only when under a trance. When Svengali dies, her masterpiece performance is a disaster and her career collapses. Ironically, today hypnosis is now so commonplace that most people can learn to hypnotize themselves without the help of a hypnotist or Svengali.

Hypnosis was eventually outlawed, or more accurately, allowed to be practiced only by licensed medical professionals. Governments in France, Austria, Italy, and the German states severely limited its use, and gradually doctors became disenchanted with its powers. Even the ultimate mentalist and one-time strong proponent of hypnotism, Sigmund Freud, stopped using it, preferring instead to plumb his patients' minds through a new kind of psychological treatment, psychoanalysis.

Although mind-body medicine has been around for centuries—what else were ancient ceremonies for casting out demons?—hypnotism was one of the first Western attempts to anchor it in science. The mind has a large say in which sensations your body feels. If you think of the history of pain medicine as a steady march along the road of consciousness, with each remarkable landmark commemorating a major reduction in how you feel pain, then hypnotism falls into place. This is one reason that as a pain doctor I sought additional training in psychiatry, so I have the tools to explore how an individual's thoughts and emotions are fueling what they are experiencing as pain. It's also why hypnotism has a place in modern pain management and why I recommend it for some patients. (I'll explain later how it's practiced.) It's one way that a person's mind and conscious thought process can take control over what the body is experiencing. While hypnosis usually cannot cure chronic pain, it can often help someone gain control over how much that pain impinges on their life. The idea of personal control is pivotal to managing chronic pain. When you feel that you can do nothing about your pain, that you're totally helpless, then the pain often grows stronger and stronger. That's when a backache becomes a back in chronic pain, and a life in pain.

SEIZING CONTROL OF PAIN: THE PCA REVOLUTION

One of the ironies of my specialty is that I am most effective when a patient is a full-fledged, active partner in the business of controlling pain. The notion that you can control your pain, or at least have a major influence on it, is a powerful analgesic. The therapeutic value of giving patients some control over their pain was the inspiration for a revolutionary approach to dispensing analgesia. In 1968, Dr. P. H. Sechzer watched a nurse give opioids to postoperative patients *when they asked for them*. Giving pain-relieving drugs on demand was a new concept. The usual procedure was to dispense drugs according to a schedule determined by the doctor in charge. What struck Sechzer was that patients who received intravenous opioids on demand felt better with smaller doses.

Other doctors were noticing and writing about the same phenomenon, especially obstetricians who let new mothers control their pain medication. It was just a short step from letting patients control their intravenous injections to inventing a device that allowed pain patients to give themselves a shot of medication whenever they wanted. The first such device, developed by doctors at Stanford University Medical Center in 1970, was called the Demand Dropmaster, which delivered a dose of analgesia when a patient pressed a button on a hand grip. The experimental Demand Dropmaster soon evolved into a drug-delivery system known as PCA, patient-controlled analgesia, that has made major inroads in controlling acute pain. My experience with Lee Smythe is typical of the kind of impact PCA can have on pain. If you're ever in the hospital on pain medication, remember PCA.

I was asked to see Mr. Smythe late one afternoon, a memorable request because the case seemed routine. He was a fifty-eight-year-old business executive recovering from gall bladder removal, a usually uneventful procedure. In this case, because previous surgeries had caused scars in the area, the surgeons had to open him up rather than employ the less invasive laparoscopic technique of using a small scope and laser knife. This larger operation required several days of recovery.

I was called in because the surgeons were unable to control Mr. Smythe's post-op pain and felt he was getting worse. I arrived at the private room to find him in bed, his wife and daughter by his side, surrounded by flower arrangements from well-wishers. He was clearly in distress, grimacing and unable to make eye contact for more than a moment. His pain centered in the area of the operation, as I expected. But I wondered why he was still in pain. He had received large dosages and many shots of morphine injected into his buttock muscle, which should have been more than enough. But he was neither relieved nor sedated. My next thought, of course, was that perhaps he was receiving too little medication.

His wife mentioned that during his last surgery he had been very frustrated that the pain medicine was never given at the right time and was never there when he asked for it. She added that he had been anxious about this operation because of the possible pain. There's nothing like a bad experience with pain to tense us up on the next go-around. As I do with any patient who doesn't respond to treatment in the usual way, I spent extra time finding out about Mr. Smythe's history. Sometimes when I am presented with unclear and incomplete information about a difficult situation, I have to put on my Columbo detective hat. In this case of "the morphine-resistant pain" the clues were coming together and evidence was mounting.

I knew he was the CEO of a large company, but his daughter offered a more telling detail. "He's a control freak," she declared. When we talked about his earlier hospitalizations, Mr. Smythe admitted that he felt helpless and at the mercy of nurses who varied in skill and concern, and doctors not old enough even to be part of his executive staff. He was used to commanding the ship and found it hard to give up the helm, even when his own welfare was at stake.

As I was leaving, the nurse pulled me aside to point out the patient's nervousness and suggest that we give him a Valium-type medication to calm him. But it seemed to me that anxiety wasn't exactly the root of the problem. I speculated that it might be anxiety's close cousin, fear. On top of severe pain, Mr. Smythe's distress was compounded by the fear of losing control and the inability to let go of the situation. He had no confidence that the nurses and doctors would take care of his pain, but he was unable to take charge of his own treatment. I had two options: either treat his fear with other medications or give him the control he wanted and needed. Since medicating his fear would only add more drugs to the mix, I chose the latter.

Some patients are frightened at first but ultimately relieved when I tell them about PCA. I explain that it's a safe approach to delivering pain medicine through a pump loaded with a drug such as morphine and a button that the patient can push when he feels pain. As you may imagine, this controlled, immediate intervention is often much better than waiting until the pain is bad enough to call the nurse, who may be tied up with another patient.

The first concern of most patients is that they might overdose themselves, a worry I take seriously because if it's not addressed, a patient may hold back on using the PCA. I explain the system's wonderful fail-safe features. For one, the doctor sets the upper limit of how much medicine patients can give themselves. Patients are given PCA doses with safe parameters that set the pump for how many doses can be given in a certain period (called the "lockout"), usually one dose every five to ten minutes, no matter how many times the button is pushed. The physician also sets the amount of drug delivered with each push, called the demand dose.

The device has an added fail-safe, which is the action of the narcotic itself. As long as it's only the patient who uses the button, it's highly unlikely that a patient will overdose himself, because if he gives himself too much, the drug will make him drowsy and eventually put him to sleep. This stops any further pushes on the button and, of course, any more medication. PCA is not only safe but smart. Its effectiveness depends on the one person who knows best how much medication is needed and when: the patient. Mr. Smythe knew from previous surgeries that other people's ideas of the right doses and good timing could be very mistaken. When I told him about the pain button, he took to it like a new car.

As soon as it was hooked up, he gave it a spin—several pushes over about fifteen to twenty minutes. His distress evaporated and his pain subsided. And this improvement happened with much less morphine than had previously left him writhing in agony. In a short time, he grew confident that he could manage almost any of the pain that might come his way. Patients often give themselves relatively small doses to find the right level and frequency. Following the pattern of most patients using PCA, Mr. Smythe needed less and less medication as he recovered from his surgery and learned more about the effects of the button on his pain.

With his PCA button close by, Mr. Smythe recovered quickly. After forty-eight hours he was eating solid food, and I shifted his pain medicine from PCA to oral pain pills. For most of us, being in pain is extremely disempowering and makes us feel helpless, if not frightened. PCA goes a small way toward offsetting this mental anguish and a long way toward defeating pain.

With PCA, the patient can give himself finely tuned pain control, particularly since the patient is the true expert about his particular pain. PCA allows patients to control the pain before it becomes a crisis in which large doses are more likely to work but bring greater risk of side effects. Patients may find they need the pain medicine only when they start to move around. For instance, patients recovering from a knee operation may give themselves a preventative dose in anticipation of the pain that is usually felt doing physical therapy. Some patients awaken at night in pain and need to push the PCA button. With nighttime pain, I may add a small amount of continuous medicine (not dependent on the patient pushing the button) through the sleeping hours. Ultimately, doctors have learned from studies that patients with PCAs may use less narcotics and may recover earlier from their surgery.

While PCA is used most commonly with intravenous opioids through a handheld button, it's being tested in other forms. New devices are applying the PCA concept to other forms of delivering pain medicine, such as epidurals that deliver local anesthetic close to the spinal cord (I'll tell you more about these later). Another system is an electrical device attached to a patch over the skin that is infused with opioids. An imperceptible electrical current drives the drug from the patch into the skin and bloodstream. In these systems, the patient controls the frequency of doses with a button.

Such advances in pain management were unthinkable to those who witnessed the birth of anesthesia 150 years ago. These new systems have revolutionized the standard of care for acute pain control that will likely impact every one of us at some point in our lives. Unfortunately, PCA cannot address all of the discomfort that comes with pain. When pain persists—when it jumps the fence and extends beyond the normal confines of surgery and postsurgical healing—different approaches and delivery systems are called for. As you will see in the next chapter, when pain becomes chronic, patients enter a new country governed by its own rules.

3

The Mysteries of Chronic Pain

When a Pain in the Back Becomes a Life in Pain

If you believe in evolution . . . you can trace all of our
lower back problems to the time when the first hominid
stood erect.

—Dr. Hugo Keim, orthopedist
Time, July 14, 1980

The formal definition of chronic pain, and one of the points I make to
patients, is that unlike acute pain, it lasts beyond the time necessary
for healing and resists normal treatment. However, if you've ever had
any sort of chronic pain, I'm sure you'll agree that this only scratches
the surface of its true nature. The best way I can give you a picture of
all that chronic pain involves is to take you back to your body's alarm
system.

If acute pain is the body's alarm system that rings when danger or
bodily damage threatens, then chronic pain is like an unpredictable
glitch in the doorbell that won't turn off, leaving a repetitious
onslaught of noise, which may be either loud or fairly quiet but after a
while drives you to a point of serious irritation. It can arise gradually
or suddenly, at any time, and frequently causes symptoms that are far
out of proportion to whatever set it off.

The primary indicator of chronic pain is not how long it persists
but whether it remains long after it should have disappeared. When I
first see a patient in pain, I always assess whether the pain has per-

sisted beyond the normal healing time. A broken arm will hurt for a couple of weeks, then begin to feel better as it heals. If it still hurts after a month or so, something's amiss. In some cases, this means that healing didn't occur, the original problem may have worsened, or another problem has arisen. But not always. Sometimes the pain remains for no clear reason or purpose, ringing the alarm over and over, long after the initial problem is resolved. Let me tell you about Roy Campbell, a patient whose low back pain typified all the ramifications of chronic pain.

TANGLING WITH A PATCH OF ICE

When Roy slipped on a treacherous patch of ice during one of Boston's worst spring storms, he was thrown several feet and came crashing down on the pavement, his head and tailbone hitting simultaneously. He lay there stunned, feeling foolish and thinking that he might be bleeding. With the help of a passerby, he slowly stood up and saw blood on the sidewalk from a cut on the back of his head. He hardly noticed that his lower back had also taken a bad hit. He had landed on the most vulnerable part of the spine, the lower lumbar region, where ligaments and tissue that hold disks in place are thinnest—exactly the area that is involved in most people's back problems.

Using a handkerchief to stem the bleeding, he returned to his office a few blocks away and stopped at the nurse's office. His head had started to throb, and the nurse made him lie down while she tended to the wound. When she saw that the gash was serious, she called an ambulance to take him to the emergency room at Mass General Hospital. The ER was teeming with people with ice-storm-related injuries, and Roy had to wait hours before seeing a doctor. Eventually, a doctor looked at Roy's bloodied head and admitted him overnight for observation. When Roy left Mass General the next day feeling better, he thought that except for the pain from the bill he would be receiving, he had seen the last of the hospital and his suffering. Little did he know how much trouble was just around the corner.

Roy went back to work as an insurance adjuster. Fifty-six years old, he was counting off the months until early retirement. He was eagerly looking forward to pursuing his passions for gardening and wine collecting. His children were grown and out of the house, and he and his wife, Ellen, would soon be completely free to travel and explore the Napa Valley wine country. But over the weeks after the fall, a dull, aching pain seeped into his lower back and buttocks. Gradually, it erupted into sharp stabs that felt like an ice pick piercing his tailbone. The pain was unpredictable, arriving at any time, no matter whether Roy was sitting, walking, or kneeling in the garden. At first, he ignored the pain, thinking it was the everyday-variety back pain so many of us get, the kind that just comes and goes. But after a month of alternating stabbing and achy pain that wouldn't let him sit still for more than a few minutes, he sought help. Back pain can be like that—creeping up on people and gradually worming its way into their lives until it has completely altered normal activities.

The orthopedic surgeon examined Roy's back, asked a litany of questions, and confessed that he couldn't determine the cause. He needed to run a battery of tests before he had any answers. Roy appreciated the doctor's candor, but he secretly worried that a mysterious mechanical glitch in his back could haunt him for years. He wasn't looking for a quick solution, but a lasting one.

The doctor gave Roy a prescription for a pain medication, Darvocet, and scheduled tests. The first was an X ray to look for broken bones. It showed nothing. Next was a bone scan to look for tumors or infection in the bone. Again, nothing. Lastly, an MRI scan explored for soft-tissue damage. When the results were in, the doctor was still baffled about what was causing Roy's back pain and suggested that he get another opinion. The Darvocet, a combination of a mild analgesic, propoxyphen, and Tylenol, wasn't helping either.

CHRONIC PAIN: WHEN SYMPTOMS DON'T MAKE SENSE

Roy's pain didn't make sense. The time had long passed for his ligaments or bruised muscles to have healed. There was no obvious physiological reason for his sensory nerves to continue to send out pain signals and for his muscles to spasm. The scans and X rays showed no tissue damage, and any touchy nerves should have cooled off by this point. This is how chronic pain attacks. It is pain that bewilders, pain that serves no purpose.

As you read earlier, acute pain is a symptom of a specific threat to the body. It alerts you to possible damage so that you can get help or treatment. Chronic pain, however, is just an ugly noise. It's a shrill alarm but serves no biological function. As the father of pain medicine, John Bonica, explains, "Acute pain is a symptom of disease; chronic pain itself is a disease."

A singular feature that makes chronic pain so distinct from acute pain, and so hard to treat, is that it usually is not connected to a specific disease and often produces effects that go beyond the bounds of the pain itself. It's usually a lot more complicated than acute pain. Of course, there are exceptions and gray areas. Arthritis is a disease that can produce chronic pain, but I consider it to be in the realm of both acute and chronic pain, meaning that it's both persistent and intermittent and it can be managed with some of the same remedies as acute pain. Cancer and multiple sclerosis are diseases that can generate chronic pain. Not only can chronic pain begin with tissue or muscle that's been injured, diseased, or somehow malfunctioning, but also it can surface without any inciting event, almost as if it came from the depths of the mind. Psychological, emotional, and behavioral forces create strong undercurrents that have a contributing role in the development and staying power of chronic pain.

I'm not implying that chronic pain is a creation of the imagination. But it stems not only from your body but from your mind. I frequently hear patients plead, "Doctor, don't say my pain is in my mind." But if you understand the whole phenomenon of pain, you know that it would be impossible to experience any pain without the assistance of the mind. It is foolish for a doctor to treat the experience of chronic pain without considering the mind as a partner with the body, just as it is foolish to ignore the body and only focus on the mind. Ordinarily, the dynamic tension between mind and body promotes health and stability—but this relationship can become diseased, and when it does, the result can be a mysterious condition.

TRIPPING THE CHRONIC PAIN ALARM

By now Roy had been living with constant pain for six months. The medication had done little for him, largely because the side effects, especially the nausea and lethargy, were so unpleasant that he ultimately threw away the pills. His doctor prescribed different medications, which Roy took for a month or so, again without improvement. Reluctantly sensing that his pain had moved in for a very long stay, he made an appointment with another orthopedic surgeon. The new doctor was much more upbeat and optimistic, telling Roy at his first appointment that he was fairly certain that he could find the root of the trouble.

On his second visit, the doctor examined Roy's back and applied mild pressure to various spots, at last pinpointing the pain in an area between the fourth and fifth lumbar vertebrae of his lower spine. Roy let out an abrupt "ouch" and then exclaimed, "You're the first person to find it!" Buoyant with hope, Roy assumed that now his pain could be eradicated because the doctor had discovered its hiding place. The orthopedist explained that the pain might be the result of inflamed ligaments that hold the bones of the spine together. He told Roy that the best course was a local injection that would halt the pain while the ligament healed and the surrounding muscles ceased going into spasms.

The initial blow to Roy's lower back probably bruised many tissues, including muscles and ligaments that run the length of the spine to the last lumbar and sacral vertebrae. Here, bones, disks, muscles, ligaments, and other tissues are connected to each other, each densely studded with sensitive nerves ready to ring out OUCH. Most low back pain is caused by musculoskeletal injuries—strains and sprains to muscles, ligaments, and other connective tissues—around the lumbar vertebrae. When Roy fell on the ice, sensory nerves communicated their displeasure, which set in motion a complex reaction intended to protect the injured area.

The nerves sound the pain alarm, which, in concert with tissue damage, stimulates inflammation that increases blood flow to the area. This increases the production of local chemicals that sensitize the area to pain and tenderness. It's a cycle that builds up over time. The muscles in the region aren't used to so much commotion and respond by becoming hypersensitive. They ultimately go into a state of sustained contraction, otherwise known as spasm.

A spasm in itself is not necessarily painful. Hiccups, for example, are the result of spasms in the diaphragm, and they usually don't hurt. But if you've ever had a bad case of hiccups, you know that spasms can be self-perpetuating, and after a while they produce their unique brand of discomfort. When muscles in the back automatically contract, you change your posture to relieve it, and this skewed position can shift weight and pressure to other muscles, disks, and nerve roots. At the same time, the spastic muscle releases chemicals that cause local inflammation and swelling, which triggers another spasm. Pretty soon, the skewed posture, inflamed muscles, and nerves are trapped in a vicious cycle of spasm, pain, and more spasm. The gluteal muscles radiating from Roy's low back—his achy butt—were undoubtedly caught in this web.

A MODERN PLAGUE: LOW BACK PAIN

Low back pain is probably the most common form of chronic pain in the modern world. I'm sure it would not be much comfort to Roy to know that millions of other people have gone through similar experiences. The medical reasons for his back pain will give you an idea of the complexity of chronic pain and help explain why relief is so often elusive. As you'll read, pinpointing the source of a particular pain is like trying to identify the one person who's booing in an entire stadium of spectators.

Lots can go wrong with your back. It's like a highly complex scaffolding held together with wire, nuts, and bolts, stabilizing guy wires, and internal reinforcements—and subject to pressure from all directions. Stress or a blow to one corner of the structure can topple another corner of it. The basic components of the back offer many different opportunities for generating pain. This includes the muscles and ligaments along the spine that hold the spinal bones, or vertebrae, together, as well as holding in place the disks that act like pillows between bones, cushioning the tender nerve roots as they exit and enter from the body into the spinal cord. Ligaments that hold the bones together, tendons that connect the muscles to the bones, and many large and small nerves and blood vessels are all capable of ringing the pain alarm. They are subject not only to the wear and tear of aging but the sprains, strains, or bruises of everyday living. And, of course, there's the wild card of back pain, bad posture. Sometimes it produces painful abnormalities in your spine or musculoskeletal system, while in other people, poor posture throws the back out of kilter but doesn't cause pain.

While many aspects of back pain remain mysterious, doctors know a lot about its anatomy. The disks that serve as pillows between the vertebrae can cause pain. These disks are usually perfectly smooth, symmetrical ovals composed of a tough fibrous outer skin and filled with thick fluid that absorbs the daily shocks of normal activity. If the outer skin of one of these pillows becomes weakened, the shape of the disk can change and bulge. Over time, you acquire bulges in your disks, but they usually don't cause any harm. In rare cases, a disk bulge, if near one of the nerve roots, can cause nerve irritation and pain. If the tough shell of the disk breaks, the thick fluid inside the pillow can leak out. This is called a herniated disk, or slipped disk. The fluid is very inflammatory, and if it leaks onto a nerve, or even near one, it can cause pain.

But a herniated disk doesn't always cause pain. Recent studies using magnetic resonance imaging (MRI) of the backs of thousands of individuals who had no back pain revealed many with disk bulges and herniations. Significant structural problems indicated by a CAT scan or MRI are no longer automatically considered cause for the pain. On the other hand, some people have gone for years with excruciatingly painful backs that look completely normal on all imaging. Most perplexing and perturbing is "failed back syndrome," an all-too-common condition of persistent or worse pain after surgery and other treatments that were supposed to help. All of these mysterious variations make back pain one of the most stubborn conditions to treat. Back pain defies simple rules and simple solutions.

Although you may feel back pain some time in your life, only a small minority of people will be confronted with chronic back pain. Most acute back injuries heal quickly, within a matter of weeks, with little or no loss of workdays or other activity. In the not-so-distant past, someone with new back pain would have been instructed to rest in bed for days to weeks. Doctors now know that low back pain usually goes away after a few days, whether or not you rest. In fact, too much rest may be harmful, while maintaining most normal activities is probably better. While back pain is usually benign and transient, it can be the alarm that calls for immediate attention. My aunt thought her back pain was nothing to worry about and would get better on its own. She tried to get on with her life and not succumb to the adversity of her pain by doing what you probably do—she ignored it. She tried many of the over-the-counter and alternative- medicine remedies. She finally called me after about six months of increasingly painful symptoms to find out whether I'd advise her to see a chiropractor. After hearing her symptoms, I immediately arranged for her to see a neurosurgeon, who quickly took a CAT scan of her back.

The CAT scan explained the symptoms that separated hers from run-of-the-mill back pain. It revealed a small fracture of the vertebral bone pushing on one of the major nerve roots to the leg. She was also weak in the leg, which, combined with the back pain and shooting sensations, indicated a nerve problem at the spine. The doctor performed surgery that relieved the pressure on the nerve and spared her from permanent loss of function in her leg. The initial injury has healed, and her leg is no longer weak. But as is often the case, surgery doesn't always fix the entire problem that is causing chronic back pain. The surgery was absolutely necessary to stop the disease. Unfortunately, it couldn't reverse all of the damage to the nerve. Had she been diagnosed earlier, she probably would have recovered more fully. But because she had suffered for so long, her back still hurts and she now has failed back syndrome. Any back pain that lasts for more than a few days or that is very severe should be seen by a physician in the unlikely case that it's a signal that something serious has gone wrong.

WHEN ACUTE PAIN BECOMES CHRONIC

You may be wondering how an acute trauma like low back pain or even a pulled muscle evolves into persistent, nagging pain that seems immune to the usual pain remedies. One of the lessons of Roy's story is that chronic pain is not simply severe acute pain but an entirely different creature. It shifts to other parts of the body and acquires, and sheds, new characteristics; it takes on a life of its own. As I consider treatment choices, I keep in mind chronic pain's deceptive nature.

I met Roy more than a year after his tumble on the ice when his orthopedist referred him to the Mass General Pain Center. During that time, he had tried a host of home remedies. He had altered his normal habits and everyday posture, cutting back on hands-and-knees gardening, always sitting on two pillows, and constantly shifting his position when he sat for long periods. And he had taken an array of pain relievers and muscle relaxants. But the pain kept coming and had mutated into a sensation that followed no rules and defied predictions.

I talked to Roy, looked at his scans, and reviewed his medical history. Although the orthopedist had located a tender ligament, this same spot was no longer tender, even to very deep palpation. Like his other doctors, I couldn't tell exactly what was making his back hurt. The possible culprits were numerous, including other ligaments, nerve roots, deep muscles, and spinal joints. But I wasn't discouraged—I knew that even though upwards of 85 *percent* of patients with chronic low back pain never receive a definite diagnosis, they can still be helped.

In Roy's case, I examined and retested, and finally we agreed that we probably were not going to find the cause. We also agreed that this was certainly no reason to give up on trying to quiet the pain. When I know exactly what I am treating, I use a procedure that specifically targets the problem. In this case, I didn't know the culprit, so I chose a broad-based attack that could simultaneously neutralize different areas. I spread a thin coat of medicine along the spine that could be absorbed into the various connective tissues, as well as bones, disks, and nerves. Unlike the standard epidural injection, Roy and I decided to proceed with a caudal epidural, which is more commonly used in children and infants than adults. I explained to Roy that this approach uses the caudal canal (*caudal* means "tail") in the tailbone, where fairly large volumes of fluid can be delivered to the entire region around the sacrum, spine, and nerve roots. I injected approximately twenty milliliters of a diluted mixture of potent anti-inflammatory steroid medication and a local anesthetic in sterile water and watched the solution spread through Roy's sacrum and lower spine via X ray. The X ray pictures confirmed the medicine had reached its diffuse target.

Steroids reduce pain in two ways: They cool inflammation, which reduces swelling and pressure on nearby nerves, and they direct the traffic of signals transmitted by the slower nerve pathways that carry pain messages between damaged tissue and the spinal cord. Steroids usually do not work instantaneously because they are slowly absorbed through membranes into tissue, taken up into the cells where they slowly turn off inflammation. After the first injection, Roy gradually felt better, but it was almost two weeks before the pain was noticeably subdued. I wasn't surprised that it didn't disappear entirely. A number of studies have shown that the longer a pain lingers, the harder it is to eradicate. Once chronic pain has moved in and sets up shop, it rarely leaves quickly.

The steroid injections worked, and Roy's pain faded. But after three months of substantial relief, it stormed back and drove him to the Pain Center for another series of injections. Roy's initial pain was now almost completely gone. But probably due to all of the changes in his posture and limited activities, his pain had changed and increased in a different area of his back. Further treatments helped quell these pains as well.

WHEN PAIN MAKES NO SENSE: IDIOPATHIC PAIN

Though much about Roy's pain baffled his other doctors—and me—I had some facts to go on. I knew when and where he first hurt himself and that the pain remained in the same general area. Not all chronic pain is so accommodating. There is a kind of chronic pain that has no particular provenance and can be mystifyingly global and attack the whole person. Called idiopathic pain, it's what doctors call pain that has an unknown cause. Doctors sometimes quip that the real definition of *idiopathic* is that the doctor is an idiot and the patient is pathetic. The sad truth is that cases in which the symptoms have no known cause make doctors feel inadequate, patients feel helpless, and both parties suspicious of each other. In the face of failed treatments and their doctor's skepticism, patients may fear that their doctors view them as fakers. Some may wonder if their physician is just another quack. When treatments don't work, which often happens, trust is severely stressed and the doctor-patient relationship is ruptured.

Idiopathic pain is more common than you might think. But it is frequently ignored or undertreated because a doctor or patient may not realize the extent of the damage and attempts what amounts to a partial repair. As my patient, Margaret, found, idiopathic pain can damage an entire life and require looking at a wide spectrum of consequences.

Margaret was waiting in the Pain Center office with her husband, John. She was in her early fifties, and her anxiety was palpable from the outset of our first meeting. As she tried to fill me in on her medical history, she became flustered and quickly frustrated. Her husband took over so quickly and seamlessly that I wondered if this hadn't happened with other doctors. John described what had been a horrendous transition from a life as a highly productive schoolteacher and mother of two adolescents who took care of everyone at home to a woman consumed with pain and suffering, no longer able to do her job or participate in most family activities.

As she listened, she quietly sobbed and occasionally interrupted to say, "I am desperate. My life isn't worth living." I heard about pain that had affected her entire body, each day changing in severity and location from one place to another. Gradually, her activities were limited, and ultimately she had to stop working. She grew progressively homebound and increasingly depressed. Depression and pain grew together, and it was impossible for her to know which came first, which was driving the other.

With a terminated career and devastated family as prominent symbols of the carnage of her life gone wrong, her thoughts turned to suicide. She thought about it daily. One day her husband found a suicide note, which she acknowledged to me she intended to use. She had been storing up pills and working on the right words to leave behind.

It was clear that Margaret knew that her story made her sound like, as she put it, "a nutcase." She said, "Even though my mind is affected, my body hurts—I know there is something wrong with my body."

Numerous visits to physicians had been frustratingly unfruitful. The pain had marched throughout her body and now was as bad as ever. None of her previous doctors found a reason for the pain, despite complete evaluations including almost every laboratory test imaginable. All too often, physicians just don't know what exactly causes some strange symptoms, particularly with pain. Sometimes the best a doctor can do is reassure a patient that there is no evidence of serious physical illness. But this was faint comfort for Margaret. Multiple doctors had concluded that nothing was seriously wrong, yet obviously something *was* very wrong. When I met her, I sensed that neither of us had the luxury of waiting for a definitive diagnosis. By the time I might discover the cause of her symptoms, if ever, all might be lost. I reviewed the extensive previous workups and accepted that, for now, I wasn't going to be able to explain why she was in this dire state. That didn't mean that I couldn't help her. Margaret felt as though she was going crazy and wondered if she was imagining her symptoms as others had suggested. She was ready to give up. As a physician, I was again thrown into the role of medical detective, with an extremely puzzling crime against a victim who had little recourse for justice. Without validity and hope, it is almost impossible for a patient to rally to her own defense. My first task was to immediately make two things clear: I believed she had "real" pain and thought there was reason to hope that her life could be better.

I reassured her that her pain was certainly "in her head" because the brain and the mind have to be involved in any pain experience. I emphasized that this didn't mean it wasn't also in her body. In her case, a body in pain had spread into a life in pain. Any signs of what started the process or clues to track the disease to problems in cells or understandable diseases had long vanished. This common feature of chronic pain distinguishes it from acute pain.

New acute pain almost always stimulates changes in the part of your nervous system that is unconscious, acting on such vital life functions as blood pressure, heart rate, flushing of the skin, and sweating. It's the part that doctors believe goes haywire in chronic regional pain syndrome. So when you get nervous, your heart may race, blood pressure may go up, and you may get sweaty palms. This is acute anxiety, and acute pain can trigger the same reaction. When pain becomes chronic, these reflex signs usually disappear, leaving little evidence to track down the crime or nail the perpetrator.

The problem with pain is that it is always an untestable hypothesis—it can never be proved and thus can't be disproved. For this reason, doctors are tempted to be skeptical or dubious of someone's complaint. Doctors who believe that pain is simply nerves transmitting a pain signal from an injury to the brain often have trouble with someone whose pain doesn't make clear sense in terms of the anatomy of nerves, muscles, joints, or other tissues. This is where strictly holding to what is known or perfectly understandable can seriously limit the help medicine can offer.

Recall the definition: *"Pain is what the patient says it is."* This may sound simplistic. But, in fact, it reflects a complex reality—pain is like a symphony conducted by the brain with major input from various instruments within the body and mind sections. The sounds can be as varied as those from an orchestra, and too often it's hard to know exactly which instruments are playing, particularly when sweet healthy melodies turn into blaring nightmarish noises. In Margaret's case, I couldn't distinguish the violins from the flutes from the drums. Have you ever listened to a stereo with the volume turned up so high that the sound just breaks down and is uninterpretable? You know there is a song playing but you just can't make out the words. This is what I often encounter when pain has been impossible to trace but has wreaked havoc for a long time. And this is when I choose to embrace the widest definition of what it might mean when someone says she hurts.

Margaret seemed encouraged that I could give a name to her condition, *idiopathic pain,* and explain some of its features. I tried to be as clear as possible about what I knew and didn't know, her possible options, and what might lie down the road. I wanted to guard against creating unrealistic expectations in her that would only lead to more problems. I impressed upon her that this was no "mental" problem but that there was likely something else wrong underneath her ravaged, fragile exterior. I hoped that by explaining the reason for how I was going to proceed, she would readily accept my approach without feeling either stigmatized or overly optimistic.

I examined her carefully and sensed that she was watching to see whether I knew what I was doing and was considerate of how much pain she was in. Idiopathic pain is frequently minimized or dismissed by medical people, and so patients can be particularly sensitive to medical professionals who seem thoughtless. Her muscles were exquisitely tender throughout her body. She was surprised when I identified several fingertip-sized spots that were somewhat harder and more tender than the rest of her muscles When I pressed on these spots, pain radiated and increased in a pattern familiar to her. I told her that these are called "trigger points" and that they're linked to certain types of pain. I wasn't sure whether or not these spots were the underlying cause or the result of chronic pain. Like so many other "cause-and-effect" questions in chronic pain, at that point it didn't matter. I first had to turn down the volume.

Patients are often reassured if I can identify a physical problem, even if there's more than a single problem at play. I explained that she and I could not focus just on her mind or her body and that her pain required multiple approaches to head off disaster. Both her mind and body had colluded against her, so opposing one and not the other would be unsuccessful. I reiterated that there would not be a quick and easy solution. The unpleasant music of her pain had been composed over a long period of time and would require time to silence.

She and I talked about the most obvious physical and personal problems surrounding the pain, leaving subtle ones for later. Our list included tender muscles with trigger points, severe depression, anxiety including panic attacks, agoraphobia, physical deterioration associated with markedly limited physical activity, and a stressed family in crisis. We discussed each and mapped out a plan. I focused primarily on ways she could restore the quality of her life. Less pain would follow if she could get back into life and do more.

Regaining function is the key to overcoming chronic pain. In treatment, I focus on function rather than pain because even when I can't decrease the pain, I can almost always make the patient feel better by improving function. Margaret and I made a pact—no more suicide gestures while I tried to make some improvements in her life.

Over the next few weeks, Margaret packed her days with visits to physical therapists, rehabilitation doctors, and a psychiatrist. I became the conductor of her revised symphony. She received behavioral therapy for reducing stress and learned new ways to relax and to take control over the sensations of her body that felt like pain. These therapies also helped with her anxiety and the phobia of being out in public and unable to move. Her physical therapist showed her ways of moving and exercising that didn't hurt and helped her begin the process of restoring strength and mobility. She got medications for depression and anxiety, while injections of local anesthetic into the trigger points began to slow the progression of pain and decrease the tenderness.

I discovered that among Margaret's other disorders she had a syndrome called myofascial pain, "myo" relating to muscles and "fascial" referring to fascia or structural connective tissues such as ligaments or other fibrous substances that hold us together. When this disorder affects all parts of the body, it is often called fibromyalgia. Although doctors don't know the cause of this or even if it is truly just one disease or many, they do know that it's rarely just physical symptoms. Margaret's many sessions with my colleague Dr. Joseph Audette, a specialist in rehabilitation medicine at Spaulding Rehabilitation Hospital, made a huge difference. He traced the trigger points and, using fine needles, released the contractions, one at a time. The procedure looks much like acupuncture, although it's different. First, he gradually released Margaret's major trigger points and later, as healing occurred, moved on to the more subtle ones. This, combined with aggressive physical therapy and psychiatric treatment, turned the tide in Margaret's life.

I don't know exactly what did it, and I'd bet it wasn't just one thing. Each treatment helped the other, and possibly none would have been of value without the others. But after about a year of treatment, Margaret was back at work and had regained her family life. While she's not the same person she was before the disorder, she is much better than when we first met, and most important, she is no longer trapped at home within a paralyzed body. She still has pain, but it doesn't interfere with her getting on with her life. I don't know if she has less pain or has found a way to lessen the significance of the same amount of pain that previously brought her life to a halt. Nevertheless, her pain eased and her life improved, which is what I hope for all my patients. Although I may not be able to cure every pain, I can almost always help a patient in chronic pain feel better.

THE EMOTIONAL UNDERTOW OF CHRONIC PAIN

I mentioned earlier that patients frequently say to me, "Please don't tell me my pain is all in my head." Patients worry that they will be perceived as a "head case" and believe that any suggestion of a psychological component to their pain reflects skepticism of how much they're truly suffering.

When a patient says that she's afraid of being thought of as a mental problem, I explain that every pain must have some psychological component because thoughts and emotions are part of every painful experience. Don't you let out an angry yell or swear word when you hit your thumb with a hammer or bang a knee on a drawer? It's an automatic and natural response.

Persistent pain can alter your thought patterns and lifestyle and create a vicious cycle of negative thinking and experiences. If you're in chronic pain, you can become conditioned to suffering, and this can cloud your entire life. When months and years of treatments and medications produce no meaningful improvement, you become conditioned to disappointment and failure. You adopt "pain behavior," which grows more pronounced over time. You curtail pleasant or fun activities that might hurt and stop productive activities like exercising or even something as routine as walking to a subway every day. You may lose interest in sex, eat and sleep poorly, and become increasingly irritable and lethargic. Constant pain may force you to cut back on work or even stop working altogether. Family, friends, and medical people unwittingly encourage negative behavior by either sympathizing with you and supporting the growing dysfunction or by isolating and avoiding you because you've become unpleasant to be around.

Chronic pain is an insidious disease that can infiltrate your entire life. It may be like a storm that suddenly floods your home or a slow, steady drip that progressively corrodes the foundation of your life. The mysterious, widespread, and intransigent nature of the pain can lead friends and relatives to wonder whether you are suffering from a mental rather than physical disorder.

Not surprisingly, if you're in constant pain you may well become depressed, or anxious and fearful. If you believe that nothing will work and that you'll always be in pain, your work life and relationships may well disintegrate. And this feeling of being damaged and debilitated can build on itself and get worse. The feeling that you've lost control of your life and body, and that not even the brightest medical minds can help, only accentuates the gloomy emotions. Dysfunction begets dysfunction. Your life gets even worse if you allow your pain to define the shape of your days and the tenor of your emotions.

Chronic pain can become an emotion as strong as hatred or love and can dominate your every thought and action. (There are sound physiological, as well as psychological, reasons for this; some theories suggest that the instructions from the brain to the spinal cord dictating which sensory signals get through have distinct emotional shading. I'll say more in the next chapter about how the brain generates the emotions that shadow pain.)

Every day I meet people whose feelings of hopelessness, rejection, anger, and anxiety rule their lives. Worse yet, these feelings become self-perpetuating and breed depression. Sometimes the depression is disguised as a change in appetite, lack of interest in activities that once were enjoyable, lack of energy, poor sleeping, restlessness, or feelings of guilt. Ultimately, the depression becomes deep and persistent.

Depression can act like a magnifying glass on pain, and pain can intensify depression. The cycle forms and the two feed each other. Patients ask me whether pain causes depression or vice versa. To be honest, I never know. But as I usually explain, it's a chicken-and-egg kind of question whose answer usually doesn't make a difference. Each condition must be taken seriously and treated aggressively, regardless of which came first. Not all chronic pain sufferers drop into depression. Nevertheless, there is no denying that chronic pain places a huge psychological burden on anyone who has it.

It's no coincidence that I combined my specialties of internal medicine and pain medicine with psychiatry. Knowing all the damage that pain can do to a person, I consider the whole individual, not just physical symptoms. You should never feel reluctant or embarrassed to tell your doctor about how your pain is affecting your life. Margaret's honesty, as well as the forthrightness of her husband, ensured that I had a complete picture of what her pain was doing to her and could fashion a treatment plan that addressed the entire spectrum of her ailments. As Margaret learned, pain can beset an entire body. There are many other varieties of pain that strike more people than the idiopathic variety. One of these directly affects the nerves and nerve pathways. As you'll read in the next chapter, this pain is frighteningly common, and if you've ever had a condition even as mundane as carpal tunnel syndrome, you've met this offender.

4

WHEN THE PAIN ALARM GOES AWRY
Traumatized Nerves and Damaged Pathways

~

Perhaps few persons who are not physicians can realize
the influence which long-continued and unendurable
pain may have upon both body and mind.

—WEIR MITCHELL,
Nerve Injuries,

Normal nerves are capable of transmitting messages back and forth
between any part of your body and the brain. The signal may be the
result of pain, or something as benign as a summer breeze or as pleasurable as a gentle massage. A healthy nervous system is an invaluable
survival tool because it sends us necessary pain signals when our body
is under assault. However, all bets are off if the nervous system
becomes injured. Malfunctioning nerves can do strange things,
including creating their own abnormal sensations. Nerve injury can
produce a distinctive type of chronic pain called neuropathic pain. It
can arise within the central or peripheral nervous system and cause a
host of conditions that can range from mildly disturbing to bizarre
and painfully disabling.

While scientists have identified some of the things that can damage
a nerve pathway, such as disease or an accidental injury, they continue
to be mystified by certain features of neuropathic pain. Why, for
instance, is the pain that lingers sometimes much worse than the pain
from the original injury? Why does it sometimes take months after an

injury for neuropathic pain to surface? By investigating the puzzle of neuropathic pain, scientists have begun to unlock some of the secrets of the human nervous system and understand some of pain's most profound dimensions. If you're one of the millions of people who suffer from neuropathic pain—neuropathic pain is involved in almost 50 percent of all chronic pain—it's important to understand what we've learned, and are still learning, about how damaged nerves cause pain and what we can do about it.

A pioneer in studying neuropathic pain was a nineteenth-century neurologist, Weir Mitchell. Writing after the American Civil War, during which he treated numerous soldiers, he noted, ". . . after lancet wounds, the most terrible pain and local spasm resulted. When these had lasted for days or weeks, the whole surface became [hypersensitive] and the senses grew to be only avenues for fresh and increasing tortures, until every vibration, every change of light and . . . even the effort to read brought on new agony."

I know well the kind of pain he describes, for it torments many patients even today. While you may not have heard of "neuropathic pain," you may be familiar with one of its many varieties, which include complex regional pain, or RSD, shingles, carpal tunnel syndrome, and pain from cancer, AIDS, stroke, or amputation. Neuropathic pain, what Weir labeled "casualgia," is the quintessential example of chronic pain from nerve damage. Not infrequently, people come to me with pain that they do not realize stems from traumatized nerves. Often, once they learn about what's going on inside them, the pain becomes more manageable.

With each new discovery about neuropathic pain, like recent findings explaining phantom limb pain, medical science gets closer to defeating it. Although Weir Mitchell's experiences may sound dated, his insights into this unique form of chronic pain are still helpful today. Mitchell worked at the Philadelphia Stump Hospital, where he treated Civil War soldiers suffering from what was called "nervous" illnesses. This was a tough group to treat because the soldiers' physical pain was so intertwined with the entire trauma of war. They had left the battlefields not only with mangled limbs and deep wounds but also with hallucinations, flashbacks, and rampant anxiety. As a neurologist, Mitchell was most interested in disorders of the nervous system. Yet he was also acutely aware of how nerve damage, especially when it persisted long after an injury had healed, could affect a soldier's pain and eventually his personality. His observations of soldiers suffering from the aftershocks of war have earned him the credit for first recognizing what's known today as post-traumatic stress disorder, or PTSD. After World War I, the chronic stress, anxiety, and emotional numbness that came with war was called battle fatigue or shell shock, and after the Vietnam War it became better understood as post-traumatic stress.

As he cared for amputees, Mitchell saw that although the men's limbs seemed to heal, some of them were still in pain. While trying to tend to their suffering, he devoted considerable attention to understanding and treating their lingering amputation pain. He saw that the chronic pain of nerve damage was not simply a creation of the soldier's scarred memories but surfaced with distinct characteristics. He labeled their pain "causalgia," a term coined from the Greek *kaustikos,* meaning "capable of burning." Today, doctors know causalgia as a signal of pain that is typical of damaged nerves or neuropathic pain. This type of burning pain, which is remarkably consistent among individuals with pain from damaged nerves, has given science important clues about the organization of the nervous system and its ever-changing connections.

Mary Lake, a patient with neuropathic pain, was miserable and mystified when she came to me for treatment. As she and I sorted through her ailment and pieced together what the pain was doing to her body and her life, she found that her condition was not hopeless and that even this awful variety of pain could be curbed. Her case helps explain how relatively minor injuries can produce dreadful and persistent sensations and sheds light on possible links between pain and the nervous system.

WHEN THE BURNING DOESN'T STOP: COMPLEX REGIONAL PAIN

Like Roy Campbell, Mary Lake also slipped on a patch of ice after a storm, but her tumble seemed fairly minor. She was leaving work, a construction firm for which she did general bookkeeping, and was walking to her car when she stepped onto a slab of black ice, landing on her right shoulder and arm. Stunned and bruised, she was slightly hurt but not badly enough to seek help. She picked herself up and continued home to tend to what felt like a bad sprain. For a couple of weeks, the pain came and went but without a clear pattern. It was a stabbing pain that could be mild or awful. Without warning, sharp jolting sensations would shoot down her arm from her injured shoulder, lasting only a few minutes. Or the pain would remain for several hours as a lingering ache and burning in her arm. From time to time, her arm turned a light shade of mottled purple and her fingers would become cold and blue, seeming to lose their circulation. The discoloration and puffiness looked like a rash that would come and go.

In her mid-thirties, Mary was the mother of an active ten-year-old and was used to a busy life of working, errands, and regular aerobics classes. She was annoyed by how the pain was cutting into the rhythm of her life. She visited a chiropractor, hoping for relief, but on seeing the discolored arm, he said it was beyond his skills and sent her back to her family physician. Mary's doctor examined her shoulder, concluded that she may have torn her rotator cuff (the muscles and tendons that hold the shoulder together), and arranged for her to have an X ray and then a CAT scan. The results showed what appeared to be a healthy shoulder, but Mary continued to hurt and continued to have the on-again, off-again flares of swelling, color change, and pain.

She went to a physical therapist, who recognized that immobility was worsening her condition and tried to help her find ways to move her shoulder without pain. Nothing seemed to help. By now she had quit her job, and her husband, Frank, a long-haul truck driver, was curtailing his trips to stay home more often and help with their child.

The next year and a half was miserable for Mary. With her arm in a sling much of the time, she couldn't cook, driving was awkward, and shopping became a one-handed hassle. Sleeping was a nightly battle to avoid placing any pressure on the inflamed arm and shoulder. And sex was impossible without pain. Although she received workers' compensation, it covered only a small part of the family's expenses. Mary and Frank were forced to dip into their savings to cover her lost earnings. Mary grew angry and frustrated, then depressed.

Not unlike an unsolved crime, chronic pain without a telltale cause can breed paranoia. Patients may sense the frustration of health-care providers who can't figure out what's wrong and are trying to help but constantly failing. They may feel as though they are letting down their doctors, or even worse, that they are seen as frauds, suspected of making it all up for some ulterior gain. Mary knew from the constant wrangling with the workers' compensation office and the tone she detected in the voices of her parents and sisters that people were growing intolerant, as though she was exaggerating or even faking her symptoms. They saw her arm sling as a needless prop or a dramatic plea for attention and suggested that she might feel better if she didn't wear it.

Mary gradually avoided the people who appeared to question the seriousness of what she was going through. The consequence was even more isolation from friends and family. Not being able to understand her doctors and the confusing technical facts of her condition left her feeling inept and powerless, so she armed herself with information and terminology. Like many patients who feel trapped on a medical treadmill of treatments that go nowhere, she tried to regain control by mastering the medical jargon of her condition. This meant not simply learning the medical system of referrals and specialists but also studying medicine. She memorized the names of the muscles and nerves in her shoulder and arms, could correctly pronounce the long chemical names of the ingredients inside medications, and learned about their chemistry. If someone asked Mary how she was feeling, she would no longer describe the burning sensation in her arm or the mottled bluish rash but would talk about causalgia and autonomic dystrophy. The words gave her a sense of validity and control over her situation.

Despite regular exercises in a swimming pool for her neck and arm, Mary noticed that her shoulder was drooping because it had become weak from disuse. An attractive, large-boned brunette who was careful about her appearance, she felt ugly and disfigured. She stopped going out in public because her arm, which was now rigged in a rigid metal contraption that she referred to as a "gun sling," made her feel like a specimen on display. Her depression and anxiety deepened. The question "Why, why, why?" kept running through her thoughts. She was angry much of the time and hard to live with. Even though Frank had quit his job for lower-paying part-time work near home, his support wasn't enough to take the edge off what had changed from a bright personality to an irritable, pessimistic gloom.

After consulting with a neurologist, who gave her a nerve conduction test, Mary attended a thirty-day inpatient pain management program at Spaulding Rehabilitation Hospital to learn nonchemical methods for easing her pain. For a month, she did stretches and exercises, applied heat and ice, and was slowly weaned off opioid medications. She began to see how much the pain had taken from her life and her role in allowing this to happen. She took the important step of not only attacking the pain but also addressing the chaos it had caused in the rest her life. She was able to take the tools she learned in the inpatient pain program and apply them at home, making her feel much more armed to deal with flare-ups. Nonetheless, the pain was still there.

The next diagnosis she received, first from a physical therapist and then from a surgeon, was a condition called thoracic outlet syndrome. This disease occurs when nerves and blood vessels are pushed by a bone at the top of the rib cage or by a muscle or a fibrous band that develops in the delicate space between the top of the ribs and the shoulder. In this very tight space, many nerves and blood vessels travel between bones and muscles, and they can fairly easily become disturbed. Pressure on them can cause symptoms that are somewhat similar to Mary's. One symptom of this syndrome is a drooping shoulder. This, at last, sounded like the answer to her pain mystery. Since it may be caused by a rib pressing on a nerve root that goes to the arm, Mary agreed to undergo surgery to remove the first rib at the top of her rib cage. This represented a big risk because there was a chance that the rib wasn't involved. But if it was, the surgery could be a cure. However, the doctor warned her that the chance of her pain disappearing was no better than fifty-fifty, and probably even less.

After two days in the hospital recuperating from the surgery, Mary returned home to wait. The numbness, tingling, burning sensation, and achiness continued to appear and disappear at random, yet she hoped that these attacks would fade. Unable to take even mild anti-inflammatory medication such as ibuprofen because of their effects on her stomach, she experimented with home remedies and herbal applications and continued to apply the techniques she learned at the Spaulding Pain Program. She meditated, did self-hypnosis, and worked hard at maintaining her spirits while she waited.

But the pain didn't go away. At last, Mary came to the Pain Center. It was the usual very busy, bustling, overcrowded day, and since all the other rooms were taken, we met in one of the rooms where nerve block injections are usually performed. Despite her cheerful tone of voice, I could hear weariness and frustration. Her smiling face shined in stark contrast to what appeared to be rigid posture held together by a metal contraption that hung from her neck and back and supported her right arm. This sort of neuropathic pain usually strikes the arms or legs, as well as portions of the trunk or face. Sometimes, I can tell it has been around awhile by looking at a person's fingernails or even the pattern of hair growth on the skin. Mary's right arm looked distinctively different from her left, with deep red and purple marks that made the limb look badly frostbitten. The pain and inability to use her hand had curled her fingers into a claw.

After reviewing her long and sad medical history, I began to understand why Mary had come in. She wanted medication, and the only ones that had helped in the past were morphine-type drugs. Though opioids had helped, her doctors clearly feared that her increasing dosages possibly indicated other problems, like addiction. Over the past months, the opioids had helped her but quickly wore off as her body developed tolerance. Not only was Mary tolerant, but she had been taking the type of opioids that are usually used after an operation or for other forms of acute, short-lived pain and last just three or four hours. These are common medicines such as codeine or Percocet (oxycodone plus Tylenol). As her body increasingly fought the drug and got rid of it faster and faster, she would compensate by taking more and more frequently.

To her doctors, she appeared to be unable to manage the drugs that were meant to decrease her pain. They hadn't factored in that the medicine was growing less and less effective. Also, they hadn't seen that opioids that work for only a brief time set up the roller-coaster pattern: The patient takes the medicine with good effect, it wears off, and the pain returns, necessitating another dose. And the cycle continues. Add to this the effects of tolerance and the perpetual focus on pain throughout the day from having to take pills every three or four hours, and you have an all-too-common destructive pain cycle. Unfortunately, this pattern can easily be interpreted as a sign of addiction. Mary quite understandably didn't want to be labeled an addict. Her behavior looked like addiction, but it wasn't. She had developed what doctors call "pseudo-addiction," first seen in patients with cancer who act as if they are addicted simply because they have been treated only partially for their pain. Once the pain is treated effectively, the troubling behaviors that worry patients, and doctors, disappear. This was the case with Mary. When I slowly shifted her from the short-acting Percocet to opioids that lasted longer and required only a few doses per day, she began to feel better. Once I found an effective dose, which decreased her pain enough for her to get on with her life but didn't cause side effects such as drowsiness, she was able to hold at the same dose for over a year. With the pain in check, she now understood that the initial disease and her unfruitful surgery had led to several others problems, including permanent loss of mobility in her right arm. Nevertheless, she was committed to recapturing a normal life.

A WOUNDED NERVOUS SYSTEM

Doctors and scientists keep uncovering new clues about neuropathic pain. Civil War doctor Weir Mitchell rightly surmised that the burning stemmed from nerve irritation because the nerve had been damaged, partially destroyed, or otherwise disturbed by an injury. But other questions remained. He observed that the burning did not appear until long after the initial wound, and he struggled to understand why an injured nerve would wait so long to turn on its alarm. Why set off the alarm long after the villain had struck?

The physical maiming of battlefield injuries provided further insights. Tending to soldiers during World War I, French physician René Leriche concluded that the condition involved not just any nerves but many of those basic for survival, controlling and constantly monitoring the body's involuntary functions such as blood pressure, heart rate, sweating, and body temperature. He suspected that its symptoms and causes might stem directly from a malfunctioning sympathetic nervous system. This would explain why Mary's type of neuropathic pain affects circulation in limbs and causes discoloring as well as sweating at odd times.

For many years, this kind of neuropathic pain was called reflex sympathetic dystrophy, or RSD. The "reflex" tag came from the belief that the pain somehow moved from the injury site to the spinal cord and back out to the body. The pain travels from one place in the body to another, away from where the injury initially occurred. Pain's ability to journey to various parts of the body explains why doctors often have a difficult time locating its source. A good example is the patient with a heart attack who, instead of pain in the injured heart, has discomfort in the left arm, a symptom that is referred from the heart to the arm. This neuropathic pain syndrome got its present name, complex regional pain syndrome (CRPS), a few years ago when pain doctors decided that "RSD" was too imprecise. They had found that the pain does not always appear to sneak through the sympathetic nervous system and isn't always a reflex pain.

A persistent mystery surrounding this pain is that there's no telling when it will strike. Nature seems to have abandoned the laws of cause and effect. As happened to Mary, it often starts with an accidental injury. I know of patients with CRPS whose condition was set off by crushing injuries, like getting hands caught in doors; by burns; by relatively minor surgical procedures, like the removal of a cyst or the wrapping of an arm cast too tightly; and even by minor cuts or drawing blood. Infections may produce the pain, as can vascular disease or apparently simple muscle disorders, like a problem with posture. Diseases such as shingles or polio are thought to possibly trigger the syndrome. Sometimes I cannot locate what incited the condition, and its cause remains an unsolved mystery. As with so many pain syndromes, science is only beginning to understand its twisted ways.

PHANTOMS OF THE NERVOUS SYSTEM: REVENGE OF THE NERVES

For centuries, phantom limb pain has baffled scientists and doctors. It's been thought to be a figment of an amputee's imagination or produced by clumps of nerve tissue at the site of an amputation. In truth, recent discoveries have found that it's a classic example of the nervous system gone wrong and one of the most intriguing but treatment-resistant forms of neuropathic pain.

Any number of traumas to the body can set off nerves—it can be a seemingly harmless fall, as happened to Mary, or a much bigger shock to the system. One of the most striking blows to the nervous system comes from amputation of a leg or arm, or loss of any body part, like a breast to cancer or a nose to frostbite. Nerves connect every nook and cranny of the body to the brain and ensure that the body's systems are communicating with each other, and with the command center, the brain. When they are damaged or severed, there are severe consequences. These traumatized nerves do not quietly cease sending signals but protest loudly. To the surprise of many patients, they don't just die off but may fight back for years. Messages traveling on a highway of injured nerves become twisted and distorted. They may scream from the slightest touch or burn even though heat was never applied. Amputation creates a new terminus of the nerve pathway, but the entire system is not completely aware of what has happened and continues to emit signals that may confuse it even further.

The question "Where does it hurt?" becomes a complex puzzle for someone suffering body-part loss. Almost everyone in this situation has felt sensation from their missing part—a breeze across an absent arm, an itch from a foot no longer there, pressure on an excised breast. Phantom limb sensation isn't necessarily pain but is any awareness of the missing part, and it's as real to patients as their reflection in a mirror. The sensation, which usually subsides within a year of the removal, may be harmless, like feeling the pressure of a shoe on a missing foot or feeling a ring on a missing finger. However, for some amputees the feeling does not fade but intensifies, changing from a benign sensation into burning, cramping, aching, stabbing, and shooting that comes and goes with little warning. A patient with a missing hand may feel like his fingernails are being pulled from his fingers, a missing leg can feel like it's cramping, or the absent part may itch horribly. The pain is unique for each person and subject to moods, fatigue, or sleeplessness.

When I first met Howard Prentice, he had been through fourteen surgeries on a knee that had been shattered in a car accident. What followed was a series of knee repairs and replacements, stemming from damage, infections, arthritis, and failed grafts. Howard was disabled, unable to leave his house because he was constantly recovering from a surgery or waiting for an infection to clear. After legions of doctors, months in hospital rooms, and years of waiting to heal, he decided that his knee was hopelessly lost and agreed to an amputation. His wife, Susan, took a picture of the swollen, blue-and-red mangled mass so that if they ever questioned the decision, they could remind themselves of how bad it was. Then they held a "funeral" for the departing limb and thought their troubles were over. They hadn't anticipated phantom pain.

A big man with broad shoulders and a natural enthusiasm for sports, Howard had abandoned outdoor activities and acquired hobbies like collecting gemstones. He hoped that someday an artificial leg might let him return to the ski slopes and woods he loved to hike through. After the amputation, the stump pain subsided, and Howard was slowly taken off heavy pain medication. He had some mild phantom sensation that he didn't mention until I asked about it. Occasionally, he "forgot" about his missing lower leg and, as he was getting out of bed in the morning, tried to stand on it or absentmindedly bent over as though to put a sock on it. But these moments of wholeness were not accompanied by pain.

Then, like a flash flood, phantom limb pain struck. It first came at night. Susan said he awoke moaning, jarred out of deep sleep by a quick shot of burning pain. It was in his missing leg, returned like a frightening ghost. Initially, he dismissed the pain, telling himself that it, too, would pass. He was a stoic and somewhat macho guy, and admitting fear didn't come easily. But months later, it was still torturing him at any moment of the day or night.

By the time Howard and Susan made an appointment at the Pain Center, the electric shocks, burning, and aching had been going on for months. The fragile life they had begun to patch together was crumbling. Howard was again housebound, tied in anxious knots waiting for the next attack, and deeply depressed. He was angry at the medical world. "I think they lied about the operation. They didn't tell me how much it was going to hurt. And since the operation, everyone I've met or talked to with an amputation says they have phantom pain. The doctors said only ten percent get it," he told me, and added, "How can it hurt so much and not be there?"

Popular science often compares the human brain to a computer, with the nervous system being the hardwiring. But this analogy is misleading; the brain is remarkably plastic and adaptable, and it can and does alter its configuration, growing new nerve connections and reconfiguring existing patterns throughout life. While much of this basic wiring takes place during infancy, scientists have found that various experiences and activities, like an amputation, can dramatically change the organization of the neurons. The brain isn't designed to understand amputation. Yet it is the command center and must deal with any major changes in the body. In the case of phantom pain, the command center is working in the dark and gets its signals crossed.

When a part of the body is removed, it's no longer there to send signals to its designated segment of the sensory cortex. And with the amputation halting signal traffic, the sensory highway shrinks from disuse. The dynamic brain adjusts and reorganizes, trying to fill the void and recover lost function. The area of the brain designed to receive signals from the missing part of the body rewires itself, teaming up with nearby sections of the brain.

Like a lush garden in which a plant has died, healthy growth nearby slowly takes over the ground where nothing is blooming. Nerve connections for a lost foot, which are no longer sending regular signals, may migrate to nearby nerves, fusing together and causing abnormal firing. No matter whether the nerves for the missing body part or the area of the brain where they operated are to blame, each continue to receive and send signals.

This adjustment by the sensory nerves may explain the phenomenon of the "trigger zone." This is a sensitive area of the body that mimics signals for the missing part. For instance, a common trigger zone for amputees is the face—wind, touch, light, or other sensory experiences on a part of the face often register as sensation on a missing appendage.

Dr. V. S. Ramachandran, a scientist at the University of California in San Diego and a leading researcher into the neurological aspects of phantom limb pain, has done extensive mapping of patients' phantom sensations. In his book *Phantoms in the Brain,* he tells about an amputee who discovered that sexual intercourse produced orgasms in his missing foot. Like Dr. Ramachandran, my colleague at Mass General, Dr. David Borsook, has also found that patients with phantom pain may have pain that is brought out by stimulating distant parts of their bodies. The areas that most likely coax the phantom to emerge seem to be the same ones that are so magnified on the Homunculus—the mouth, tongue, and genitals. This is not surprising, since these areas correspond to the parts of the brain that have disproportionate shares of sensory perception.

TRYING TO KILL THE PHANTOM

When Howard came to the Pain Center for better ways to control his phantom leg pain, he was in bad shape. He rarely complained—I once suggested that he was a "silent sufferer"—and we talked many times about the difficulty he had asking for help. Now he desperately requested medication for the constant burning, aching, itching, and "breakthrough" pain, the instant zings and surprise jolts that came unexpectedly. He said that the sudden electric shocks would almost lift him out of his seat. He never knew when they would strike—when he was sleeping, or eating a quiet meal in a restaurant—so he was always braced for an attack.

He arrived in a wheelchair pushed by Susan. Unlike what often happens with many other couples, their ordeal had brought them closer together even though they admitted that their sex life had virtually vanished because of his medications. It was obvious that they were finely attuned to each other's moods. Some people would become bitter and pessimistic in the face of such adversity; these two were clearly determined to triumph. They were a formidable team, making sure all questions were asked and all vital information conveyed.

Howard wanted to understand what was happening. I explained how his nerves were still irritated and excitable, and still delivering pain messages even this far out from the operation. As I described these details, Susan framed her questions. If nerves were sending old messages, she surmised, why not just stop the transmissions? Since medicine could not change the messages, why not attack the messenger?

A common misconception about pain is that it can be sliced off like a frayed wire. People with pain stemming from an injury to a limb or other part of their body frequently wonder whether cutting the nerve, either close to the injury site or where it enters the spinal cord, will eliminate the pain. The idea of severing the pathway that carries pain signals makes sense. It's sometimes effective early on, and neurosurgeons have long looked at this possibility. However, in the long run, pain is usually too sneaky for the surgical knife. More often than not, the severed nerve grows back, makes new connections, and may even transmit more intense pain than before.

As I told Susan and Howard, "You can cut nerves, but they usually come back, and they can come back angry." Also, while severing nerves may initially make pain better, relief can come at the cost of losing feeling in the involved area or paralysis in the specific muscles that the nerve may also serve. For this reason, surgical procedures to cut pain nerves are usually reserved for patients with cancer or terminal diseases. Burning pain that comes on suddenly, months after an injury, like the spontaneous combustion of something that has been smoldering a long time, cannot be cut away. The surgical knife would surely not eradicate Howard's pain. Eventually, his pain was calmed by drugs used to treat other conditions involving malfunctioning nerves resulting from seizures, like epilepsy or cardiac arrhythmia.

Solving some of the riddles of phantom limb pain has shined new light on the causes of other kinds of neuropathic pain. Armed with the knowledge that pain can be the result of the brain rewiring its sensory nerves, scientists have shifted their attention to the brain's role in generating not only neuropathic pain but an entire spectrum of physical discomfort. As you will read in the next chapter, the brain adds new layers to pain beyond the purely physical, influencing our emotions and promoting suffering.

5

DECODING THE NEUROMATRIX

How Pain Changes the Brain

~

You don't need a body to feel a body.
—RONALD MELZACK,
The Challenge of Pain

Howard Prentice felt pain in his amputated leg because his brain had crossed its wires and was mistakenly receiving and sending pain messages. His brain had compensated for the loss of sensation from his lower limb by making new connections, but they were the wrong ones. In short, his brain was causing all the trouble.

In the past decade, as neuroscientists have learned more about the brain's structure and chemistry, they have found that pain can have a profound effect on the brain's very architecture. Their findings are of more than academic interest. By following pain into its lair, they are providing doctors with more clues on how to fight it. Let me give you an example that you'll be reading more about. One of my most prescribed medicines is a class of medications called psychotropic drugs. These are drugs that are normally used to combat mental illnesses such as depression, mania, and psychosis. But because they affect the brain's chemistry, they are also potent weapons against pain.

Everything you think, feel, and do produces an imprint on your central nervous system. Your brain is highly impressionable, so much so that scientists consider it virtually "plastic" or changeable. Scientists have known for decades that the human brain changes with age. As you learn, memorize information, and acquire physical skills, nerve cells in your brain (neurons) send out new branches to connect with other neurons. The neurons can strengthen weak or barely used pathways or make new ones—it's as if you started to regularly visit a neighbor you've never spoken to before, wearing a path between his house and yours. Over the years, your brain accumulates layers of information stored within thousands of nerves. If a layer or region becomes disabled, another one may take over or a new one can be developed. This is how someone with a stroke, which is basically damaged neurons in the brain, regains lost function.

Every thought and experience activates chemicals and electrical charges at different rates and concentrations, and these events shape your unique neural network. Although your brain does not grow new cells, it does sprout new connections called dendrites, the microfibers that deliver messages to a cell, and axons, the longest microfibers that send electrical charges from one neuron to the next. At the end of each axon is a slightly swollen knob, the synaptic bulb, and from here chemicals are released across a microscopically thin gap, or synapse, and are "caught" by a neighboring neuron.

When an experience involves your senses, as happens when you feel physical pain, sensory nerves flash a message to the Homunculus's headquarters, the brain's somatosensory cortex. From here, the communiqué about exactly what was felt is relayed to other areas of the brain. When the experience is especially intense or repeated, the synaptic connection and ensuing neurochemistry becomes heightened and embedded.

It's only been in the past couple of decades that scientists have uncovered proof of how the brain can change. In the early 1980s, University of California at San Francisco professor Michael Merzenich began experimenting with monkeys. He was searching for evidence of changes in the brain, or as Merzenich called it, "cortical reorganization." (Monkeys are often used in brain studies because their cerebral organization is very similar to that of humans.) Merzenich and his colleagues mapped the monkey's Homunculus, pinpointing exactly where signals from individual fingers linked to the cortex. They then cut the nerves that carried signals for particular fingers, which silenced the part of the brain (the somatosensory cortex) that would register activation of these nerves prior to being cut. To Merzenich's surprise, the neurons in that patch of brain began firing again, apparently managing signals from other fingers. The brain had adjusted to the change and shifted its configuration of neurons within hours! This was not the end of Merzenich's investigation; more startling discoveries were to come.

The neuroscientist next designed an experiment to see whether training the monkeys in a test of motor function might alter the nerve configuration in the sensory section of their brains. He taught an animal to touch a rotating disk repeatedly with only its three middle fingers. When he later examined its brain, he found striking growth of the synapses for the trained fingers and shrinkage of synapses of unused fingers. Now he had evidence that the brain can rewire itself not only when there's been traumatic damage to a nerve pathway but also as the result of training and learning.

The idea of the human brain continuing to alter its nerve patterns long after infancy and childhood surprised many people. David Hubel, who won a Nobel Prize in 1981 for experiments with vision showing that areas of the human brain are "hardwired" in infancy, has since concluded that the brain "is much more modifiable than we ever suspected."

The new growth patterns that Merzenich detected were admittedly microscopic, but they signaled the beginning of more dramatic breakthroughs. Perhaps one of the more astonishing involved the infamous "Silver Spring monkeys," which in the early 1980s were at the eye of a hurricane of international controversy between animal rights activists and medical researchers. The crab-eating macaque monkeys were residents of the Institute for Behavioral Research in Silver Spring, Maryland, and the subjects of studies on spinal cord and brain alterations. The lead scientist in the study, Edward Taub, was investigating whether animals could be trained to use an arm even though its nerve connection to the brain had been severed. But Taub never finished his experiments because one of the institute's lab workers, who was also an active animal rights advocate, accused him of mistreating the animals. Police seized the animals, and the institute was shut down.

Learning about the Silver Spring monkeys made me very uncomfortable. The monkeys were subjected to radical experiments that severed their arms or forearms. Harder still to stomach was that instead of being put to sleep at the end of the study, the animals were isolated and vanished into legal limbo for ten years as various organizations argued over their fate. Ironically, however, if the animals had been put down, scientists never would have learned about their brains' phenomenal mending capabilities.

Twelve years after the monkeys were removed from the institute, neuroscientists at the National Institute of Mental Health received permission to examine them to see how their central nervous system, especially their brains, had adjusted to absence of sensation coming from their arms. They looked at seven monkeys and, based on their map of the primate Homunculus, tested the electrical activity across various regions of the monkeys' brains. To their astonishment, the scientists discovered that the nerves for the severed arms, rather than having withered from disuse, were quite lively and responsive to stimulation. According to the sensory maps, the animals' nerve connections for their upper limbs were bordered by trunk and facial nerves. True to design, the nerves that once received messages from the arms were now responding to stimulation from areas on the face. The monkeys' brains showed, in the scientists words, "massive reorganization" that far exceed what had been found in any other studies. The Silver Spring monkeys proved not only that pain and trauma do alter the brain's wiring but that the brain can recoup many functions. While scientists will surely argue for ages over the ethical dilemma of learning about human neurology at the expense of animals, the Silver Spring monkeys dramatically revealed the dynamic, plastic nature of the brain.

What does this mean for someone in pain? Remember a few chapters ago when I talked about the subjective nature of pain and how it defies definition? For centuries, scientists have considered pain to be an emotion as much as a physical sensation. Now, the discoveries of neuroscientists are leading to hard proof of the physiological basis of pain. These discoveries contradict old notions of the brain as a fixed organ that, after we reach adulthood, is set for life. On the contrary, the brain is always changing—always trying to adjust to do the best job for each of us. When the brain is barraged by pain signals, particularly when the barrage is chronic, the brain tries to adjust. Sometimes, the changes aren't effective and the brain gets locked into a dysfunctional pattern. This is likely how chronic pain sets in and offers hope that doctors can find ways to unchange the perpetually hurting brain.

How Pain Changes the Brain

Ages ago scientists and philosophers believed that the body generated pain and that the brain was a passive receiver and announcer of pain signals. Pain originated not in the brain or mind but somewhere in the body. If you've ever studied philosophy, this may sound familiar, for this is a pure mechanistic philosophy that depicts the human body as a kind of machine that can be fixed, or healed, by attending to its various parts. The most famous mechanistic philosopher, René Descartes, had much to say about pain. His declaration "I think, therefore I am" suggested that only mental ability determines who you are and nothing in your physical being contributes to your sense of self. Of course this is a flawed theory. We are all much more than pure thought, and nowhere is this more apparent than when it comes to experiencing pain.

According to Descartes, pain started at some point on the skin and traveled along a dedicated pathway to a "pain center" in the brain, causing a person to react. He drew a picture of how this happened: A young man bends beside a fire, his foot is burned by the flames, and the pain runs up his leg into his spine and then into the brain. Descartes envisioned pain as a rope pulling on a bell in a steeple.

As you now know, the brain is not a passive receiver of pain signals. Instead of functioning as Descartes proposed, like a mechanical announcer of pain sensation, the brain is an active participant in the process, constantly adjusting and initiating messages. Pain does more than ring a bell—it hammers the bell into a new shape to produce cacophonous sounds. Once rung, the bell never sounds exactly the same again.

Scientists now know that unrelenting pain can alter the way neurons handle information; it can make sensation more intense, twist its character, create additional sensations like stabbing pain, or set off other neurological events common with stress. Lasting pain can produce a cycle of chemical and electrical action and reaction that becomes an automatic feedback loop—a chronic, self-perpetuating hurting that persists long after the original trauma has healed.

Pain can reconfigure the architecture of the nervous system it invades. It can be stamped so deeply as to make a permanent impression. This is why phantom limb pain may feel exactly like the pain experienced before a limb was removed, and in the same place. The earlier pain experience leaves an indelible imprint on the brain. Even patients who have had other types of surgery tell of feeling old pains. There's an account of a patient tormented by an ingrown toenail after his spinal cord had been injured. There are reports of women continuing to feel menstrual cramps after total hysterectomies and patients who feel hemorrhoid pain after having their rectum removed.

What's known as "referred pain" offers solid evidence of the extraordinary organization of the nervous system, with all of its elaborate connections, way stations, and signals. "Referred pain" is pain that pops up far from where the related injury took place. For instance, symptoms of a heart attack frequently occur in the arms. I have heard of cases of pain from cardiac trouble even erupting in a patient's ear or lodging itself at the site of an old back fracture. Similarly, patients have complained that changes in barometric pressure from high-altitude flights have generated new pain in old painful spots, such as where a damaged tooth had been extracted. Neuroscientists believe that the initial pain made the central nervous system of these individuals more sensitive to later pain and perhaps lowered their pain thresholds.

Ronald Melzack, one of the psychologists who developed the gate-control theory of how the spinal cord handles pain, says there is ample evidence of the brain's ability to generate pain independent of the body. He marvels at how quadriplegics, whose spinal cords have been completely severed above where sensory nerves attach, still feel sensations in their bodies, including pain. "You don't need a body to feel a body," says Melzack. "The brain itself can generate every quality of experience which is normally triggered by sensory input." He theorizes that there is a "neuromatrix" in your brain, a network of nerve connections between different areas, such as the thalamus, cortex, and limbic region, that not only receives and processes pain signals but also generates them. This neuromatrix produces a "neurosignature" of how and what you feel that is unique. The signature usually remains unique to each person, but, like your written signature, it can change with time.

I would add to Melzack's theory another important element of individual pain: the "neurosignature" of suffering. Just as you have an individual response to physical pain, you also possess individualized ways of feeling and expressing suffering. By "suffering" I mean the entire spectrum of possible emotional and psychological reactions associated with discomfort. A death in the family is invariably experienced differently by each member of the family. So is the experience of pleasure, love, or happiness. Every person possesses a unique combination of genes and personal chemistry that, combined with years of life experience, determines how they respond to the world. These aspects of your physical and psychological makeup affect how you deal with stress and feel pain and ultimately how you experience any emotion, from joy to suffering.

WHEN THE NERVOUS SYSTEM IS TRAUMATIZED: CENTRAL PAIN

Unfortunately, many people have firsthand experience of what it feels like to have their nervous system traumatized and altered by chronic pain. When pain lodges in any part of the central nervous system—which consists of the spinal cord, brain stem, and brain—it can cause unbearable discomfort. The source of the pain is usually an area of nerves that has been damaged, or what is called a lesion.

Pain from a wounded central nervous system is unlike any other kind of pain. It's an insidious case of the enemy having infiltrated the fortress and sabotaged the command center. The twisted nature of central pain has to do with the problem occurring within the same brain that must then try to make sense of it. It's like being fooled by a horrible hallucination.

The most common victims of central pain are people with injured brains, such as victims of multiple sclerosis, spinal cord injuries, or stroke. Almost any disease affecting the central nervous system can bring it on, including cancer, Parkinson's disease, AIDS, epilepsy, or vascular diseases. Experts say that more than 100,000 people in the United States and a million worldwide are afflicted. Although central pain has not reached the epidemic levels of other varieties, it's one of the most difficult to treat. According to medical records, fewer than 30 percent of its sufferers are able to live a normal life, and suicide among its victims is not uncommon.

One of central pain's most distinctive features is that it doesn't strike immediately. There's usually a delay of weeks, sometimes months or even years, between the event that caused the lesion and the resulting pain. Six months is a common lag time. Central pain generally involves a burning sensation and alters a person's sensitivity, either heightening or dampening reactions to touch. For someone with central pain, mildly cold temperatures, a pinprick, or even the feel of clothing may be excruciating. It may include a steady feeling of aching, squeezing, or stabbing, and any body movement can aggravate it.

HOW CENTRAL PAIN DOES ITS DIRTY WORK

If you bear in mind the alarm analogy for pain, central pain is akin to the system sounding the alarm even though no door or window has been opened; the alarm wires are damaged and the alarm is falsely tripped. Let me tell you briefly how doctors and scientists first encountered central pain, which may help explain how the brain becomes the ring leader in this crime.

The condition was first recognized in the early nineteenth century when neurologists noticed pain that spontaneously erupted in patients long after brain damage had occurred from vascular disease. French physicians noticed that some stroke patients were afflicted with varying degrees of pain. It was apparent that their reaction to pain had changed, causing greater sensitivity—or even transforming something that was normally not painful such as a breeze across the skin. The pain was called "thalamic syndrome," named for a part of the brain that is crucial for sensing the world, and particularly for sensing pain.

The thalamus is two walnut-sized bundles of nerves deep within the brain that acts as a relay station for sensory information coming from the spinal cord and brain stem—and again out to the body from the brain's outer layer, the cortex. The word *thalamus,* Latin for "inner chamber" or "master bedroom," was coined by the Greek doctor Galen, whose revolutionary medical knowledge was gleaned from his examination of dead Roman gladiators in the catacombs of the Colosseum in Rome. If you think of the thalamus as the main switching center of your sensory "home," then Galen's "master bedroom" metaphor appears very much in sync with medicine's contemporary understanding of the brain's anatomy.

In fact, the thalamus is probably the closest spot you have to a pain center in your brain. One of the first physicians to notice what happens when the thalamus is damaged was the renowned English neurologist Dr. William Gowers. He was treating a patient with a bullet wound and noticed that the patient was no longer able to sense pain or temperature below the location of the wound. Gowers went on to describe what doctors now call the "pain tract," or the spinothalamic pathway, the largest highway of nerves that carry pain signals from the spine to the brain—all of which funnel through the thalamus. This path is pain's major route—two-thirds of Descartes' rope, if you will.

Today, technology that allows doctors to take pictures of the brain and advances in neurosurgery have enabled them to learn much more about the thalamus and the pain it controls, and even creates. Studies with both animals and humans have revealed fascinating insights into how the thalamus and pain interact. Using electrical stimulation of precise spots on the nerve bundles of the thalamus, scientists have been able to touch off a wide spectrum of sensations, from instant shots of burning, shooting pain anywhere in the body to intense emotional feelings.

Brain studies involving healthy, living people are unusual for obvious humanitarian reasons, making the recent findings of Dr. Frederick Lenz of Johns Hopkins University and Dr. Richard Gracely of the National Institutes of Health so extraordinary. While operating on the thalamus to correct a patient's motor problems, they uncovered secrets about its role in magnifying the physical sensations of pain and suffering. Dr. Lenz was performing brain surgery directly on the thalamus to quiet particular nerves in a patient with crippling hand tremors who also had a history of panic-anxiety attacks. The patient was a thirty-six-year-old man who in the months before the surgery had experienced paralyzing panic attacks with chest pain, heart pounding, ringing in the ears, shortness of breath, and even fainting. Before the surgery, the doctors inserted a thin wirelike device called a microelectrode into the patient's thalamus to pinpoint the exact source of his hand tremors. The young man stayed awake the entire time and could tell the doctors what he was feeling.

As they explored the portion of the thalamus that receives input for the hands, they stimulated neurons that produced a deep, painful tugging feeling in the forearm. Zeroing in on their target, their probe hit a spot that generated chest pain identical to what the young man felt during a panic attack. Normally, stimulating this area produced only mild tingling, but this time, the man cried out in pain and reexperienced the panic. The pain was electric, he felt as if he were suffocating, and he had a strong urge to flee. The physical and emotional parts were meshed together as one.

Doctors Lenz and Gracely say they have rarely seen this before. This operation sheds new light on the highly individual nature of pain. In this patient, the thalamus had constructed a unique network that integrated input and output, including both physical and emotional sensations. Although the input in this surgery came from the doctors' probe, it could have easily arrived under normal conditions via the patient and could even have been triggered by the pain tract.

The thalamus does much more than regulate your sense of pain and temperature. It also juggles other complex signals that can be grouped together to form any human experience—from pleasure to suffering. The thalamus is thought to act like an executive secretary for the higher centers of the brain, screening calls and forwarding information to other parts of the brain. The brain may then add its special blend of flavor and color to the information, which may again pass through the thalamus as it travels back to the rest of the body— all of this occurring in the instant of a thought.

One of the prime recipients of thalamic signals is the cortex—the outermost, most developed part of your brain. This "thinking" part of your brain contributes memories, attention, and suggestion to what you ultimately feel as pain. Scientists know by studying the results of surgeries that severed connections in parts of the cortex that other parts of the cortex add to pain. Patients who had a lobotomy, the infamous surgery of the frontal cortex that was too commonly performed in the 1950s to treat mental illness, reported that they still felt pain but that it no longer bothered them. Not only was the element of attention gone, but also the prominent feelings of anguish or suffering.

Another regular recipient of pain signals via the thalamus is the part of your brain that handles your moods and instincts, the limbic system. Depression, anxiety, irritation—even such seemingly vague emotions as a bleak outlook on the future—very probably involve neuron activity in this region. (I'll talk much more about the limbic system's role in feeling pain in the next chapter.)

STROKE: WHEN STARVED NERVES CAUSE CENTRAL PAIN

Not all central pain stems from lesions in the thalamus. A large portion of my patients with central pain have had strokes that have damaged other parts of their brain stem or brain. A stroke damages brain cells by obstructing necessary blood flow—because of a blockage, a clogged artery, or even a blood vessel that leaks because of head trauma from a violent accident. How a stroke affects a person depends on exactly where in the brain it occurs. A stroke is not usually painful, but when pain does erupt, it often appears with a strange pattern that can initially confuse doctors. When the pain is caused by a defect in the central command station, all bets are off. It can look like any possible array of symptoms because a sick brain can create its own experience.

When Mr. Genovese first visited the Pain Center, I knew relatively soon that his central pain had been caused by a stroke. All of his pain was on the right side of his body, from his shoulders down to his toes. This was an important clue, because while a collection of problems might cause such widespread yet one-sided pain, it was highly unlikely. It's like Jesse James's famous explanation for why he robbed banks: "That's where the money is." From there, I worked backwards and put together the otherwise perplexing pieces of the puzzle.

The pain made no sense to Mr. Genovese. How could his arm and leg hurt when there was absolutely nothing wrong with his arm or leg! He was so frustrated that he wanted someone to operate on his arm and leg, and the sooner the better. After I explained the situation and we talked about it, he realized the rotten trick his brain had played on him. It was as though a trusted old friend had betrayed him. He became quiet and sad, muttering, "At least we know the truth."

Central pain from a stroke is like other varieties: It burns, aches, tears, and is fairly constant, but it can rise and fall in intensity. It can pop up virtually anywhere in the body, including the face, or deep within your organs, which is called visceral pain. One of the wicked features of central pain is its tendency to suddenly and unexpectedly attack. The pain may explode when a patient moves or changes posture, hears a loud or startling noise, or feels emotional stress such as sudden fear. Two other common causes of these outbreaks are cold and light touch. The pain generally settles into one side of the body and produces some kind of abnormal sensory reaction. Most often, there is diminished sensitivity to extreme temperatures, especially cold. A Swedish study by Dr. Doran Lejon at University Hospital in Linköping reported that about three-quarters of his stroke patients with central pain could not distinguish between freezing and warm temperatures, and almost all of them reacted more strongly than normal to being lightly touched by the tip of a pin.

STRIPPING THE WALLS BETWEEN NERVES: PAIN AND MS

Stroke is not the only condition that can generate central pain. People with multiple sclerosis are too often familiar with the agony of central pain. Despite what people unfamiliar with multiple sclerosis (MS) believe, extreme, persistent pain is not a standard feature of this degenerative disease. Nevertheless, surveys show that about 43 percent of MS patients are affected by some kind of pain. Hannah Post had MS, but when she came to my office I did not immediately assume her discomfort was central pain. A fifty-year-old woman who had developed MS when she was in her early thirties, her shoulder hurt and, as in so many cases, the pain could have signified anything from a sore shoulder joint to a sore brain.

MS is a cruel disorder that disrupts the spinal cord and brain by contaminating nerve cells and interrupting normal nerve transmission. Despite her pain, Hannah appeared to have adjusted remarkably well to MS. Although she had gradually scaled back her work teaching high school, she did so because of fatigue and difficulty getting around rather than pain. Within the limits of her disease, she had a fulfilling life. She and her husband, Jeff, a successful computer executive, were raising two daughters, were active in their church, and, after moving near the Massachusetts shore, had become avid bird-watchers.

When I met Hannah, the pain was beginning to unravel her tranquil life. She complained that her shoulder had been bothering her for three years. She had had MS for eighteen years, and what she was feeling now was entirely different from the low-level discomfort that had occasionally intruded on her life. It had started three years before with vision problems; as is common with MS, her eyes seemed to bounce around out of sync with each other, so she had difficulty focusing, which made her dizzy and nauseous. Around the same time, bouts of burning pain in her hand became so bad that her hand turned red and swollen. The pain then crawled up into her shoulder, acquiring a skin-ripping, jabbing quality. When the pain swept over her, Hannah had to stop whatever she was doing and retreat to a soft armchair and deploy a succession of ice packs and a book on tape to distract her. (She couldn't read because of her eyes.) For the first time in her illness, her limitations were making her depressed and irritable. Normally outgoing, she had stopped socializing with her church group because she was embarrassed by her frailty and didn't want to be seen in public. She was exhausted, run-down, and, according to her husband, unusually argumentative. It was as though her personality had changed.

The pain was achy and burning, but it stayed in her shoulder, so that's where I focused my attention. She winced as I carefully palpated and moved the joint through its normal range of motion. The shoulder muscles were clearly tender, and the joint had lost a lot of its normal flexibility. This exam was among the scores of tests, scans, and evaluations other specialists had performed, all aimed at finding out what was wrong with her shoulder. The possibilities ranged from dislocation due to muscle weakness, to disk degeneration in her spine, to arthritis, to central pain from MS.

Hannah had another medical complication that caught my attention because it affected her attitude toward doctors and treatment. Many pain patients have a history of conditions that seem unrelated to their pain yet color their outlook. Years before, Hannah had had bouts of Crohn's disease, an inflammation of the small intestine that slows absorption of nutrients and can causes spasms, diarrhea, weight loss, and anemia. She consulted a number of doctors, and treatment took many months. She had lots of pain but resisted using pain medicine. Although it had been years since a flare-up, Hannah admitted she had felt guilty about "pestering" specialists who couldn't help her and leery of dependency on narcotic medication. I'm sure this added to her feelings of helplessness and doubts about whether anyone could relieve her pain.

The numerous visits to other doctors had not helped her pain. So far, she had found the medical profession somewhat unsympathetic. "It wasn't *their* pain," she told me with a note of bitterness. Even though I couldn't discover the source of the pain, I focused on treating the pain as if it were a problem in the shoulder, even though I suspected that it could be a creation of her diseased brain. I tried anti-inflammatory and anticonvulsant medications, and mild narcotics. I even did a procedure called a stellate ganglion block in case her pain was due to complex regional pain syndrome. Alas, nothing helped.

Finally, I attempted to treat the pain by directly injecting her shoulder joint with a local anesthetic that temporarily blocked the nerves in her shoulder. It soon became clear that even turning off the pain nerves in her shoulder wasn't stopping her pain. In fact, after the injection, she said the pain was worse than ever for a few days. There was only one other culprit that could rear its ugly head in such a way—disease in the central nervous system. While I knew that Hannah's shoulder had deteriorated from disuse and required physical therapy, I turned to the real perpetrators: the nerves in her spinal cord.

Multiple sclerosis is a disease of the central nervous system that destroys the protective outer coating of nerves, called the myelin sheath. Doctors don't know what causes MS, although some genetic, viral, and geographic factors appear to be at work. Once the process begins, the body's immune system attacks the protective outer coating of nerves in the spinal cord and brain. Not unlike frayed wires, as the coating melts away, nerve fibers are unable to conduct impulses normally, and this impairs body functions. Loss of function, however, does not necessarily mean excruciating pain. Hannah's pain was most likely caused by damage to the coating of her nerves within her spinal cord in the exact area that handled sensation for the shoulder. Finally, an MRI scan of the spine in the region of Hannah's neck confirmed this.

As Hannah found, central pain is often confused with other medical conditions. However, the sensation is usually distinctive—steady burning, aching, numbness, and tingling in a limb or part of the body that hasn't been injured is the unmistakable calling card for damage to the central nervous system. As with Mr. Genovese, the pain usually affects only one side of the body and may cover too large an area to be explained by another single disorder. After her shoulder pain developed, Hannah could not stand to have anything touch her skin, and she even slept sitting up, leaning against her other shoulder.

There's a psychic dimension to central pain that, like all chronic pain, goes well beyond the physical realm. Hannah said that her attacks felt "like the skin was being ripped from my body." Hannah's comment suggested a nightmarish experience that, were it played out in a horror movie, would probably make any of us squirm. She eloquently described her physical sensation but also the terror, fear, and destruction of one's self-image that central pain can wreak.

Patients often describe central pain as baffling, vexing, perplexing, and frustrating. As is the case in many with chronic pain syndromes, patients sometimes use emotional words such as "cruel," "ruthless," "unkind," "grim," and "relentless" to characterize their symptoms. Central pain can be so psychologically devastating that sufferers are willing to try any treatment, even risk total paralysis or death, to relieve it.

In recognizing the combination of overactive nerves in her spinal cord and brain, as well as the emotional effects of the pain on her psyche, Hannah and I were finally able to find a combination of medications that kept the demons at bay.

A SURGICAL STRIKE ON THE COMMAND CENTER OF SUFFERING

There is a rarely performed and extraordinary surgery that does reduce a patient's suffering. This neurosurgery, called a cingulotomy, has been successfully used to treat certain psychiatric illnesses such as obsessive compulsive disorder and depression that have resisted all other known treatments. Its impact on people for whom no other therapy has worked offers a telling perspective on that fine line between the mind and the body.

While a cingulotomy is brain surgery, its effects on the mind and mental functioning have earned it the name "psychosurgery"—a term with such a controversial history that few hospitals perform these operations. In the 1940s and early 1950s, psychosurgery was used as a last-resort treatment for many different kinds of psychiatric disorders. These operations, notably the infamous lobotomy, deadened nerves in patients' frontal lobes and had the unfortunate side effect of not only quieting their illness but also disconnecting their emotions and virtually dousing their personalities.

Psychosurgery was abandoned as psychiatry developed much less harmful and more effective treatments. Nevertheless, doctors have continued to perform psychosurgery on patients with intractable psychological disorders. As you might expect, this is a dramatic operation performed only on patients for whom no other treatment has worked. It's almost never used solely to treat pain but only when pain is tangled up with severe problems that the operation is known to help— namely, the most severe forms of depression and obsessive compulsive disorder.

Following a devastating work accident, Montana farmer Robert Evans suffered from chronic pain and suicidal depression—both of which proved intractable and untreatable by his doctors. As a last resort, he underwent psychosurgery. His story reveals how an operation that doesn't directly impact the brain's pain centers can be a potent pain reliever when the brain and mind have been crippled by certain combinations of physical and emotional illness.

It was the middle of harvest time on Mr. Evans's wheat farm. On the day of his accident, he was rushing to beat the rain when he got caught between a truck and a moving tractor. He felt his back crunch and crumpled to the ground in pain. He let his son finish for the day and went to bed, assuming the pain would pass. Like many people who work with powerful machines, Mr. Evans accepted cuts and bruises as a daily occurrence and rarely raised a complaint. But this time, the pain did not abate, and the following Monday Mr. Evans visited an emergency room for X rays. Upon seeing the results, the attending physicians sent him immediately to the hospital for a series of interventions for multiple spine fractures that left him in a large body cast covering most of his back.

Mr. Evans was devastated by this turn of events. Unable to move or walk, he felt totally helpless, "As if my world had come to an end." And his back pain was unremitting. His son couldn't harvest alone, so he had to hire help, which strained the family finances. Over the ensuing months, Mr. Evans got out of the cast, but the pain worsened. Desperate for relief, he launched a sweeping search for effective treatment. He visited doctors and clinics in California and Colorado, and even checked into the Mayo Clinic. He tried reverse traction, surgery, electrical stimulation, and many unconventional cures, such as having his teeth removed as a treatment for his back pain. The medical doctors he saw couldn't find a specific cause and, concluding that his pain was in his head, sent him to a psychiatrist.

The pain persisted, becoming so intense that he wondered if he had had a stroke. With each treatment came hope and failure, and Evans slipped further into deep depression. He was angry, bitter, unreasonable, and impossible to live with. The pain had transformed his personality. His wife, a geriatrics nurse who encountered misery every day, reached the end of her patience and left home, telling him that he was no longer the man she married. Evans's daughter, who had been helping take care of him, grew more distant and, over time, stopped coming to the farm. He was left alone with his son, who was forced to run the farm alone while Evans sat at home, barely able to get around. With each passing day, Robert Evans considered suicide more seriously.

He continued to search for a cure, scouring the libraries and reading all he could about pain and depression. In a book on depression, he found a one-sentence reference to neurosurgery; if all else fails, it said, this sometimes helps. Evans telephoned the author for details and was told that only one place in the country was performing such surgery: Massachusetts General Hospital. Evans began to research psychosurgery.

The procedure he was investigating was a cingulotomy, which—unlike its horrific predecessors that were performed on cognitive areas of the frontal lobe—involves deadening nerves in the area of the brain that, among many other functions, gives pain its emotional coloring. The operation does not alter the pain signal; it alters how the brain reacts to this signal. It doesn't stop pain, but in some cases of severe depression it seems to reduce the impact of the pain. A patient may still hurt, but the pain matters less—reduced from a loud, harsh noise to light, white noise that can almost be ignored.

Evans applied to Mass General for the procedure. Even though the cingulotomy is one of the least invasive and least risky of all brain surgeries, it is still brain surgery and never done lightly. Psychosurgery changes how the brain functions, so doctors are extremely cautious about undertaking it. And despite technological advances, no one knows precisely which nerves control depression, which may be one reason it does not always work or that surgeons often have to repeat the operation. Given all these risks, Evans was told that before being accepted for psychosurgery, he would have to exhaust every possible conventional therapy, beginning with a full course of an antipsychotic medication.

Mr. Evans complied. After the antipsychotics failed to work, and after a great deal of review, a team of neurosurgeons and psychiatrists at Mass General declared him an appropriate candidate for a cingulotomy, to be performed by Dr. Rees Cosgrove.

In a cingulotomy, a neurosurgeon inserts a small instrument through a fine hole in the skull, reaching the anterior cingulum of the brain. This small area of complex fibers sends and receives messages within the limbic system—one of the brain's main centers for integrating emotions. When the instrument reaches its target, which the surgeon can see via CAT scan, it heats and destroys a very small area of brain tissue. The small lesion created by this procedure blocks the transmission of nerves in the area. It is much like blocking an exit on a busy highway and rerouting traffic elsewhere.

This surgery is surprisingly safe and remarkably devoid of long-term side effects. While a cingulotomy has profound effects on emotion, it causes no paralysis, numbness, motor incoordination, or thought impairment. The surgery does not present the same risks as cutting nerve pathways because it doesn't go near them. In other words, it doesn't directly affect pain signals, so there is little risk of nerves returning angry. After a short period of recovery, most patients have almost no evidence of having had the procedure other than a small scar, which is usually covered by hair. While pain is not a primary target of the surgery, chronic pain can become the beneficiary of what might be call "referred healing."

Before the surgery, Dr. Cosgrove spoke at length with Mr. Evans, making it clear that he could offer no guarantees. He said that it was an extremely safe operation, with rarely any complications, and that it would likely do nothing for his everyday pain and probably very little for his chronic back pain. Dr. Cosgrove also cautioned him about expecting miracles for his depression. "If it does anything for your depression, it'll be four to eight weeks until you'll feel a difference," the neurosurgeon warned. Mr. Evans anxiously asked about post-surgery pain medication and requested a special bed for his bad back.

The operation didn't take long. Prior to surgery, precise measurements were made with MRI scans so that once in the operating room, Dr. Cosgrove knew where to enter the skull and the brain. Given only a local anesthetic while holes were drilled into his skull, Mr. Evans was awake for most of the procedure. He fell asleep toward the end and awoke in the postsurgery unit. He remembers immediately searching his body for pain, starting with his neck and back. "I was totally pain free," he says. "There was no pain, and no depression." He felt stunned, even euphoric.

Robert Evans was discharged from Mass General four days later and returned to his farm in Montana. He is now remarkably improved. Although he never totally reclaimed his health, the only pain he experiences today are strains that come from overdoing. "If I spend too long on the tractor, I know my back's going to hurt," he says. And his depression has faded, though he has some sadness about the consequences of his nightmare. "In hindsight, I'd do the surgery sooner. I lost my wife, my kid . . . such a wasted life. . . ."

While the eradication of Robert's back pain was not expected, it was not entirely surprising. Dr. Cosgrove had hoped that the operation would dispel his agonizing depression and preoccupation with suicide that almost overwhelmed him "like a primitive drive." And although Robert Evans still has some back pain, and it's quite possible that as many nerves as before are transmitting pain signals, he no longer suffers as much. With the intense, crippling depression being literally cut away, the intensity of his physical pain was probably also excised.

This unusual case illustrates one of the most difficult challenges in trying to understand pain. If pain is a sensation and the sensation is not altered, then how can the pain be changed? Has pain relief occurred if the pain persists with the same intensity but with lessened emotional impact? I think if a patient is less bothered by pain, there has been some pain relief, regardless of what any particular nerves are doing. Pain relief without changing the sensation that initially caused the pain is hard to understand, but this paradox underlies what is most perplexing about the chicken-or-egg nature of many chronic pain syndromes.

Pain is more than a sensation—it is the individual interpretation of various sensations and emotions that allows each person to experience it differently. For most people, any unpleasant stimulation—such as touching a hot stove—can cause pain. But another way of understanding pain is that any stimulus—painful or otherwise—can become painful if your ability to cope with it has been diminished. Pain can also be modified by changing its prominence in your consciousness, that is, changing how meaningful or incapacitating it is to you. Adjusting any of these variables can offer important tools for controlling pain. Consider how some individuals walk on hot coals or endure superhuman amounts of pain; I am certain that the way they control their thinking offers a strategy for recovering from chronic pain.

The success of Robert's surgery vividly shows how suffering and physical pain are inextricably bound together. They are not exactly the same, but they rarely travel alone. One of the pervasive obstacles I encounter in pain medicine is the troubling relationship between pain and depression, each antagonizing the other and neither doing any good. Fortunately, doctors have found that when they defeat one, the other is severely weakened.

As medical science has gradually pieced together the puzzle of what pain does to the brain, it has also been investigating how the brain, and the mind, can alter a person's reactions to physical sensations. Neuroscientists are fairly certain today that not only does pain change the brain but that the brain, and its thoughtful inhabitant, the mind, can alter the pain experience. In the next chapter, I'll tell you about some enlightening discoveries involving the brain's ability to regulate, and at times defeat, pain.

6

THE MIND FIGHTS BACK

Placebos, Endorphins, and
Other Miracles of Consciousness

> Pain is an experience subject to modification by many
> factors: wounds received during strenuous physical exer-
> cise, during the excitement of games, often go unnoticed.
> The same is true of wounds received during fighting,
> during anger. Strong emotion can block pain.
>
> —LT. COL. HENRY BEECHER,
> "Pain in Men Wounded in Battle," 1946

Most of us are aware of how our emotions influence the intensity of pain. When a headache strikes, we intuitively know that a good way to fight back is to calm our mind and quiet our emotions. We may seek out a dark room to lie down, meditate, or try to drift into a nap. Somehow we know that feelings of peacefulness can help defeat the pain in our head.

The emotional center of the brain is a series of nerves and tissue called the limbic system, which form a ring beneath the gray matter. From here, signals are beamed out that influence our memories and moods, creating a rainbow of emotions stretching from anger to euphoria. Not incidentally, the limbic system also influences pain sig-nals and adds emotional texture to them.

Although pain always hurts, it comes in infinite styles and colors. The variations may be effected by spontaneous situations or predeter-mined by personality, genetic makeup, and past experiences. This is much the same for many of our other behaviors and sensations. Pleasure, comfort, security, fear, and fun are all affected by factors that are very difficult to pin down, largely because they occur outside awareness. How often have you been unable to enjoy something because of a "bad mood" but been unable to put a finger on the cause? Somehow, something from somewhere ruined your experience—but how, and from where?

The coloring of pain is part of what makes our behavior nonrobotic, or in other words, human. Without the limbic system, we would be more like Mr. Spock, our cognitive ability intact but without animation, spirit, or personality. The influence of the limbic system is clear when patients describe their pain in emotional terms such as cruel, grim, unkind, or savage. I don't mean to imply that pain is merely a product of the emotions. However, as we learned from the previous chapter, pain is never purely physical. Remember the words of Ronald Melzack: *"You don't need a body to feel a body."* As you read on about placebos and the chemicals your brain and body generate that can act as powerful analgesics, you will have a better picture of the complex and powerful role the mind plays in the way we experience pain. And you will begin to see that pain can be calmed by harnessing your own pain-fighting powers.

FIERY EMOTIONS STIR UP FIERY PAIN

When I think about how a person's emotions and pain can magnify each other, I remember Mark Hamilton, whose crippling physical pain and overpowering emotions fed his discomfort like wind blowing on a fire. Mark had been in terrible pain for months when he came into the Pain Center demanding that something be done. In his late fifties and head of a large construction firm, he wasn't rude, just insistent that surely there was something that would stop his misery. And, he was clearly accustomed to getting his way.

Mark Hamilton, like most patients I treat, was at the end of his tether. I was the latest in a long line of doctors who had tried an assortment of drugs and procedures with only modest results. I took notes as Mark methodically recounted his story. His pain, an electric shock through his mouth and jaw, had burst into his life when he was having a lunch meeting at his desk with his company accountant and sales manager. It was a tense discussion about financing, and Mark recalled being upset and yelling. When the pain seized him, he stopped eating and fell silent. With his tongue, he gently explored his teeth and gums and sensed that the pain was coming from the left side of his lower jaw. He assumed that he needed a dentist and possibly a root canal.

The pain had faded in minutes but made an impression, and Mark told his secretary to schedule a dental appointment that afternoon. The dentist poked around Mark's mouth, took X rays that revealed no tooth problem, and concluded that he had had an attack of trigeminal neuralgia. Although Mark would later consult an internist and neurologist looking for other explanations, I shared this diagnosis.

Mark had never heard of this type of pain, which is an abnormal firing or seizure of the largest sensory nerve in the face, the trigeminal nerve. This nerve has three large branches that fan out on both sides of the face. It is both a sensory and motor nerve, so when it malfunctions, it causes pain and a physical reaction, such as twitching or muscle seizure. The nerves in Mark's lower face were firing abnormally or seizing, not unlike what happens with an epileptic convulsion of the brain or with an arrhythmia, a sudden change in the way the heart beats. The abnormal nerve can make a whole face twitch, so the condition has also been called *tic douloureux*.

Mark's case was classic. Like many sufferers, his pain appeared when he was eating. Other triggers are brushing teeth, shaving, or washing the face. Perhaps a more forceful stimulus for Mark was emotion, in particular anger, which was compounded by the yelling that usually accompanied his agitation. Anger and stress set off a chemical tide of hormones and neurotransmitters that destabilized his nerve, and his face convulsed.

As soon as Mark described the pain and what brought it on, I knew he had trigeminal neuralgia, so the mystery was not the nature of the disease but what caused it and why other remedies had not worked. Although soft-spoken and respectful, Mark sounded defensive about my questions surrounding the medications the other doctors had prescribed him. While I was seeking a pharmacological history, he later told me that he thought I was looking for signs of drug dependence. The idea had not occurred to me because his pain and symptoms were so clear-cut, but like many pain patients, Mark was sensitive to people's opinions about painkillers. Being the son of an alcoholic father had made him extra aware of the stigma of addiction.

I pushed forward. "Indulge me," I asked him. "I'd like to get to know you and know about your life. Tell me more about what you do for a living, who you live with, your family life, and what gives you the most stress." An important part of my medicine is listening, which I think of as my collaboration with a patient. Hearing what the pain had done to Mark's life helped me not only to understand it but, more importantly, work with him toward a treatment to restore the treasured activities that he had surrendered.

A beefy man with a flushed complexion, Mark put on a stoic, gruff exterior that easily could be intimidating. A no-nonsense business-man, he seemed taken aback when I asked about his emotional life and what made him angry, something his other doctors hadn't explored. We later struck a deal. "You have trigeminal neuralgia," I told him, "but I'm not sure why the drugs you're taking are not work-ing. I promise you this, though: Help me understand the source of your pain and I'll follow up with whatever it takes—whatever proce-dure, whatever drug, whatever experimental therapy—until we have succeeded."

Mark's personal story contained numerous clues about his pain. Of Irish descent and one of eight boys, he grew up in a rough neighbor-hood outside Boston. Because his father was an alcoholic and his over-whelmed mother was depressed, his parents could not keep the family together, and the boys were sent to foster homes. Foster care was a nightmare—Mark was in and out of twelve different homes before he was fifteen—and in some he was neglected and underfed. He has a vivid memory of sneaking out from a home at night to find food. Poverty and emotional deprivation had eroded a gaping hole in his psyche that he was spending his adult years trying to fill. The hunger that Mark felt as a child remained with him and, over the years, developed into an unrelenting drive for success and financial security. Mark described all the years he was obsessed by what he called his "back of the bus" syndrome. Having felt discarded first by his parents and then by a succession of foster parents, he assumed that the whole world regarded him as inferior.

These feelings had likely spread through his teen years and young adulthood into a pervasive anger against the world and a raging deter-mination to prove everyone wrong. I inferred from hearing him talk about people at work that his anger flared often and that he could be a bully when he felt that his will was ignored or his financial health threatened. He was also proud of what he had accomplished and marveled at his good fortune as he described his palatial new house and eighty-five-foot yacht.

As he built up his company, he acquired the lifestyle of a compulsive workaholic. He devoted long days to meetings and expansion projects. Work was his constant companion—his car, with a multifeature cell phone, and his new home, with thirty separate phones, were extensions of his office. His phone lines, operating as a kind of shadow nervous system, enabled him to keep in touch with the office but also delivered pain in the form of stress and problems. Unable to relax, he rarely took a vacation, and when he did, his anxiety abated only when he was back in cell-phone range. Given the cyclical nature of the construction business, Mark was driven by fear of losing everything. Impatient and short-tempered at work, his tirades around the office were legendary. He had been seeing a psychiatrist for years for anxiety and depression, but there seemed to be little carryover from those sessions to his daily life.

After the first attack and the visit to the dentist, Mark sought help from a neurologist, who confirmed the diagnosis and put him on Tegretol (generic carbamazepine), an anticonvulsant medication that's frequently prescribed for trigeminal neuralgia as well as for psychiatric distress, particularly manic depression and aggression. But Mark did not improve with Tegretol; in fact, his pain got worse and his daily life deteriorated because the drug sedated him. For pure pain caused by a seizure, the drug should have worked. But pain is rarely "pure," and chronic pain especially is blended in with large doses of emotional discomfort, which can aggravate the pain and be a by-product of it. Unfortunately for Mark, his treatment aggravated his anxiety and explosive temper, which predated the pain, and didn't make the pain any better.

The side effects of the Tegretol, coupled with attacks of facial pain, reduced Mark to whispering and barely eating. When the pain hit, it marred his home life as much as his work life. Normally animated and lively, Mark slipped into a stupefied funk. He was always sleepy due to the Tegretol, and when he couldn't concentrate, he felt helpless. One evening, his wife, Laura, found him in his study asleep at his desk, the phone off the hook with his lawyer on the other end wondering what had happened. Laura was terrified that he would fall asleep at the wheel, so she called him in his car every evening on his drive home.

The pain of eating made dinner with friends so awkward for everyone that the couple stopped going out. At work, Mark felt trapped and unable to control what was happening to him. Facial seizures reduced him to whispering or mumbling, and as a result, he was angry and impatient over work not getting done and fearful of the next pain attack. Listening to his story, I was not surprised when he told me that some employees had quit because of his unpleasant moods. Pain transforms people. Mark's life had been like this for six months by the time he came to the Pain Center. The more I learned about what he had been going through, the more I understood his desperate need for a miracle.

Although I could not give him immediate relief, Mark was encouraged. I said that I had never seen a case of trigeminal neuralgia that I had not been able to help, and I had a battle plan for combating it. The only way to attack his pain was on both physical and emotional fronts, which included not only quieting the hyperactive nerve but also subduing his anger and stress as well as reversing the listlessness, sleepiness, and slow thinking.

"Stress is a major part of your pain," I said. "It's your joy but it's also your hell. I'm sure you would probably find it impossible to give up your work, and I'm not suggesting a 'personality transplant' or giving up the drive that makes you happy and successful. But if I am to change what ignites your pain, you and I need to find ways to help you adapt to stress—and that means changing how you live your life."

Aside from adjusting his medications and starting some new ones, I contacted his psychiatrist to make sure that the new drugs would not adversely affect the old ones. I chose drugs that would simultaneously calm the hyperactive trigeminal nerve and decrease anxiety. Certain antianxiety medications are often used to fight pain, working both directly on the pain and indirectly on the anxiety that magnifies it. One drug, Klonopin (generic clonazopam), was particularly useful in someone like Mark, where anxiety can actually trigger a pain episode. In many people, anxiety and stress are two faces of the same attacker. They feed on a person's pain, intensifying the physical discomfort and mental distress. I also prescribed a different anticonvulsant, which slows down the abnormally firing nerve. I told Mark that I was not trying for a quick fix but for a permanent fix, so his progress might be slow and incremental but it would stick. If the drugs did not work, there were numerous other treatments and therapies to try.

Mark's telephone number popped up on my pager a month later. His whispery voice sounded discouraged. He had done very well with the first drug he tried, Klonopin, which completely stopped the attacks. He thought it was a miracle, but success was fleeting. He now knew it wasn't going to be defeated overnight, as he had originally hoped.

Mark never used the word *suffering* to describe his pain, but that's what it was. People suffer when they lose control over their lives and access to what is most pleasurable to them—whether it's work, intimate relationships, or everyday personal interests. Mark began learning to control his anger—some employees had even commented that, without his temper outbursts, he seemed like a changed man—and he was learning not to work all the time. He and Laura had taken a couple of long weekend vacations, and, he announced proudly, some days he left the office early to spend the afternoon on the golf course. His life was beginning to improve.

SYNCHRONIZING LIMBIC MUSIC

Although Mark was clearly beset by physical disease (a malfunction of his neurological system that was generating seizures in his face), his suffering seemed linked to raging emotions. His pain was never just emotions or only the outgrowth of psychological distress. Nor was the connection between his physical pain and emotional suffering a coincidence.

Pain often occurs with alterations of mood or behavior, particularly when it becomes chronic. This overlap of mind and body is vividly revealed by the kinds of drugs in the pain medicine arsenal: *There is not a single class of drug used in psychiatry that is not also used to treat pain.* Patients, however, misinterpret the presence of psychiatric medication in pain medicine. When they find out that they are receiving a drug for pain that is also used for psychiatric purposes, they usually think that the doctor believes their pain "is all in their head." On the contrary, these drugs, such as certain antidepressants, are used directly to treat pain. Although they may be the same chemical, the analgesic pain-relieving properties of some antidepressants are different from the properties that make them useful for depression. Nevertheless, if depression is present, or anxiety as in Mark's case, treating this problem will also decrease pain because it will demagnify it. But while pain and emotional states are closely related, it's not so clear how. Undoubtedly, the limbic system plays a large role in meshing physical signals with emotional character.

One of my favorite teachers at Mass General, a renowned psychiatrist named George Murray, described the relationship between the limbic system and the thinking part of the brain, the cortex, as like a musical composition. While the cortex is in charge of analytical or concrete thoughts, the limbic system adds color and texture—the cortex forms the words of a song while the limbic system forms the melody. Mark Hamilton's trigeminal neuralgia demonstrated that the words may be a loud "ouch" but the background tune may be quite different, ringing out depression, anxiety, fear, anger, or even sadness.

According to Dr. Murray, the more developed cortex of the brain is responsible for the intellectual parts of your thoughts, and the older limbic system takes care of the less conscious, more primitive emotional parts of your thinking. Together, these parts fuse into coherent and human expressions of your mind. Dr. Murray could detect when a patient's brain was not integrating these two ways of thinking. To test the two systems, he would tell a patient about his friend Frank Jones. In a deliberately unemotional tone, he would say, "Frank Jones has very large feet. In fact, his feet are so large that he has to put his pants on over his head." The normal reaction to this is to laugh—or at least crack a smile. This is because the limbic part of the brain immediately registers the information and helps translate the usual human response, humor. No wonder the words *humor* and *human* are so close.

Mr. Spock would not laugh at such a story because he is not human, although he would probably recognize the illogic of trying to put on pants over one's head. This is the second part of the test, a test of the cortex of the brain, which is responsible for analytical or concrete thinking. Most of us recognize it is both funny and physically impossible. A patient who thinks it's funny but doesn't quite know why may have disease in the cortex, such as from a stroke. A patient who understands the physical impossibility but can't appreciate the human quality of the story may have normal cortical function but a disease elsewhere in the brain. For these patients, Dr. Murray might conclude that the words and the music don't go to the same song.

When I hear persistent pain, I listen for Dr. Murray's limbic music. Mark Hamilton's words and music didn't go to the same song, and if I had not recognized this, I might have missed the presence of the emotional stress that was ringing his pain alarm.

A MIND THAT HURTS CAN ALSO HEAL

The link between pain and emotion is not always destructive. You also possess emotions that can reduce pain. It's only logical that if strong emotion can magnify pain, it can shrink it, too. Researchers have produced encouraging evidence of the power of positive thinking. One such study involved people who were subjected to a measurable type of pain in a "cold-presser test," which you may remember from chapter 1 as a test for pain tolerance. Emotion plays a part in pain tolerance, and in this test, volunteers were told to place their hands in ice-cold water until the pain became so intolerable that they had to withdraw them. The researchers found that by instructing the volunteers to apply imagery to create positive feelings such as pride, confidence, and humor, they could postpone the point at which the temperatures became unbearable. The ability of the mind to postpone pain is vividly evident in accounts of superhuman feats of tolerating enormous pain during stressful emergencies such as lifting a car off a trapped leg or walking barefoot on hot coals.

Not too long ago, unexplainable chronic pain was called "psychogenic" pain, meaning that it was somehow not physical but largely a creation of the mind. Medical people assumed that what they now call idiopathic pain was generated by personal psychology and skewed emotions. This kind of pain was regarded as a manifestation of psychiatric trouble with no reality beyond the patient's imagination, moods, and feelings. Doctors no longer use the term "psychogenic pain" because they know that all pain has a psychogenic or psychological component. And they realize that labeling a pain condition that they don't understand with a name that highlights the mental component can stigmatize a patient.

Ironically, as medicine has acquired more knowledge about the biology of pain, scientists have also learned about the biology of emotions. The emotions that accompany pain, they have found, are not a fabrication of the psyche but a full-fledged partner in the neural processing that generates uncomfortable sensation. Certain emotions are so embedded in the pain experience that they are inseparable. It's like notes and music—you can't have one without the other. Chronic pain *always* stirs up emotion. Pain is derived from the Latin meaning "punishment," and painful experiences always evoke the feeling of being punished. Imagine being punished without any emotion attached to it—it wouldn't be experienced as punishment at all. If there is no unpleasant emotion, there can be no pain. Conversely, pleasant emotion or feelings of relief from stress can provide powerful pain relief. This was graphically shown in a landmark study of World War II soldiers.

"I'm Wounded, Thank God"

The study was undertaken by Lieutenant Colonel Henry Beecher, an anesthesiologist in the army during World War II who later became the first chairman of the Department of Anesthesia at Massachusetts General Hospital. He also was a pioneer in placebo research. Beecher interviewed 215 soldiers who had been badly wounded on the Italian front and were being treated in a combat hospital. He talked to them within thirteen hours of their injury, hoping to learn something about the relationship between how much pain they felt and the severity of their wounds and to assess whether their pain could be better treated. For this reason, he talked only to those with the worst injuries.

Soon after the soldiers were brought into a front hospital, they were asked, "As you lie there, are you having any pain?" Keep in mind, these men had compound fractures, extensive tissue damage, and/or wounds that had penetrated their throats, abdomen, or heads. In addition to interviewing those with the severest wounds, Beecher made sure that the men were mentally coherent and that none was in shock. At the end of his interviews, forty-eight said that their pain was bad and they wanted morphine. Yet, 157 soldiers said they either had no pain or only slight pain and wanted no medication. A full 75 percent of these terribly wounded soldiers reported that their pain was not just tolerable but *insignificant.*

Beecher was puzzled by the soldiers' apparent lack of pain. There was nothing special about their ability to withstand pain. He had watched many of them complain loudly when they were given inept injections that caused much less discomfort than the battle wounds. He knew from private practice that civilians with similar injuries, such as from a car accident, would react much differently to their condition. The most logical conclusion, he believed, was that the circumstances surrounding the injuries added potent emotional overtones that overpowered the pain. Although battle normally heightens soldiers' anxiety and fears, as they worry for themselves and friends, the soldiers in this study were so badly wounded that their combat commitment had clearly ended and instead of fear they felt overwhelming relief.

"Strong emotion can block pain," Beecher wrote about the men. "Consider the position of the soldier: his wound suddenly releases him from an exceedingly dangerous environment, one filled with fatigue, discomfort, anxiety, fear and real danger of death, and gives him a ticket to the safety of the hospital. His troubles are about over, or he thinks they are. He overcompensates and becomes euphoric. Whether this actually reduces the pain remains unproved. On the other hand, the civilian's accident marks the beginning of disaster for him." In 1946, when Beecher's article was published, medicine and science had no inkling of the tangled web inhabited by pain and emotion. He was one of the first modern scientists to explore our innate pain-fighting system and to suggest that somehow complex feelings have a decisive impact on how we feel tissue damage in the body. Beecher's research opened many doors for later science.

Medical science now has reams of studies that demonstrate how strong emotions can silence the severest pain. There are now hundreds of studies into the immense power of the placebo effect and how it influences all aspects of medical treatment. Although few people like to think of themselves as being subject to placebo effects, everyone at any time can be affected. Surely you have heard of human dramas that give strong credence to the power of mind over matter, like stories of parents ignoring life-threatening burns in order to save a child, athletes oblivious to broken bones while in the heat of competition, and participants in religious ceremonies eagerly enduring flesh-cutting initiation ceremonies.

In Beecher's time, strong emotion, or the "powerful placebo," as he called it, was a marvelous mystery of pain medicine. Somehow, the emotion that came with a potentially painful injury at times relieved the physical discomfort and mental suffering. Today, science has clearly demonstrated the effect strong emotion can have over physical sensation. In the same way your immune system can protect you from disease, your emotions can be stimulated to form a natural defense against pain. Such powerful tools can also go awry. As any chronic pain sufferer knows too well, pain rarely brings waves of soothing emotion. The very fabric of persistent pain is woven throughout with extremely noxious feelings. That pain is so difficult to define attests to its elusive place between your body and mind. Discounting or ignoring the emotional facets of pain simply allows them to do more damage. Although patients usually fear that psychological explanations of their pain will devalue their suffering, the emotional component does not always work against you. Just as in Beecher's remarkable study, the mind plays an invaluable role in helping us cope with any adversity, including pain. Learning how placebos tap into pain relief is one of the most dramatic and promising areas of modern medicine.

THE POWERFUL PLACEBO

Lieutenant Colonel Beecher knew he was onto something; ten years after his study of soldiers in pain, he was still mulling over how their emotions had muted their pain. He wondered if perhaps the findings were not isolated results of combat experience but reflected a universal phenomenon. The horror of the battlefield had triggered self-defense emotions. Perhaps there were other ways to stimulate people's ability to conjure up feelings that suppressed pain.

Beecher left the army and was doing research at Harvard Medical School while practicing at Massachusetts General Hospital. One of his next major publications, an article in the *Journal of the American Medical Association* entitled "The Powerful Placebo," is credited with introducing psychosomatic analgesic into modern medicine. For this study, he analyzed the findings of fifteen drug tests involving placebos and other medications as tested on more than a thousand patients. The patients were trying drugs for a variety of conditions, from severe postoperative pain to headaches, seasickness, and the common cold. Some were given their medication in tablet form, others received it by injection. Nevertheless, despite the diversity of the patients and their ailments, their reaction to placebos was remarkably consistent.

The range of people responding to placebos was as low as 15 percent and as high as 58 percent. Beecher saw that on average, about 35 percent of the participants responded to placebos. He also noticed that people reacted better, feeling more relief, when they received more doses and that some patients experienced unpleasant side effects from their sugar pills or saline injections. The sicker patients, those with more serious ailments, experienced greater relief from placebos than the mildly ill.

When your doctor claims that on average one-third of all patients get better or worse on placebos, he or she is harking back to Beecher's findings. Beecher pointed out other conclusions that have also held up over time. For instance, in his own studies with patients, he found little difference in reactions to placebos between men and women or according to intelligence. And he saw a large spread depending on people's attitudes, habits, education, and "personality structure," presumably meaning their reaction to stress. Beecher is rightly considered the first modern pioneer into the science of placebos. He offered persuasive evidence that placebos "can produce gross physical change" and debunked the myth that only unsophisticated people "fall" for them.

Despite all that science knows about placebos, I regularly encounter medical professionals who believe that placebos are a clever way to prove that some patients are faking it or that it's "all in their head." At the Massachusetts General Hospital Pain Center, I supervised a steady stream of newly minted doctors receiving additional training in pain medicine. Called fellows, these doctors were exceptionally bright and accomplished operating-room anesthesiologists who chose to get advanced training to become pain specialists. Like most physicians, they were more accustomed to grappling with the raw pain of a surgical patient than with pain that had been woven into a person's personality. Coming from the best medical schools and residencies around the country, they had in common only their general medical and anesthesiology training. Each fellow brought a unique personal background and bag of professional experiences with him or her, so I was always amazed when virtually every year one of the fellows would declare that he had used a placebo to uncover the "truth" about a patient he had been treating.

Time and again, a fellow would tell me that he had proved that a patient did not have "real" pain. The fellow would sound embarrassed for the patient, as if he were revealing an unpleasant secret. My reaction was always mildly raised eyebrows: How do you know it's faked? The fellow would explain that he had injected a water solution instead of lidocaine and a few minutes after the injection, the unknowing patient, who had been suffering, was ecstatic; the pain had been significantly reduced or even disappeared.

I would listen to this story without interrupting and then explain, "You have proved something very important, but not whether the pain is real. What you've proved is that the patient responds to a placebo. What you don't realize is that that patient could be any of us at any time." I am always reassured when I hear that a patient has shown a placebo response. It just confirms that the mind has much to say about pain.

CURES, NOT TRICKS

I recently treated a young woman suffering from migraines who had been receiving large amounts of narcotics from other doctors trying to control her horrendous pain. Doctors now know that repeated dosages of many analgesics, including narcotics such as Demerol, may eventually make the pain worse. This is called the rebound effect.

Jane had been hospitalized for some time, but her pain and behavior had both deteriorated; she appeared relatively comfortable during the day but consistently demanded narcotics in the middle of the night when the house staff was most tired and stressed. Later, even a headache specialist could not break her confusing pattern of pain.

Weeks after she'd been admitted, the treating team asked me to meet with Jane and assess her medication. Although I knew that some of her nurses suspected something was unusual about this case, perhaps involving drug-seeking behavior, I assumed that the headaches were quite real. From reading her chart, I saw that she had been using narcotics in a self-defeating pattern. So my goal was to understand why and find a better way to help her cope with the headaches. It was quickly clear that making any sudden changes was not going to be easy. To say she was resistant to the idea of reducing the narcotics is an understatement. The only way I could get her to agree to any other course of treatment was by negotiating with her about what other kinds of drugs might work—essentially wondering with her why only one single pain medicine among all that were available was doing the job. She was well aware that I had been called because her other doctors and nurses had become frustrated with her, and she with them. She seemed resigned to my being involved but didn't exactly welcome my efforts to help.

As in most difficult cases with patients who have had difficult interactions with other caregivers, I try not to take sides. I want to find solutions, so I focus on the facts that everyone can agree upon. As clearly and dispassionately as possible, I laid out for Jane what I understood about her case and explained that I could only act as her consultant and offer advice based on my experiences with similar

cases. I told her that from my point of view, her situation had esca-
lated to a crisis and treatments were not only failing but making
things worse. As part of this discussion, I had to explain that the staff
would soon be denying her demands for pain medicine, particularly in
the middle of the night.

Jane accepted that her situation had reached a stalemate. Despite
all the emotionally charged personal interactions between her and her
doctors and nurses, her distress was still palpable. I could not tell
whether her pain was worsening from rebound narcotics or, as some
had suggested, from the stress of her impending wedding. Either way,
I'm sure no one would willingly go through what she had experienced. She deserved help; how to help was far less clear.

So, in the face of strange behaviors, deteriorated relationships with
caregivers, suspicious theories, and broken-down communications, I
aimed for the truth. I candidly shared with Jane my lack of clear
answers. I emphasized that while this was a real mess with many possible causes, probably no one single cause was at fault. She reluctantly
agreed to try an experiment with several active medicines as well as a
placebo, although she would not know which she was getting.

During the first procedure, I was helped by several nurses and two
medical students. With much flourish and medical ceremony, I started
to give her small injections of either active medicine or water solution.
The first was saline solution, essentially sterilized salt water. All the
while I watched intently; the nurses took vital signs as the students
manned the machines at Jane's bedside. After a few minutes, she said
that her pain dropped from most severe, or a ten (on a ten-point scale),
to a five. Ten to fifteen minutes later, I changed the injection to a mild
sedative, Ativan. This drug has minimal direct effects on pain but does
have other noticeable effects like sleepiness and loss of concentration.
Her pain again dropped by half. Lastly, I gave her lidocaine, the short-
acting local anesthetic, and the last of her pain disappeared.

For the first time in weeks, her migraine vanished. I explained that
I had given her a combination of active and inert chemicals and that
her pain had decreased substantially without a strong pain reliever.
She was not surprised—which surprised me—and she suggested that
perhaps the saline fluid worked by hydrating her. It was a good guess.
When I told her that the saline was purely a placebo, I also cautioned
her to resist the natural tendency to feel "tricked." I declared that this
was an important finding that held an optimistic message: She clearly

possessed within herself the capacity to manage her pain, and do so with far fewer side effects than with any narcotic.

After several nights of meeting her nighttime pain attacks with the same drugs or placebo that had worked in her experiment, she broke the headache cycle and was able to go home. A few months later she was hospitalized again with headache pain. This time the doctors stopped the rebound from starting by immediately repeating the multiple drug-plus-placebo infusion treatments. Forty-eight hours later, she was discharged and has not been back since.

A medical student later asked me if I hadn't just fooled Jane and not really treated the problem. I understood his sentiments but pointed out that I had no other way to show Jane that she had the power to heal herself. I explained that this treatment was far safer than the others that worked far less well. Jane consented to being given a placebo, and its use was not only ethical but possibly the only answer to her crisis. The key was to clearly help Jane know that she was neither tricked nor considered a fraud. Jane needed to feel that she was in control, whether it be control of her pain or over a possibly doomed marriage. Maybe she needed an "excuse with honor" to release the pain, or maybe the treatment was a direct hit on pure nerve pain. All I knew for certain was that the previous treatments of throwing one drug after another at her had proven counterproductive. So, I went the other way and found a pain-relieving solution within the patient rather than in the pharmacy.

Virtually every facet of medical care can evoke a placebo response, from the smell of a waiting room to the size of a bandage. The universe of possible placebo effects can arise from a host of procedures, including surgery, injections, biofeedback, psychotherapy, physical therapy, and hypnosis, as well as a patient's expectations and attitudes toward pain and medical people—even his or her feelings about the medical surroundings and equipment. The placebo effect reaches beyond inert medications or pseudo-procedures—it arises from any sight, sound, action, or treatment that produces an effect wider than a treatment's direct effects. It's part of every treatment.

DOSES OF THE MIND: CUPPING TO COPPER BRACELETS

Placebos are as old as medicine itself and have become more refined as medicine has learned more about their actions. The placebo effect explains the widespread popularity of such ancient remedies as temple sacrifices, water cures, leeches, bloodletting, cupping (putting hot glass cups on the skin to produce a blister and draw off harmful humors), and patent medicines. Historical accounts report that the discoverer of homeopathy, Samuel Hahnemann, gave his patients pills emptied of all their medicinal ingredients and convinced them that the pills would "remember" the strong medicine they had contained and so cure their ailments. Although these remedies may have an unknown force that promotes health, I am certain that believing in Dr. Hahnemann or believing in the promise of the remedy boosted, if not created, the positive effect on patients.

In the eighteenth century, Swiss doctor Anton Mesmer, the father of hypnotism, designed a novel device to treat pain: He filled a tub with water and magnetic material that purportedly helped him induce a hypnotic trance in his patients. Yesterday's mixtures of powdered mummies, frog sperm, lizard tongues, and animal dung have given way to modern concoctions of apricot pits and the like. Other treatments that probably contain a hefty dose of placebo power include copper bracelets, colonic irrigation, shark cartilage, and megadoses of vitamins. Many accepted medical treatments may also be fueled by placebo power, which is why medical science continuously studies the effects of drugs compared to a known placebo.

It seems that regardless of what's in a particular placebo, large capsules are generally stronger than small capsules, yellow capsules may produce greater antidepressant or stimulant effects, white capsules evoke more analgesic or narcotic responses, and injections are more potent than any pill. A placebo response can be created by something as intangible as a caregiver's attention and concern; doctors have found that a patient is more likely to have a placebo response if they take a full medical history and perform an examination. A symbol of aggressive treatment, like the hospital pomp-and-circumstance of surgery and a visible scar afterwards, can also generate a placebo response. Amazingly, some studies say that placebos are more effective with severe than with mild pain.

The placebo response is not always positive. Occasionally I see a patient who displays a negative placebo reaction, such as showing unpleasant side effects like palpitations or diarrhea from a treatment that normally does not generate such reactions. These adverse reactions, called "nocebo effects," can worsen a patient's symptoms. Just as a placebo effect may explain an otherwise baffling positive effect, nocebo effect can explain otherwise unexpected negative effects. Placebos and nocebos are really one and the same.

It is a myth, however, that some people are particularly susceptible to placebos. There is no such thing as a "placebo personality." Doctors have found that certain attitudes make people more open to placebos, namely expectation that a treatment will work or that a doctor will make them better, willingness or ready compliance with whatever is recommended, and anxiety over their situation. Time and again, doctors have seen that placebos help reduce a patient's anticipatory anxiety, that is, fear of pain to come. Another misconception is that a third of any group of patients receiving treatment shows a placebo response. In fact, in various large studies, anywhere from one-quarter to three-quarters of patients react to placebos.

Why is the placebo response so pervasive? One explanation is that placebos themselves do nothing while the pain or disease they supposedly treat runs its course regardless of what drugs or procedures doctors apply. Many conditions and illnesses have a predictable course of incubation, onset, peak, and gradual disappearance. People tend to call on medical help when symptoms are at their worst, at the illness's peak, so time alone may well bring improvement, regardless of treatment. "A tincture of time" is a common and often effective prescription. However, this "natural history" theory doesn't account for the frequency and intensity of placebo effects. I am much more convinced that placebo effects reflect the natural interaction between the mind and the body. As a potent system with significant influence on how you feel, the placebo response is also prone to malfunctioning, which may account for mysterious diseases that make little sense.

YOUR BRAIN'S OWN PHARMACY

Morphine is the gold standard of pain relief. Even biotechnology has not been able to improve substantially on this ancient pain reliever. Medicine has numerous chemical variations, but these are modifications, not radical alterations, of the basic structure of the morphine molecules.

One of the Holy Grails of modern science has been to learn why morphine and its derivatives affect people so strongly. Why, scientists have asked, is morphine able to eradicate the severest pain, produce the loftiest euphoria, and generate debilitating addiction? Is there a reason that the human brain, when exposed to large amounts of the drug, craves it to the point of self-destruction? This question launched one of the most remarkable scientific races in modern neuroscience.

The answer is that perhaps the brain contains not just a chemical affinity for morphine but is uniquely designed to use it. Given morphine's influence, perhaps the brain possesses its own source of an opiate-like chemical. Perhaps the brain even manufactures it.

Morphine is the most famous member of a large family of drugs medical professionals call opioids (*opium,* which means "juice" in Greek, is a poppy extract). Historians assume from the *Odyssey* that the potion Helen of Troy gave Ulysses to bring forgetfulness contained opium. The panacea created in ancient Rome by Galen around 158 A.D. and used in Europe into the nineteenth century contained more than a hundred ingredients, with opium's contribution perhaps rivaled only by that of snake venom. The Renaissance marked the flowering of opium as well as the arts. The famous fifteenth-century healer and mystic Paracelsus mixed opium with alcohol to make laudanum, which became a popular antidote for everything from melancholy to surgical pain.

Morphine, the active ingredient in opium, was not isolated until 1817, but its effective use was limited until doctors came up with an efficient delivery system when the hollow needle and syringe were invented in midcentury. Today, doctors have a large medicine chest of opium-derived drugs at their disposal. After thousands of years of using opiates, chemists now know how to make semisynthetic versions, such as heroin, and synthetic versions, such as methadone and fentanyl. Codeine and morphine are natural forms. Even more natural are the ones you make inside your body.

The firing gun for the race to discover the brain's natural morphine sounded in the early 1970s when Avram Goldstein, a professor of pharmacology at Stanford University, devised a chemical test for locating where such opiate-like molecules might be found. The brain is a big place. As Joel Davis aptly put it in his book *Endorphins, New Waves in Brain Chemistry,* "There are more brain cells at a dinner for ten than there are stars in the Milky Way galaxy." So to narrow the search, scientists like Goldstein went looking for binding sites or receptor cells, which are like baseball mitts designed to catch chemicals. In this case, they hunted for the receptor that would catch only molecules that work like morphine. Once they found the receptor, a new question emerged: Wy would the body have this specialized baseball mitt if it didn't have its own baseballs?

Scientists from Sweden, Scotland, and the United States joined the hunt, which largely consisted of grinding animal brains into a soup and filtering the mixture through radioactive chemicals that would attach to and highlight the specific receptors. The winners of the first leg of the competition were the well-known professor of psychiatry and pharmacology at Johns Hopkins University, Solomon Synder, and a young graduate student in his lab, Candace Pert. In 1973, they announced in the journal *Science* that they had found opiate receptors in the brain cells of mice. Three years later, Scottish scientists found what scientists now refer to as the key that fit the opiate receptor lock, the brain's naturally manufactured opiates. They named the opioid chemical "enkephalin," a Greek word meaning "from the head." American scientists on the trail of similar innate opioids called their version "endorphin," a combination of *endogenous,* meaning "produced in the body," and *morphine.* In the ensuing war of words, the American term gained general currency. There are really three kinds of natural opioids—endorphins, enkephalins, and dynorphins—but the term "endorphins" has come to be used to encompass all three.

The discovery in 1976 that your body produces a chemical that, like morphine, mutes your pain and heightens pleasure set off a worldwide quest to learn how to harness this fabulous substance. Scientists everywhere wanted to know whether particular activities or conditions cause the body and brain to produce more endorphins. Were there other ways you could deliberately unleash their power? Was there a chemical or drug you could take to stimulate their production? What was nature's purpose in designing endorphins? Was there a downside to producing too much of the chemical?

An intriguing aspect of the endorphin discovery was that scientists found opioid receptors all over—in intestines, the stomach, glands, the central nervous system, and the brain. This prompted speculation on how endorphins might be involved in all sorts of body functions, from the physiology of dependency to why humans feel pleasure and pain. Evidence that endorphins suppress the body's production of Substance P, a chemical that washes through damaged and inflamed tissue, may explain why morphine injected into inflamed joints provides long-acting pain relief and how endorphins can mute other types of pain. A major place where endorphins circulate is the pituitary gland, which may partly explain how exertion and exercise can change pain and even produce moods like "runner's high." There are also opioid receptors in the sex glands, and Pert reports that in animal studies, endorphin levels jump 200 percent between arousal and orgasm.

Pain is a warning system that alerts you when you are threatened with bodily harm or have an injury that needs immediate medical attention. In the face of imminent danger, the best protection is either to fight or flee, and in both cases, endorphins earn their keep. While endorphins are definitely not the entire reason why we can produce our own pain relief and pleasure, they are certainly an important part. When your body needs to override pain to survive, endorphins, in conjunction with many other chemicals that the body uses to manage stress, can come to the rescue, perhaps as an evolutionary survival mechanism. People who ignore their seared skin to drag themselves from a burning building or lift a car off their severed leg may well be awash in pain-numbing endorphins. Endorphins may also explain how people triumph over one of the most common experiences of pain; studies of pregnant women during labor have found that their endorphin levels rise significantly and may enable them to endure the pain of labor long enough to give birth.

The uncovering of endorphins helps explain, at least in part, the mystery of placebos and offers strong evidence of the biological underpinnings of the mind. It appears that some placebo responses may involve endorphins. In certain cases where placebos reduce pain, studies have shown that blocking endorphins with naloxone also blocks the pain relief. This implies that physical chemistry is at play in some placebo effects and even more compelling evidence that there is a physical, neurochemical basis to the mind. Sometimes, if you think that a painful sensation is going to ease up or even disappear, this can stimulate neurons to change your neurochemistry and possibly raise endorphin levels. The placebo acts like a drug that triggers the release of your body's inherent analgesia. It's not the placebo substance but the belief in and expectations for treatment that somehow turn on the chemical faucet. Despite their reputation as a psychological ploy, placebos likely release of a symphony of potent neurochemicals, probably including the endorphins. But the exact instruments and music of this symphony still remain to be discovered. The Nobel Prize, among other rewards, is waiting for the scientist who figures out exactly how the mind controls specific chemicals and interacts with the rest of the body.

TREATING WITH PLACEBOS

As we have seen, many people have a simplistic notion of placebos, embracing the outdated idea that they are sham treatments, "sugar pills" designed to trick patients. To me, a placebo is a profound sign of the mind's enormous power over the function of the body. Although scientists do not have a clear explanation for how placebos work, the placebo effect is a potent pain modifier. Its only drawback is that doctors don't know enough to harness its power consistently. They don't know when the analgesic impact will occur, how forceful it will be, how long it will last, or what kind of patient will be most affected. Nevertheless, placebos can so dramatically subdue pain that I would gladly use them first, and almost exclusively, if I could always make them work and make their effects persist.

Even though medical science has not advanced to the point where doctors can harness the power of placebos, I still have a large arsenal of mind-body therapies as well as medications, procedures, and surgeries to apply in the war against chronic pain. In the next section of this book, you will hear about these treatments—how they work and who they work for—and get a glimpse of how technology and discoveries about neuroscience are generating innovations that are helping turn the tide and eventually win the war.

PART II

STRATEGIES
FOR
HEALING

The State of the Art in

the War on Pain

By now you have a fairly good picture of what pain does to your body and how your body reacts in response. If you're in chronic pain, you know from personal experience that understanding the science beneath your discomfort is only part of the solution. Now you want to know what to do about it.

For the remainder of the book, I am going to take you to various pain centers to show the many ways we pain doctors are attacking pain. Pain medicine is a young specialty, and multiple medical disciplines are contributing new ideas and techniques. To show you current and future pain treatments, I will take you to my previous home base, Massachusetts General Hospital, and my present pain center at the University of California at Davis. And we will go beyond these sites to other medical centers, hospitals, and clinics around the country that are on the frontier of pain management.

A truism about chronic pain is that treatment is as much an art as a science. Given all the dimensions of pain, it should come as no surprise that chronic pain has many facets and many treatments. While any given treatment may be useful for a specific condition, it's usually not the only therapy needed. Often, the best treatment is a coordinated attack of medications, procedures, and other therapies. In addition to standard treatments, I often suggest that patients try nonsurgical and nondrug therapies such as biofeedback, physical therapies, hypnosis, behavioral medicine, and acupuncture. A treatment plan should reflect the personal nature of what a patient is feeling rather than follow a fixed formula. When I am choosing and contouring combinations of treatments, the needs of the individual patient are foremost. Two patients with exactly the same symptoms may do better with different approaches. So much depends on who the patient is and what the illness has done to his or her life.

The first chapters in this section are organized by the cause of the pain. Chapter 7 investigates treatments for pain that is triggered by aggravated tissue. The angry tissue signals the nerves that something is wrong and pain results. This happens with many types of pain, including back pain and arthritis. At first glance these two ailments appear unrelated, but in both conditions the nerves that signal pain are doing their job properly. Chapter 8, which describes what happens when your nerves are injured and misfiring, highlights treatments for such nerve pain conditions as diabetic neuropathy, trigeminal neuralgia, and complex regional pain.

Chapter 9 looks at a kind of pain that almost everyone knows first-hand—headaches—and chapter 10 offers a slightly different perspective by exploring the world of mainstream treatments that are effective but not well understood as well as some so-called "alternative" treatments and the conditions for which they are most effective. In chapter 11, you'll read about the extraordinary measures demanded by end-of-life pain and the absolute necessity of reckoning with the suffering that besets someone with a terminal illness. In the final chapter I look ahead to the future of pain medicine and offer a preview of innovative treatments just beyond the horizon.

7

NORMAL NERVES, DAMAGED TISSUE

Low Back Pain, Arthritis, Joint Pain, and Other Common Aches

The cure for this ill is not to sit still,
Or frowst with a book by the fire;
But to take a large hoe and a shovel also,
And dig till you gently perspire.

—RUDYARD KIPLING

A common scenario at pain centers throughout the country is a story I hear almost weekly. If you are one of the millions of Americans who suffer from chronic low back pain, you know the tale well. It's most often told by a middle-aged or elderly man or woman, and the tales are strikingly similar. The patient was at work or home, doing something he or she does every day, like lifting a box or a child or turning quickly, and felt a wrench in the lower back. The back seemed to catch on something, sending gripping pain that seized the back, freezing the person in mid-motion. Over the next couple of minutes, the pain subsided and the patient slowly resumed moving, even though there was a lingering soreness where the hitch occurred. But the pain was not bad enough to sideline the person, and he continued with normal activities. The patient was sure that it was a passing incident, like a small burn, and tried to ignore it.

However, the back remained tender, and over the following weeks the soreness deepened to a spreading ache. He saw his primary-care physician, who prescribed mild pain medicines like ibuprofen and suggested rest with a critical dose of the most common healer of such problems, "a tincture of time."

The patient made small adjustments in his posture and the way he sat and walked, but relief was elusive. The pain grew, stemming not only from the lower back but also the buttocks and upper thighs. Sleeping became difficult, as did sitting for any length of time, like during a movie. The back and buttock muscles grew irritable and frequently erupted into spasms. When the pain became severe enough, the patient cut back on work, curtailed doing things around the house, halted leisure activities and exercise, and spent most of his day on the couch. Usually at this point in the story, the patient returned to the primary-care doctor, who tried other treatments or sent him on to an orthopedist or to someone like myself at a pain management clinic.

Given the structure of your back, with all its nerves, nerve roots, joints, muscles, and ligaments, and the hurried pace of modern life, it's no wonder low back pain has reached epidemic proportions. I'm sure you've read the staggering figures about the incidence and cost of low back pain. It is the leading reason for office visits to primary physicians and the main reason for workplace disability, and it is responsible for twenty million sick days each year. Doctors have also learned that traditional ideas about telling patients with low back pain to rest—essentially on their back—in bed or on the couch for days is not always helpful, and may be harmful.

What makes low back pain thorny to treat is the constellation of possible causes. The patient with the twisted low back could have a dizzying variety of possible problems. These include a mechanical injury, such as an overstretched ligament (strained or sprained); a problem with one of the many joints that make up the back, such as the facet or sacroiliac joint; or spondylolisthesis, which occurs when a vertebra slips forward, or sometimes backward, over the one beneath it. You could have a slipped disk, otherwise known as a disk bulge or, if it is more severe, a disk herniation. Or you may have worn-out tissues, which doctors simply call degenerative disease. Other possibilities are spinal stenosis, a narrowing of the spinal canal, or a pinched nerve, which is any problem in the spine that constricts the nerves that exit the spine. And then there's that deep well of unknown causes of back pain—an injury of mysterious origin or symptoms that don't make clear anatomical sense or respond to conventional treatments. Such "idiopathic back pain" accounts for a staggering majority of all chronic back pain cases.

A further complication is the possibility that symptoms that look like they're stemming from the low back are not, but are migrating from elsewhere. For instance, the piriformis muscle deep in the buttocks crosses the sciatic nerve and can bring on pain known as sciatica. Some ways of moving can cause the piriformis to squeeze and crowd the sciatic nerve and trip pain that seems to begin in the lower back and radiate down the legs. At other times, this small muscle irritates the sciatic nerve because it has formed scars or has otherwise become overcontracted. So when a patient comes to me because of a hurting back, I have to remember that there are many possible causes and that even the likeliest suspects can be deceiving.

If you've been treated lately for low back pain, you may have noticed the absence of some terms traditionally associated with back pain, like "lumbago." The language of low back pain has evolved in recent years away from terms that broadly refer to symptoms—lumbago simply meant soreness in the lower back—to labels that indicate the underlying cause or nerve activity. For instance, I frequently encounter a type of low back pain called radiculopathy, meaning that the pain radiates from a compressed or disrupted nerve root somewhere along the spine. The same symptoms may be called "sciatica," but this is now a much less used term because it means simply that the sciatic nerve is involved for any number of reasons. The word says nothing about what's causing the aggravation, which could be from joints, disks, or muscles anywhere in the region, whereas "radiculopathy" clearly identifies the nerve root as the culprit.

With the spinal cord being home to key segments of your central nervous system, it's not surprising that nerve injury or malfunction is the cause of much low back pain. Nerves along the spinal cord that have been provoked by tissue damage, such as from a pull, bruise, tear, or inflammation, can generate pain almost anywhere in the body, and most certainly in the lower back. Low back pain can begin suddenly and severely or gently, rising gradually to a crescendo of acute pain. Usually, even the worst back pain can be treated, and sometimes cured, as long as its source can be identified, as Kitty Marshall learned.

A Special Kind of Band-Aid

I knew Kitty Marshall as a vibrant young nurse in the pediatric unit at Mass General Hospital, so I was shocked to see her hobbling into the Pain Center like an old woman. A trim twenty-five-year-old blonde with rosy cheeks, she had changed dramatically since I had seen her last. She did not walk so much as lurch in a crouch, propelling herself from chair to chair or using the hallway wall to keep upright. I immediately suggested that she might be more comfortable lying down on a stretcher, and I sat beside her as she recounted what had happened.

Kitty had contracted meningitis, a serious infection of the brain linings, most likely from one of the kids on her unit. To diagnosis this, her doctor had done a routine spinal tap that involved passing a thin needle into the low back and through the spine to collect a sample of cerebrospinal fluid. As the term suggests, the needle penetrates the spine in the lower lumbar area. Kitty said that the lumbar puncture did not hurt and she went home afterward with a slightly sore back, hopeful that her troubles were over.

The pain started several hours after the spinal tap and slowly made its way to her head, where it produced a thunderous, god-awful headache. "I spend my days on the couch," she said, "barely able to move. My head hurts so badly when I stand up that I crawl to the bathroom. I haven't been able to take a shower or bath in days, I can't eat, and I've lost about seven pounds." In the knowledgeable tone of a professional nurse, she added, "I'm taking two Percocet every six hours, but it's not making a dent." What Kitty didn't know was that her headache was coming from her back, or more precisely, it was a result of the spinal tap.

Usually, new patients to the Pain Center go through a series of exams and assessments, beginning with a medical history and pain evaluation, then on to an exam by a resident or fellow, and finally, my questions and physical examination. My goal with virtually every patient is to make an accurate diagnosis as quickly as possible, covering the entire gamut of possible causes for the pain. But there is not always a straight line through an unambiguous diagnostic tree in which "yes" or "no" answers lead to a certain conclusion. Objective signs can be interpreted in many ways, and a patient's subjective feelings and stresses add further complications. But sometimes, the cause and treatment are obvious. Such was the case with Kitty's lumbar puncture headache.

The tip-off in the case was that Kitty had a very unique kind of headache that was painful only when she was upright. Almost no other headaches behave this way. The diagnostic spinal tap was almost certainly the source of her misery. The needle used to extract spinal fluid punched a hole in the lining around her spinal cord through which fluid was now probably leaking into the surrounding tissue. The change in fluid pressure caused by this leak made her head ache.

When Kitty said that her head hurt especially when she tried to stand up, I was certain that the lumbar puncture was causing her pain. Standing upright exacerbated the pressure on the tender lining of the spinal canal and damaged tissue, understandably accenting her pain. Young people get these headaches more often than older people, probably because they have more spinal fluid and so more pressure changes when that fluid is disturbed.

Back pain like Kitty's is highly treatable. Pain medicine has an assortment of procedures and medications that can swiftly and efficiently correct the damage and calm damaged tissue and protesting nerves. With a lumbar puncture headache, the remedy is so rapid and perfect that it seems almost miraculous. I explained to Kitty that I wanted to do a procedure called an epidural blood patch, and that I could almost guarantee that her pain would vanish soon afterwards. In my business, I am rarely able to offer such guarantees.

On that day in the Pain Center, I had Kitty lie comfortably on her side and numbed her lower back with a tiny shot of lidocaine. I then guided a thin needle into the epidural space the same way anesthesia would be given for childbirth. Instead of anesthesia, I was going to use Kitty's own blood as a kind of Band-Aid. Using a syringe of blood from a vein in her arm, I injected it into the layer that had been punctured, right where she had been stuck for the lumbar puncture. In essence, I was inserting a patch of her own blood to stem the pain-producing pressure from the puncture. Her blood would make a healthy clot and stop the leaking. The procedure lasted about fifteen minutes, and when she slowly sat up to move into the wheelchair that would take her from the hospital, her headache and back pain had disappeared.

Kitty's type of back pain is not widely seen because it usually only follows spinal injections. Yet it offers a wonderful example of how sensitive the back can be and how quickly it can become aroused to painful irritation. And, her story shows how quickly and completely pain can be eradicated if the cause is clearly understood and the treatment strategically delivered.

BLOCKS FOR BAD BACKS

Nerve blocks are a prominent part of treatment at many pain centers. They comprise an array of injection therapies that are especially useful for pain that's local and pouring forth from damaged tissue. Nerve blocks are a fairly simple concept, and doctors have been performing them since the early 1800s when they learned that nerves are like a highway that carries pain signals. To block pain and prevent the signal from reaching the central nervous system, doctors found that a variety of solutions did the job, including cocaine, adrenaline, saline solution, mild opioids, and anti-inflammatory agents like steroids. The use of nerve blocks multiplied as early patients, mostly those undergoing eye or limb surgery, benefited from their pain-numbing powers. Undoubtedly, part of the success of blocks stems from their regular use in childbirth, which started around 1900 and is now a part of most hospital births. Today, many patients are frightened by the thought of being injected with a needle, but some come into the Pain Center knowing the exact injection that helped in the past and request a particular nerve block.

A nerve block acts like a roadblock on the pain highway, or like those sand-filled safety barrels for runaway trucks. While originally developed for surgery and often used to make diagnoses, their widest use today is to relieve pain emanating from an identifiable nerve. Many pain doctors use the term "block" to refer to any injection procedure that stops pain signals or cools off inflamed nerves. Keep in mind that nerve blocks are not a universal treatment for all pain: They're best for reining in pain from an identifiable place in the body, whether it is the back, legs or arms, or face. While sometimes they work like a one-shot cure, blocks often give only short-term relief. Most patients tolerate them well, they are over quickly, and when specially trained doctors perform them in the right environment, they are very safe.

For most nerve blocks I give a shot of medication, typically a local anesthetic or anti-inflammatory drug, to halt the signal traveling along the affected nerves or cool off inflammation in the area. When the block contains a local anesthetic, it's usually at a low concentration so that only sensation such as pain is reduced while other functions such as movement are preserved. In other words, the dose is low to avoid temporary paralysis. With either a local anesthetic or anti-inflammatory drug, the chemical washes through the body within hours to weeks, and the pain-relieving effects may be equally short-lived or lasting. However, the effect of turning off the nervous barrage of pain signals or decreasing inflammation can last longer.

Blocks are tricky this way—it's hard, if not impossible, to predict the length of their impact. Whenever I do a block, I usually counsel a patient to keep an optimistic and realistic outlook and to plan on complete pain relief but not be surprised if the pain returns. If it does, the block either worked temporarily or not at all, but even this development usually helps me focus more clearly on what's causing the pain.

The blocks and treatments for Cameron Rogers's aching back are typical of what pain medicine now offers. He slipped in his bathroom getting out of the tub and landed on his tailbone, and for the next year visited doctor after doctor looking for a reason why his buttocks ached. He couldn't sit still for more than twenty minutes at a stretch. When I saw him more than a year after his tumble on the tile, his back continued to hurt even though none of the diagnostic tests and scans found a physiological reason for so much discomfort. Although I didn't know why his back ached, I saw that the pain was concentrated in his low back and that the best remedy might be an epidural injection with an anti-inflammatory drug. I injected a cortisone type of drug in the sore spot with a procedure called a caudal epidural steroid injection.

For most forms of low back pain, I rarely use the caudal epidural block that Cameron received for the very reason I gave it to him. A caudal injection spreads medication throughout the region, offering wider coverage but less exact targeting. With Cameron, I could not tell where his back was injured, so I applied medication as broadly as possible. I much prefer to aim the medication at a precise nerve or tissue space.

Firing at a Narrowing Spine

A somewhat more precise block is the traditional epidural steroid injection, one of the workhorses of pain medicine. Jack Russo's back pain looked like the sort of pain that anyone over forty can imagine— the ache from the wear and tear of aging. The primary-care physician who had referred Jack to the Pain Center had initially thought the sixty-two-year-old accountant had run-of-the-mill low back pain. Although he was thirty-five pounds overweight and had smoked since college, this accountant had not seen many specialists before. Other than arthritic joints, he had been relatively free of medical problems, and his back pain had been a nagging, gradual discomfort over several years. He had successfully ignored the symptoms for as long as he could recall and couldn't remember if the pain in his back came before or after the troubling ache in his legs.

Jack's doctor thought his legs ached because of old veins that didn't circulate his blood as well as they should, a condition called vascular claudication. But tests of his veins were normal. So he concluded that the culprit was most probably degenerative arthritis—in other words, wear and tear from aging. But Jack's back pain didn't respond to any of the usual approaches, namely rest, physical therapy, and pain medications. The failure of the surest approach to back pain—waiting it out—was a definite sign that Jack's back pain was not garden variety.

Jack came to the Pain Center because he had become frustrated when walking. When he first started having leg pain, he could walk only about twenty or thirty minutes before his legs hurt. Now, he had to stop every five minutes and felt better only when he sat down.

This pattern of painful walking and brief relief was my key to understanding what had happened to his back. As his primary-care physician suspected, problems with circulation in the legs can cause similar symptoms. But if Jack's discomfort arose from circulation, then stopping walking would make it better. Why then, I wondered, did he need to sit down to get relief? This wouldn't happen with a circulation problem. It was possible that he had both vascular and back problems, but not likely.

Doctors know that most of the time any given set of symptoms can usually be attributed to a single cause. So they always try to think of the one condition that would account for all of the symptoms. In Jack's case, his need to sit to relieve the pain was the answer. Sitting down released the pressure on Jack's spine. So, even though his symptoms were primarily in his legs, it was his back that caused the problem. When he showed me where he felt his leg pain, I saw that it corresponded with the nerves that spread out from the spine in his low back to his legs. His condition was classic spinal stenosis, a common cause of back and leg pain due to narrowing of the tunnel in which the spinal cord and nerve roots live.

The spinal cord protects the body's major nerves by suspending and bathing them in a fluid-filled sac that adheres to the inside walls of spinal bones. This arrangement protects the cord as it moves and adjusts to every change of your posture. However, even the smallest change in this space can markedly affect how you feel.

In Jack's back, irritation and inflammation in the spinal canal had resulted in narrowing around the spinal cord. Over time, the narrowing encroached on what had been more than adequate space for his spinal cord. At rest, Jack's back still had enough room and he didn't hurt. But when he walked, the increased pressure on his spinal fluid and blood flow tipped the scales. The result was pain in the legs from walking, and as the condition worsened, it took less and less time for the symptoms to flare up.

My first goal with Jack was to reduce the inflammation that had probably caused the problem in the first place. There are numerous ways to douse the fires of inflammation. One of the first steps is to apply ice. Ice cools the injured tissue and slows the inflammation. As the body tries to heal itself, it summons new cells to the damaged area by first increasing blood flow. This increased blood flow heats the area and prompts swelling, which ice will slow down.

For inflammation that has become entrenched, you often need medicines like the anti-inflammatory drugs aspirin or ibuprofen (Advil or Motrin), the class called nonsteroidal anti-inflammatories (NSAIDs). As the name implies, these drugs are not steroids. You may have heard of steroids in reference to athletes who abuse them to build muscles. Steroids are a large group of chemicals your body generates and that are manufactured synthetically for many purposes. For instance, the sex hormones estrogen and testosterone are steroids; cholesterol is a steroid. Cortisol, a hormone that, among other functions, regulates your body's reaction to stress, is also a steroid. Some help with bodybuilding, but others have absolutely no impact on muscle size. Pain medicine uses steroids that are potent anti-inflammatory drugs. With some types of back pain, these drugs can help stop the cycle of chronic inflammation, acting like a shot of WD-40 to loosen a tight nut on a bolt. But to prevent the problem from reoccurring, the back has to be strengthened and stay healthy.

With Jack, my hunch was that decreasing the inflammation in his narrowed canal might just make enough extra room for his nerves to function better. Even the space of a hair's width could make a difference. I wanted to get potent anti-inflammatory medication to the area. While there are many ways to do this, the most common and direct is an epidural steroid injection (ESI).

The ESI is one of the most common procedures performed by pain doctors, but even so, a needle in the spine is a terrifying thought for many. I explained to Jack that the injection usually does not hurt and he would probably look back on the anxiety he was feeling as needless fretting.

Jack came into the nerve block room at the Pain Center and asked if he could speak with me first. He was so wound up about the injection that he wanted to be "knocked out or something." I told him that, since it was a quick procedure, I didn't want to sedate him too much because he would be going home soon afterward. I assured him that if he had any discomfort at all, I would give him an instant sedative. I also reassured him that I thoroughly numbed the area with local anesthetic and the most pain in the whole procedure is usually just the little bee sting from the first numbing shot. I also explained that I use a special type of X-ray machine, called a fluoroscope, to show me exactly where the thin needle will pass without resistance.

I layered on a lead apron to protect me from X rays, and gathered equipment and drugs. Jack was helped onto the block table and lay on his belly. Like many people, Jack found it hard to turn over his body to someone else. Some patients come to these procedures with enormous fear, but others don't. Some allow intervention without the slightest concern, and others become so tense that it is almost impossible to proceed. Some wish to know everything that is happening to them, and others don't want to be involved at all until "it's all over."

I reassured Jack that I was thinking about his comfort and would explain everything I was doing throughout the procedure. He would be able to speak and could also watch the video monitor that showed the pictures of his back. After sterilizing and numbing his skin and finding a clear path to the right spot, I injected the steroid between two vertebrae into the epidural space, and the needle passed without a peep from Jack.

Since the epidural space is just one layer of tissue lying against another, it's called a "potential" space because it becomes a real space only when expanded by adding air or fluid. To find the epidural space with a needle, doctors use a technique that requires substantial skill and practice. As the needle slides inward, I gently press the plunger so that once the epidural space is entered, air or water from the syringe escapes into the epidural space. I can tell by the feel of the needle and the release of the air exactly when the epidural space is encountered. With fluoroscopy, I then inject a small amount of contrast dye to confirm that I am in the right place. Jack watched the monitor as I slowly injected the steroid medication and then gently removed the needle.

After a couple of days, Jack was able to walk for a noticeably longer period of time. Over six weeks or so, he had some improvement but wanted to see if he could do even better, so I gave him another epidural steroid injection, which helped. For Jack, the injections not only soothed his pain but, most importantly, improved his function. Jack understood that if the injection was to hold, he would have to change his lifestyle, enlist in a regime of physical therapy, and lose weight. Fortunately, the success of the injections had spared Jack the real possibility of requiring surgery to take the pressure off of the spinal nerves.

Striking at a Weak Spot in Our Armor—the Facet Block

One of most accurate assaults for back pain is the facet block, which homes in on a minute nerve fiber that can be the source of lots of suffering. Although the word "facet" (accent on the second syllable) may not sound familiar, the sensation is well known to many back pain sufferers. It's possible that you've felt a bum facet joint if you've ever had low back pain caused by degenerating disks, arthritis, radiculopathy, spondylolysis, or muscle spasm radiating from the low back into the butt and leg.

Further down the spine, the lumbar facet joints may be an accomplice—if not an instigator—in much low back pain. The facet joint does for the back what the knee does for the leg—provide an essential pivot for stability and movement. If you did not have facet joints, you'd walk like a broomstick. Facet joints bracket each vertebra, connecting one to the other and running the length of the back. At the end of the line are lumbar facets, which are particularly susceptible to being compressed and shoved out of alignment. Facets, being very small joints that have fat padding and cartilage to smooth their movement, are also subject to wear and tear. Like most joints, they are well endowed with nerves that sense problems and signal pain. It is these very small nerves, two for each facet joint, that doctors can find with a needle to diagnose whether or not the joint is the problem. It's also the very same anatomy that makes treating a painful facet joint so controversial.

Typically, low back pain caused by a problem with the lumbar facet joint is a dull ache that spreads into the buttocks and, at times, the upper thighs. But the pain can migrate across the region, not following a set pattern. When I'm examining a patient with low back pain, few clues expose the facet joint as the offender. Some doctors believe that facet joints may be involved if there is tenderness around the lower vertebrae, increased pain when the back is rotated or bent back-ward, or pain in the groin or upper thigh. But I'm never 100 percent sure from an examination that an irritated facet has caused someone's low back pain, so part of my treatment involves identifying whether the facet is really at fault.

Pain from a tender facet is transmitted by two small nerves called medial branch nerves, and the injection to block this nerve is a medial branch block. This nerve can be set off by compression or inflamma-tion from damaged tissue in the area. Many forms of back pain can stem from facet joint problems, and often the only way to know for sure is to turn off the joint's nerves with a block.

When I perform a facet block, I aim for the small area around the joint where the medial branch nerves live. Using a fluoroscope to guide the needle, I inject the space with a local anesthetic such as lidocaine to see if there's quick pain relief. If there's relief, this sug-gests that the trouble is probably coming from the facet. The lido-caine lasts for a short time, so later on I may reinject with a longer-lasting medicine such as an anti-inflammatory steroid, but this too may not be a permanent fix. The beauty of the facet block is that the structure of the joint allows me to direct the pain relief at a few nerves. There's nothing scattered about this approach—it's target shooting at a bull's-eye.

A patient may feel quick relief, but unfortunately it can wear off and the pain can resurface days, weeks, or months later. When the pain does return, I can't be certain whether or not that means that the pain never did arise from the facet. The initial pain relief could always have been a placebo response. For such reasons, doctors disagree about treating back pain with a facet block. Many believe that these blocks are best for diagnosing the source of low back pain and offer only modest, and temporary, pain relief. Others feel that injections or alter-ing the facet joint can cure certain forms of back pain. The best recourse for the confused patient is a trusted physician and carefully discussing the issues and options.

For some people, temporary relief from the pain makes a big differ-ence, but the local anesthetic or cortisone injections don't last long enough. When this happens, I may raise the option of radio-frequency lesioning, which zaps the offending nerve and tissue with heat. As with the facet block, the physician uses a fine probe to reach the aggravating nerve and delivers a quick burst of heat through radio wave frequency. The size of the lesion is controlled by the placement and temperature of the probe.

Like blocks, radio frequency does not require general anesthesia. However, it's not without risk. Trying to kill nerves to quiet pain is usually only a temporary cure. These delicate fibers often grow back, and the average pain-free time from a facet radio-frequency lesion is about eight months. So, doctors do them with genuine concern about whether the benefits truly outweigh the risks, wondering whether the relief justifies the trouble of an invasive procedure. How does one judge the value of eight pain-free months? This is one of the current dilemmas in pain medicine. Even the best trained, most respected pain physicians have differing opinions about what to do with these tough cases.

A cousin of this technique is cryoanalgesia, or freezing unruly nerves. Cryoanalgesia has been around for centuries. In its crudest form, it's using cold temperature to numb nerves. Its current, sophisticated form involves freezing and destroying nerves with a needlelike instrument, a cryoprobe. It, too, zeros in on a single nerve and incapacitates it with intense cold from liquid nitrogen. If you've ever had a wart frozen, then you're familiar with the freezing action of liquid nitrogen. Other chemicals also destroy nerves, such as solutions of alcohol or phenol. Nerve-destroying techniques such as radio frequency, cryoanalgesia, and alcohol are usually reserved for critical cases—patients with serious if not terminal illnesses, like cancer, or when pain is so severe that there are few other choices.

SEARCHING FOR PAIN IN ALL THE WRONG PLACES

It's a popular myth that the sacroiliac joints—the meeting of the pelvic bones and the sacrum—is prone to going out of whack. In truth, the sacroiliac joint is rarely the source of low back pain except with unusual kinds of arthritis or pelvic dislocation. The SI joint is a very stable intersection, and the ligaments on either side are some of the strongest in the body. In fact, by the time you have reached adulthood, your sacroiliac joints have pretty much fused and, unlike other large joints, don't move much.

Identifying this joint as the source of low back pain is also tricky business; there aren't any absolutely accurate diagnostic tests, and even a scan that reveals a misaligned joint does not necessarily mean it's causing the pain. As the imaging experts say, "Taking a picture of a telephone does not tell you if it's ringing." This is especially true for all the nooks and crannies of the lower back. A CAT scan illuminating a slipped disk doesn't necessarily mean that the disk is actually the problem. Many people with no back pain have CAT scans or MRI images that show ruptured disks appearing so severe that, were they also to have pain or other neurological symptoms, they might be considered for surgery. A positive CAT scan or MRI isn't always the smoking gun it was once believed to be. Because of this, doctors can't rely too heavily on technology and must talk to patients and consider their history and physical examination.

Years ago, doctors believed that the sacroiliac joint generated most low back pain because the area around it is often sensitive to touch. As a result, surgical fusion of these joints became a regular occurrence. But as low back pain has persisted over the decades and become more widespread, doctors have realized that surgery in this area is usually not a lasting solution. They found that much of the tenderness did not signal problems at the sacroiliac joint but was often the product of other disorders such as a herniated disk further up the spine. Or sometimes the pain emanated not from the joint but from muscles in the back and buttocks that had been strained by heavy lifting, sudden motion, or exertion.

It is often a challenge to tell whether the sacroiliac joint is the ultimate source of pain. One scheme for identifying a clue is to turn off the nerves that control the joint and see what happens. To do so, I inject local anesthetic into the joint to see if that temporarily erases the pain, which would point to the sacroiliac being at fault. With confirmation in hand, I may then inject a steroid into the sacroiliac joint to cool off inflammation.

For most of these back conditions, more than just blocks are needed. A complete menu of treatments is usually called for, including aggressive physical therapy and interventions for lifestyle changes, like losing weight, exercising regularly, quitting smoking, and lowering personal stress. Too often, I can temporarily ease a particular pain, while the underlying problem persists. For permanent results, I need to look at the whole picture.

THE SURGERY ROUTE

Low back pain is a somewhat modern creation. In the nineteenth century, it was considered a specific disease caused by an "irritated" spine or accident or trauma. The advent of the social security system, first in

Germany and later in the United States, made low back pain a work-related condition and a reason for compensation. It also shifted the emphasis of treatment away from remedies to eradicate the "disease" to rest and inactivity. The discovery in 1934 that disks could rupture added a whole new dimension to low back pain, pushing it into a realm that seemed to be a good candidate for surgery.

If you suffer from chronic low back pain, you may have entertained the idea of a surgical fix. This supposed magic bullet can be very tempting, especially if X rays or magnetic resonance scans picture herniated, worn, or otherwise abnormal disks and joints. Pain alone is usually not the sole reason for a back operation. Occasionally, though, it may point to a necessary, even urgent reason for surgery. My aunt's backache, which you read about in chapter 3, looked like run-of-the-mill pain but really signaled a broken bone pressing on a major nerve in the back. For her, immediate surgery was critical; otherwise, she risked paralysis. Less urgent reasons for cutting may include relieving pressure or firming up weakened structures. And every now and then, surgeons decide to operate on a patient's back because the pain responds to no other type of treatment.

Bad disks are a frequent reason people opt for surgery, even though studies show that bulging disks usually shrink over time and that disk problems clear up in 90 percent of these patients. Nevertheless, more and more people are opting for surgery. In fact, surgery for spinal stenosis, especially among people over sixty-five, is the most rapidly increasing back operation. *Scientific American* reported that between 1979 and 1990, these operations increased by 343 percent.

The most common back surgeries—laminectomy, discectomy, and spinal fusion—focus on structural repairs to disks or vertebrae. Any of these surgeries may be done alone or combined, depending on the patient. A laminectomy is spine surgery that removes one of the lamina, a bony segment of the vertebrae, to relieve pressure on the spinal cord or nerve root. Usually, just one lamina is removed, but if a couple need to be taken out, a spinal fusion may be called for. Spinal fusion tries to eliminate abnormal spine movement by binding together two vertebrae, usually with a bone graft from another part of the body. A spinal fusion may be performed because of instability in the spine, perhaps as a result of an injury or disease. A discectomy removes a disk because it has become ruptured or herniated. Herniation means the disk's jellylike interior has squeezed through the harder outer layer. This jelly substance, which is kept separate from other tissues by its strong outer coating, is extremely irritating to the surrounding bones and nerves. Surgery may attempt to clear out the irritating leakage. It often clears itself, which may be why most people ultimately get better from a disk rupture over time without surgery or any other particular intervention. In fact, it now appears that maintaining normal activities is the best approach to common low back pain.

If someone's back is hurting badly enough to contemplate surgery, I may be asked to see him or her in the pain clinic with a referral from a neurologist, neurosurgeon, or orthopedic surgeon who wants first to try less invasive remedies. The people who eventually undergo back surgery have either rapidly progressing problems that only surgery can fix, have probably been through a series of blocks or other treatments, or also have more than pain wrong with their backs. Back surgery today is rarely conducted solely to treat pain. By and large, there is usually another medical reason for surgery, perhaps neurological symptoms such as decreased sensation in the back or down the legs, abnormal reflexes, or weak or numb muscles. Pain may be in the picture, and while doctors hope that surgery will resolve the pain, most surgeons acknowledge that many back operations are much more successful at solving other problems such as nerve compression.

I have seen cases of back surgery that have miraculously cured long-standing pain. I have also seen people feel worse after the surgery than before. Interviews with patients months and years afterward have shown that upwards of 90 percent still feel pain and more than 70 percent still can't do normal activities. Others say the success rate for pain-free surgery is either better or worse, depending on the source of the pain.

While surgery usually does the job as promised and removes bones or tissue, or welds them together, the pain may not be fully abolished. Many of the same patients that come to the clinic before surgery may return after the operation, but now their pain has changed shape. While the underlying cause of the previous pain may have been resolved, these patients can be left with chronic back pain with a much murkier cause. The new problem may have as much to do with the old problem as with having had an invasive operation on their back. A patient coming into the Pain Center after surgery may actually return with a different kind of pain because the operation has stirred the soup and produced a new flavor.

A PERISCOPE INTO PAIN

Scarring is a natural part of the healing process after surgery, and I always wonder if scar tissue may be the cause of a lot of postsurgery back pain. So medicine has long been exploring ways to dissolve scars in the back. An interesting but yet unproven technique ventures into the epidural space, right next to the delicate spinal cord, where scar tissue may be pressing on nerves. Epiduralysis, as it is called, is a serious procedure and requires careful consideration, not to mention a sterile operating room. The treatment is new, can generate serious complications, and hasn't yet been performed widely enough to have a track record. But for patients with nowhere else to turn, this approach offers hope while giving pain medicine a window into the inner workings of some types of back pain.

Epiduralysis, or breaking down scars in the space where nerves exit the spine, employs new tools for visualizing the trouble spot and breaking down the scar. It seems that every medical specialty is now developing specialized scopes that enable doctors to peek at the most hard-to-reach, microscopic areas of the body. In one form of epiduralysis, pain doctors use a tiny scope not much larger than a spaghetti noodle to peer, as with a periscope, into the fine outer layers of the spinal cord to find scar tissue and break it down.

Epiduralysis can be done two ways. One uses a Racz catheter, named for the doctor who designed it. Gabor Racz from Texas Tech University in Lubbock introduced the use of a thin tube with the consistency of a stiff piece of string. The most novel feature of this catheter is that it can be steered around the area next to the spinal cord to view the nerves that might be injured. Before the Racz catheter, most catheters were used solely to deliver drugs. Now, this and other catheters are threaded into the epidural space and maneuvered around the layers overlapping the spinal cord. Doctors can inject dye, which contrasts with the scar tissue, while watching the area through motion X ray (fluoroscopy) and see scarring. Once the catheter has found the right scar, injected enzymes or other fluids break up the troublemaking tissue. The same procedure can be done with the doctor looking at the offending area through an epiduroscope instead of a Racz catheter. Both instruments can be steered to the scar. With an epiduroscope, once the scar has been spotted, it can be gently and repeatedly nudged until the tissue breaks up. At present, doctors don't know which is better or if either will bring long-term benefits. Neither is a trivial intervention nor a proven remedy. But such advances offer hope and new insights into the cause of chronic pain.

So far, the results of epiduralysis have been tantalizing, producing good results in some patients. While it is an effective way of removing scarring, the technique does not yet combat the continuing scarring process. Thus, after employing the Racz catheter or epiduroscope, it's possible, and some say likely, that scar tissue will form again. Pain medicine does not yet have the right tools to prevent scarring, but this is an area ripe for improved treatments, and several are under investigation. Soon, doctors may well be able to prevent scars from returning or, better yet, halt their formation before or soon after surgery.

Another revolutionary surgical technique for low back pain applies the technology of modern plastics. Percutaneous vertebroplasty is a mouthful of a term that refers to injecting medical-quality glue around broken vertebrae. In essence, this gluelike substance fills in cracks in bone or repairs other deficits that make bones ache. This technique provides back stability for people who have compression fractures, which are typically caused by the bone loss of osteoporosis. The epoxy is injected into the center of a collapsed spinal vertebra, then quickly hardens. The procedure takes less than an hour and patients can go home the same day. For many, vertebroplasty is a welcome addition to current treatments, which include spinal fusion and bone graft.

WHEN BACK PAIN BECOMES INTRACTABLE

When I see a patient whose back pain has persisted despite a smorgasbord of treatments, including surgery, the underlying problem has often become undeterminable and pain and dysfunction have usually become the prominent feature of the disease. I try to look at this condition with a fresh eye and make few assumptions based on earlier experiences. I do a complete evaluation and search for immediate neurological or other physiological causes as well as studying patients' posture and the way they move or sit. I look at how the years of pain have affected their health and changed the way they live. Patients with failed back syndrome need a comprehensive evaluation from multiple perspectives, often requiring a team of medical professionals. This is the core of the multidisciplinary approach to pain management.

Failed back syndrome is not a single disease but a collection of conditions that emerge after any number of surgeries or other treatments. The sensations that crop up after surgery include diffuse dull and achy pain, pain that radiates into the hips, buttocks, and thighs, or sharp stabs of pain in the back and legs. It may result from scarring on the nerves and so be categorized as a radiculopathy, meaning that it radiates from an overactive nerve root. The surgery may have cut tissue that became damaged and caused neuropathic pain. The failed back pain may come from a joint that's become irritated and inflamed because the surgery altered the person's posture, gait, and way of moving. Another possibility is that the surgery has disrupted the usual way muscles are positioned or function and has triggered muscle spasms or myofascial pain. A host of things can go wrong with back surgery, either because of the surgery or from the healing that follows, such as from the scar tissue that always forms. Any surgery is going to change the back's configuration, which always raises the possibility of new developments. That is why no surgeon can ever give an ironclad guarantee of long-term success.

Medicine's recent understanding that spinal disks and structural weaknesses probably have less to do with some low back pain than previously thought has significantly changed the way doctors view back pain and back surgery. This is one of the lessons of failed back syndrome and another compelling reason for approaching back pain first by looking to treatments that change the way you use your back rather than changing the back itself.

FIGHTING BACK: PHYSICAL THERAPY

Despite a series of nerve blocks, Cameron Rogers's pain came roaring back. He showed up in the Pain Center more than a year after I had seen him, walking slowly and laboriously. He later told me that he had been in pain much of this time but was too discouraged to get on the treatment treadmill again. I understood well what he was saying—many people living with chronic pain give up trying to find relief. One survey reported that 90 percent of back pain patients stop seeing their doctors after three months. Cameron and I had a heart-to-heart over what to do next. I reassured him that we still had many arrows in our quiver and explained why I believed that concentrated physical therapy could do much for his back.

Increasing function and improving quality of life through movement is the heart of physical therapy. In the past, physical therapy was seen as simply a side dish on the menu of pain treatments. Today, it is often the main entrée. For example, pain doctors are increasingly using other treatments, like nerve blocks, which may have only the short-term effect of opening a window of opportunity for physical therapy to make crucial progress.

I referred Cameron to a physical therapist at Spaulding Rehabilitation Hospital in Boston who has worked with hundreds of back patients and helped many learn to move and live again. Physical therapy for chronic low back pain centers on teaching patients how to manage pain rather than promising yet another treatment that may well fail. It revolves around educating patients about ways to cope with pain and what they can do to minimize its effect on their life.

I sent Cameron to Penny Herbert, the clinical supervisor for physical therapy at the chronic pain unit at Spaulding. With more than twenty years' experience behind her and a specialty in therapy for pain, she is the first to acknowledge that physical therapy does not work with all patients. Patients do best when they accept that they need to manage their condition and don't overfocus on a possible miracle cure or medical savior. "Sometimes, a patient has to realize that a pure medical approach isn't working, that one more surgery won't do the trick," she says. But once a patient recognizes that exercise is not the last resort but the best resort, and can help both treat and prevent back problems, improvement soon follows.

For Cameron, the first day of physical therapy is devoted to assessing his back pain. Penny asks him to fill out the Health Status Survey, a questionnaire used by most pain centers, and gives a hands-on examination, looking for how his back pain has altered his gait, posture, sitting tolerance, flexibility, and muscle strength. The Health Status Survey gives her a good idea as to how much the pain has affected his overall health and attitude and what it's done to his daily routine, such as whether he can carry groceries, walk, or do light housecleaning. It provides a baseline from which she can judge Cameron's progress and growing control over his pain.

During the physical exam, she looks for limitations or changes in normal movement and posture. She watches him walk and sit, checks his muscle tone and range of motion, and asks how much, if any, aerobic activity he can do. Cameron's back pain, like that of many patients, has created a cascade of changes in how he moves, sits, and stands. For instance, he has tight hip flexors, limiting flexibility in his lower back, hips, and legs and making walking difficult. He has lost muscle strength in his lower abdomen and developed a misaligned posture. His weakened muscles have also curtailed his aerobic capacity. Lastly, his achy back has curtailed how long he can sit at a time. The upshot of all this weakness is that Cameron, like many low back pain patients, has ceased many of his usual activities. So Penny's goal is "to nudge him toward activity." If he does too much too soon, he'll almost certainly fail if not get worse. If he doesn't make progress, he'll also fail. So Penny is his guide through what can be a tricky if not treacherous journey to rehabilitation.

One of the biggest obstacles to normal activity, she says, is disorganization. "Patients' lives become lost and unstructured," she observes. As a result, they don't pace themselves, either overdoing it when they feel good or going inert when they hurt. Jobs, daily routines, social lives, and hobbies are sidelined by their pain. "Back patients frequently retreat," she says, "doing less and less, until they're virtually cloistered. I try to feed them back into the world." Thus, the centerpiece of physical therapy is a program and schedule for managing pain while gradually returning a patient to an active life.

Together, Penny and Cameron map out a schedule and activities designed to address each of the impairments caused by his bad back. He must sit every day, starting with sixteen minutes and adding a minute daily; he must ice his back four times a day for a minimum of twenty minutes; he has to walk ten minutes twice a day and add a minute to his walk every day; he has to do hip flexion exercises, three for each leg, three times a day and extending the amount of time he holds his leg out by a minute a day; and he has to do pelvic tilts three times a day, holding a certain position starting at five minutes and adding a minute daily. It's serious stuff, and much like a coach working with an elite athlete preparing to improve physical performance, Penny asks him to keep track of his progress on a quota sheet, a chart outlining the five activities and how long he's to spend doing each every day over two weeks. She and Cameron also lay out a schedule with fixed times every day for when he needs to stretch, ice, walk, or do exercises.

Penny escorts Cameron into the hospital's rehab gym to instruct him on how to do his exercises. Sitting sounds simple enough, but she points out unbalanced postures that aggravate the lower back: slumping with the head forward of the shoulders, not sitting up straight, or sitting in chairs without low back support. Ideally, he should sit with both feet on the floor or on a footrest, and if at a desk, in a position that allows him to rest his forearms without having to bend over. She devotes a lot of time to his posture, not only for sitting but also walking. A balanced, neutral posture is essential, she cautions; otherwise, the back continues to be stressed and is not freed or relaxed enough to heal. Tight hip flexors cause the back to go into a swayed posture, and so Cameron is shown how to bend one knee, then the other, up to his chest to stretch the flexors. The pelvic tilt exercise, called a crunch involving a partial sit-up, is to strengthen his abdominal and buttock muscles. At a later appointment, Penny will videotape Cameron doing his exercises so he can watch it at home and correct any distortions in his movements.

Occasionally, Penny uses traction to aid low back motion, particularly when there are signs of disk degeneration. As she explains it to patients, traction isn't necessarily a pain remedy or treatment but a way to ease back stress and enable a person to move more freely. The traction device tugs on the lower back, gently pulling apart vertebrae that may be pressing on nerve roots. Lumbar traction may relax the muscles around the spine and open the space between vertebral joints. There's also some evidence that traction reduces the electrical activity of pain nerves in the region. By easing the pressure on the spinal system, Penny wants to interrupt the pain–muscle spasm–pain cycle that is so often at the core of low back pain.

Before applying traction, Penny always begins with slight manual tugging to gauge how a back will respond before putting someone into a harness and weight system. Though there are a couple of ways to do traction, Penny uses a harness and weight system in which a patient lies down on an exercise bed with a harness around his shoulders and chest and a cummerbund belt around his waist, his lower legs hanging at a ninety-degree angle over the end of the bench. At the end of the ropes and pulleys are weights calibrated according to the size of the patient and never more than 50 percent of the patient's weight. The traction process, which is a gradual tug that rarely raises any discomfort, lasts for ten to twenty minutes, with a continuous or intermittent tension. Over the course of traction therapy—typically twice a week for the course of the therapy, which is usually a maximum of six weeks—the weight will be increased and the length of time extended ultimately to thirty minutes. Lumbar traction creates pockets of pain-free time when a patient can begin to experiment with activities and movement that had been curtailed.

With any therapy that involves movement, Penny strongly recommends initially applying ice afterward and later, heat. Changing skin temperature between cold and heat relaxes muscles underneath, controls swelling, and increases blood flow to stimulate tissue healing. When ice is applied to a painful area for twenty minutes and then removed, veins first constrict and then dilate. Over time, this produces a milking effect that removes metabolic waste as well as reduces swelling. Applying heat to a painful area, with hot packs, infrared lamps, or hydrotherapy, usually comes after ice treatment because heat can increase swelling by quickening blood flow. Heat therapy increases tissue temperature and makes connective tissue more pliable. The best combination of these therapies, says Penny, is a daily regimen of cold, numbness, and heat, with each segment taking ten to twenty minutes.

Massage is not only another avenue to better back flexibility, it also gives Penny an opportunity to reinforce her message. (You may know this treatment as "soft tissue mobilization," which is the bureaucratic, reimbursable term for massage.) This kind of massage is intended to help calm overcontracted muscles and to assist with all of the many other facets of physical therapy. It is a rare passive part of what is predominantly an active process for the patient. Patients can even learn to massage themselves. This is far from the massage found at a resort, and there are no piña coladas afterward.

Massage is a part of the process, but it's not the whole shebang, as Cameron found out. While Penny's softening and flexing soft tissue and breaking up scars, she has the captive ear of her patient. Many of her patients are first-time physical therapy users who tend to be skeptical of her advice. Exercises are forgotten, regimens are dropped, and suggestions about applying cold or heat are dismissed. And given the current tempo of modern medicine, with managed care limiting the amount of time any specialist spends with a patient, she rarely has time to explain fully and repeatedly the physiological or anatomical reasons underlying her recommendations. She has discovered that her best talking time is during massage.

Initially, Cameron saw Penny in the Spaulding outpatient gym twice a week. There, with her coaching, he progressed through his flexibility, posture, and strengthening exercises. After about a month, she saw progress, both in his chart and in the way he walked and sat. One of the best signs was when he resumed gardening again, learning how to bend properly and carefully over his flower beds. From here on out, Cameron continued his rehab program without professional supervision, although he called Penny every six months or so to "buff up" his program and progress.

If the experiences of other low back pain sufferers are any indication, Cameron's chances for getting his pain under control and resuming a normal life are good. Just a few years ago, a government panel of twenty-three doctors, physical therapists, nurses, chiropractors, and back experts reviewed thousands of studies of low back injuries and compared the results of three approaches to treatment. For at least three months, patients relied either on bed rest and special stretching exercises or ignored their discomfort and resumed normal activity. Overwhelmingly, the people who stayed active, even though their backs sometimes hurt, did much better than the patients who went to bed or tried stretching as their sole remedy.

ATTACKING ARTHRITIS

Like low back pain, arthritis crops up when tissue has been damaged and nearby nerves send out painful messages. Arthritis is the crabgrass of pain medicine, an almost universal complaint that strikes someone in virtually every family—one in seven Americans. It can be mildly annoying or totally crippling, and in its worse incarnation, its power to twist joints, halt simple movement, and prevent people from leading normal lives adds a profound layer of suffering to its damage. Regaining lost lives, rather than cure or eradication, is often at the heart of treating it. To date, there are no cures for the forms of arthritis that take the biggest swipe out of the population, osteoarthritis and rheumatoid arthritis. Treatment is largely symptom control, although lately researchers have cooked up new drugs that seem to slow and even halt the corrosion. The pain of arthritis, because it comes from the disfiguring of tissue, including nerves, can be cooled with an assortment of analgesics, including anti-inflammatories, acetaminophen, and even opioids.

If you know that the medical suffix *-itis* means "inflammation" and that *arth* indicates the involvement of a joint, you have a clear outline of the disease. Arthritis is a general term encompassing more than a hundred diseases that cause swelling and restricted movement of joints and connective tissue anywhere in the body, including skin and organs. The two garden varieties are osteoarthritis and rheumatoid arthritis, and the more unusual forms include gout, lupus, and scleroderma.

Rheumatoid arthritis is activated by the body's immune system—it goads the immune system into attacking the tissue it's supposed to protect. It can strike at any time of life. On the other hand, osteoarthritis results from the wear and tear of joints and tissue, degeneration that usually appears in middle age, although aging itself is not necessarily the cause. Given their distinctive features and separate paths over time, these sister diseases are treated in different manners.

Osteoarthritis is an unfortunate infirmity that usually comes as you age, like hardening of the arteries. Although it can show up in young people, prompted by an abnormal metabolism, heredity, or injury, most of its victims tend to be older and female. Despite the popular image, your joints are not like wheel bearings on a car that wear out after a certain number of miles. Osteoarthritis is not the inevitable result of years of activity, and regular exercisers are no more prone to getting it than couch potatoes. In fact, they may be less prone. Inactivity may be as much of a culprit as overusing a joint. Scientists have found that arthritic joints have a high concentration of cartilage-corrosive enzymes and believe that it may be caused by joint injuries, muscle weakness, and being overweight, among other factors. Its favorite targets are knees, fingers, feet, and hips, which, as they lose the lubricating, soft cushion between hard bones, become inflamed and cause pain. Pain may also stem from the stretching of the bone coating, stretched membranes between joints, or from trapped nerves. Yet another source of pain can be the achy, knobby, bony growths that develop in hands and fingers, giving them a clawlike appearance.

Rheumatoid arthritis is also an insidious disease, being a reaction of the body's immune system against its own tissue. For unknown reasons, the immune system attacks the joint's soft tissues as if they were invading bacteria or viruses. Many fewer people suffer from rheumatoid arthritis—around three million Americans, two to three times more women than men—and it also assails people at any age, although it tends to appear between the ages of twenty and fifty. In most people, it usually attacks the hands and, being a disease that travels throughout the body, any of the body's more than three hundred joints.

The assault sets off a chain reaction with a type of white blood cell latching on to the cells that produce the lubricating fluid between joints, igniting inflammation. Gradually, as more and more of these white blood cells gather, the joint begins to swell and feel stiff, and the unfortunate owner starts to feel tired and worn out. As the disease gains momentum, it spreads to cartilage, tendons, and bone, the swelling worsens, and tissue is transformed. In its full fury, the disease destroys so much cartilage and bone that the simplest motion becomes an excruciating ordeal. But not everyone comes to this point, for the disease may slow, even halt on its own, or treatment may impede its incursions.

Moving Sore Joints

Perhaps one of the first reactions to a bout of arthritis, regardless of the type, is to avoid aggravating the inflamed joint or body part with movement. But some type of exercise, whether it's modest stretching or conditioning, goes a long way toward lessening the devastation. Exercise builds muscles around crippled joints (as well as other muscles and bones), helps lubricate bone and cartilage tissue, and helps you resume normal activity and improve general health. And the price of not exercising is frequently more stiffness and pain. In extreme cases, when people avoid using bent, arthritic joints, they can lose the ability to ever straighten them. So while exercise does not directly fight pain, it does protect against further incursions of the weakness and discomfort that fuels pain. If you are in the middle of an arthritic flare-up, you have to find a balance between protecting and supporting an ailing joint and doing exercises that will strengthen the joint and add to your range of motion.

The exercise that works best depends on the damage the arthritis has done. No single type of activity helps all patients. Too much, or the wrong activity, may only aggravate a condition. A physical therapist can assess what kind of movement will do the most good. Regardless of which activity a therapist recommends, warming up before moving by gentle stretching, applying some kind of heat, or massaging the joints starts to relieve soreness and improve movement.

Exercise for arthritis falls into three categories: *Range-of-motion activities* include moving limbs through their normal arcs to keep joints flexible and ease stiffness. *Strengthening exercises* can be either isometric activity, which is the tightening and releasing of muscle groups, or isotonic exercises, moving joints with or without very light weights to build up muscles. Lastly, *endurance exercises* like walking, water exercises, and riding a stationary bicycle beef up the heart and improve stamina. Another standard feature of physical therapy is cooling down, which may mean ending the activity very slowly or with gentle stretching.

To reap the benefits of exercise, people with arthritis need to do something every day. Physical therapists usually recommend doing range-of-motion activities daily and strengthening and endurance exercises every other day. Knowing that most people with arthritis feel stiff in the morning, they suggest first "oiling and lubing" joints with ice or warm water (if joints are very inflamed, heat only adds congestion) or light massage. But exercise should not be put off, and all therapists say that even painful flare-ups should not stop a person from exercising, but just limit how much you do.

Cooling the Flames

Treating any variety of arthritis quickly becomes complicated because it doesn't advance at a steady, predictable pace but lurches. It's given to flaring, with times of extreme inflammation, and remissions, when it's fairly quiet, so it's hard to know when symptoms subside whether that's from treatment or its natural, quirky course. Treatment can take two routes: pain-relieving drugs alone or in combination with physical therapy to root out painful symptoms, and for the autoimmune variety, drugs that restrain or slow the cannibalizing of joint tissues.

All varieties of arthritis may succumb to more or less the same pain relievers. And there are a lot of options. For years, the customary treatment for arthritis has been anti-inflammatories like aspirin and ibuprofen. These do a good job soothing the symptoms, but consumed over time, they stir up unpleasant complications. Taken month in, month out, these drugs can cause stomach ulcers, kidney problems, or up the odds of bleeding problems. Regrettably, other drugs that treat pain and inflammation, such as cortisone-type medications, are hazardous when taken steadily for a long time. Over time, these drugs, commonly referred to as steroids, can weaken bones, exhaust the immune system, and have many other serious side effects. So arthritis patients have always faced the predicament of trying to find pain relief and avoid intolerable side effects.

Acetaminophen (Tylenol) is another familiar arthritis drug that, while effective, is not as trouble-free as its over-the-counter availability suggests. In low doses over short periods, it does a good job. It rarely irritates the stomach and kidneys and doesn't cause ulcers like aspirin and other anti-inflammatory drugs. But it can be hard on the liver, especially when mixed with alcohol. Taken in high doses or for a long time, it can even produce outright liver failure and, in the extreme, necessitate a liver transplant.

Despite the widespread use of Tylenol, scientists do not know exactly how it suppresses pain. Researchers are intrigued by its pain-relieving potential and think it possesses unknown properties that could lead to a more effective analgesic. It's possible that it harbors special properties akin to other novel analgesics that may help make angry pain nerves less irritable.

Yet another sphere of soothing remedies are the numerous over-the-counter medications that are touted to make achy joints and muscles feel better. My patients often find relief with products such as Aspercreme, Ben-Gay, Vicks VapoRub, and other ointments. Their effectiveness can be traced to the gate-control theory of pain sensation. As you may recall, that widely accepted notion describes an area in the lower brain that determines which sensations pass through to be felt in the brain. I think of this gate as a toll booth, and when the body sends along competing sensations, namely a painful joint followed by a distinctive warmth or tingling from a cream, both can't pass through. The pleasant countersensation may well be prominent enough to shove aside some of the pain sensation.

An overlooked class of drug for arthritis is opioids. When I talk to physicians about pain management, I often tell them of my unusual experience with rheumatologists, the subspecialists who most commonly treat arthritis. While doctors are typically cautious, if not averse, to giving opioids such as morphine for any extended period of time, I have found, to my initial surprise, a different perspective from many rheumatologists. Rheumatologists who have years of experience battling arthritis are acutely aware that taking NSAIDs and other anti-inflammatory drugs for a long time can produce serious, even lethal, complications. In light of these problems, they are becoming much more willing to prescribe narcotics. They often tell me that although narcotics are believed to be more dangerous than anti-inflammatories, the opposite seems to be the case. While many doctors worry about the repercussions of long-term use of morphine-type drugs, many rheumatologists view them as less risky than long-term daily doses of many over-the-counter pain relievers.

Nevertheless, while opioids can offer substantial relief with, in many cases, less severe long-term side effects than chronic anti-inflammatories, they're not widely prescribed. I think the reason is fear on the part of patients and doctors and outdated ideas about addiction and concerns about social stigma. Even though pain medicine is introducing new ideas and methods that are changing the way people think about many medications, a cloud continues to hang over the medicinal use of narcotics.

A REVOLUTION IN ANTI-INFLAMMATORIES

Traditional anti-inflammatories like aspirin and ibuprofen, the NSAIDs, are excellent pain relievers and pack an extra punch by reducing inflammation. This double-barreled effect comes from divergent chemical actions and timing. Analgesia arrives first, while the anti-inflammatory agents can take many days. As happens with many drugs, each ingredient may tackle a couple of tasks. In the case of NSAIDs, one of their assignments is to suppress the COX (cyclo-oxygenase) enzyme, the chemical that transforms other substances into a potent player in inflammation—namely prostaglandin, which produces pain, swelling, and redness. Unfortunately, these drugs check the COX enzyme throughout the body, not only in inflamed joints but also where it provides protection as in the gastrointestinal tract, kidneys, and in the blood, where it boosts clotting. While COX drugs quiet pain and inflammation, they can also leave the stomach, kidneys, and blood defenseless against dangerous erosion and bleeding. For years doctors have wished that they could block the COX enzymes in the joints and leave alone all the good COX in the rest of the body, so that patients could take these drugs for months and years without all the problems.

The universe of drugs that tinker with the COX enzyme has been expanding for decades, with a steady stream of new members of the same basic family. They're all related, differing in potency, how long each dose lasts, and possible side effects. Just recently, however, scientists have discovered an entirely new type of NSAID that is much easier on the body.

In 1991, researchers were looking into why drugs like corticosteroids stopped inflammation but didn't trigger bleeding or hurt the kidneys. They uncovered two distinct COX enzymes. The first, COX-1, was their old friend and considered a "housekeeping" enzyme that acts to maintain a healthy stomach lining, kidney blood flow, and inflammation-fighting prostaglandins. Researchers realized that when NSAID drugs suppressed COX-1 production, this not only halted inflammation but also removed its safeguarding qualities and opening the door to nasty side effects. The second enzyme, COX-2, the newcomer, quickly turned heads because it was not as widespread, appearing to multiply and fuel inflammation when there was tissue damage. But it seemed to leave healthy tissue alone. Put another way, the COX-2 enzyme fueled pain-causing inflammation chemistry without stirring up the usual unpleasant side effects. Blocking COX-2 might offer the benefits without the risks.

Naturally, as soon as the scientists identified this special enzyme, they teamed up with pharmaceutical researchers to design a drug to suppress only the COX-2 enzyme. They succeeded and have hustled these drugs into clinical trials and the marketplace. These next-generation NSAIDs, COX-2 inhibitors, have come out under the trade names of Celebrex and Viox, with other versions sure to follow. They have been called super aspirin because they may deliver a double whammy, knocking out both inflammation and pain without gut-wrenching side effects. However, even if these drugs are as wonderful as the previews suggest, they probably will not be any stronger than the regular NSAIDs already available. Their appeal is not potency but less collateral damage. Nonetheless, muting arthritic pain with fewer side effects would be a great step forward. On the other hand, there is a chance that these safer agents might also have diminished pain-relieving power. But this is a small price to pay for safety over the long haul.

Knowing something about pain's complexities, I tend to be skeptical of new wonder drugs and remind myself, and patients, that the jury is still out on the COX-2 inhibitor drugs. The annals of medical science are full of high hopes and dashed dreams, with magic bullets coming and going. Declarations that the pain war has been won are too often followed by realizations that the battlefront has simply moved.

Slowing It Down

While the COX-2 breakthrough could benefit all arthritis patients, other research has been investigating ways of slowing the erosion from a diseased immune system, as happens with rheumatoid arthritis. One avenue of success involves drugs that have a track record of restraining the body's immune system, drugs that are also used for chemotherapy against cancer. Methotrexate, an established cancer drug, has been found to quiet rheumatoid arthritis's too-busy immune system and slow its relentless attack on joint tissue. It received renewed attention lately when researchers found that combining it with a new, genetically engineered drug, Enbrel, significantly boosts its effectiveness. Yet, like all powerful drugs, methotrexate, too, raises the specter of potentially dangerous and possibly devastating side effects.

Any drug that messes with the immune system presents a delicate balancing act by weakening one system in order to pump up another. The negatives often make these treatments hard to tolerate, and so they must be chosen with care and expertise. As with chemotherapy, using a strong drug involves a precarious strategy of simultaneously fighting for and against fragile systems within the body and betting that the benefit to one system will be greater than the damage done to another.

Advances in biotechnology have recently delivered hope to people with rheumatoid arthritis. Building on a growing wealth of knowledge about the body, scientists are devising drugs that zero in on particular molecules instead of employing the old-fashioned method of drug development, trial and error. They are developing so-called "hypothesis driven" drugs that attempt to correct a skewed area of human chemistry. For rheumatoid arthritis, new insights into the immune system have prompted scientists to create drugs aimed at one of the essential molecules for launching an immune attack.

Tagged with the deceptive name of tumor necrosis factor (it is not predominantly related to tumors), these molecules stir up the immune reaction, and so the new drugs are intended to inhibit their activity. Unfortunately, by defanging the immune system, these drugs may leave patients vulnerable to other diseases. And they are not cheap, costing more than $5,000 a year for regular injections. Still, they're generating excitement among doctors and patients. The versions recently approved for public sale by the Food and Drug Administration are Enbrel and Arava. The drug Remicade, which also constricts the tumor necrosis factor, has been approved for Crohn's disease, another autoimmune disease, and its manufacturer has begun to test it with rheumatoid arthritis.

An over-the-counter food supplement has been drawing attention for its apparent ability to stimulate cartilage growth and relieve osteoarthritis pain. Glucosamine has held its own in tests comparing it with ibuprofen and other NSAIDs, and it has produced fewer side effects. But none of the studies went beyond eight weeks, so I'm going to wait and see. Another newcomer, with good early results, is a drug that is injected into joints, particularly the knee. This drug, called sodium hyaluronate (trade name Hyalen), represents a new treatment strategy called viscoprotection where drugs are placed within a joint for the purpose of helping with shock absorbency that has been lost through deterioration. These drugs are in their infancy and need a longer track record before they can be accurately evaluated.

Treating the discomfort of a chronic low back problem or arthritis is obviously complicated, and always requires looking at what the pain has done to a patient's ability to function and live a normal life. Not all chronic pain is as transparent as these, with their normal-acting nerves simply reacting to damage nearby. With many other varieties of pain, the nerves themselves become damaged and compromised or malfunction for unknown reasons.

8

WHEN NERVES MISFIRE
Diabetic Neuropathy, Trigeminal Neuralgia, Complex Regional Pain

> Pain upsets and destroys the nature of the person who
> feels it.
>
> —ARISTOTLE

As I explain to my patients, nerves can cause pain in two ways. Sometimes the nerves that carry pain signals fire too loudly or too often. The nerve system itself is not the problem; something else is triggering the alarm. The other kind of nerve pain occurs because the nerves themselves are injured or malfunctioning. The crippled fibers can be found anywhere along their long chain, from the tip of the toe to the brain.

Why does this happen? Sometimes the reasons are clear, sometimes not. Drugs or diseases can injure nerves. Usually the smallest nerves are the most vulnerable. At the tail end of the circulation system and the farthest away from the heart, they are the last to receive nutritious blood. A particularly destructive disease is diabetes, which eats away at the thread-thin blood vessels that feed delicate nerve cells. This is why diabetes pain usually strikes first in the hands and feet. Unfortunately, the reason for other nervous system malfunctions is more obscure.

Despite the mystery surrounding the origin of some nerve pain, I have learned that aggressively controlling pain early, regardless of its genesis, offers the best chance of preventing an acute injury from becoming chronic pain. Nerve pathway pain can erupt anywhere in the body. Pain syndromes like herpes zoster (better known as shingles), postherpetic neuralgia (chronic pain after shingles), trigeminal neuralgia, and even extreme itching usually come from injury to nerves in the central or peripheral nervous system. When the sympathetic nervous system is hurt, the result is another sort of nerve pain, complex regional pain. Diseases like diabetes, AIDS, alcoholism, and cancer, as well as drug treatments like chemotherapy, can also harm nerves, generating substantial discomfort.

Direct trauma to nerves, like from a car accident or complications from surgery, can incite pain. As we have seen, an especially odious type of post-op nerve pain is phantom limb syndrome, the feeling of pain in a limb or body part that has been amputated. It's not uncommon among women who've had mastectomies. It may even be possible to have phantom pain from an excised gall bladder or a kidney. This peculiar type of pain may account for the strange abdominal or pelvic pain after surgery that can plague patients and mystify physicians.

Regardless of which nerve pathway has been injured, the pain is usually surprisingly uniform and almost always distinct. Nerve pain, otherwise known as neuropathic pain, has characteristic features—you know when you have it. Perhaps the most distinctive quality is a feeling of burning or intense heat on the skin. Other common sensations are extreme sensitivity to normal stimulation, like cool air or the light touch of clothing. Moderately painful sensations, like a needle stick, can hurt even more than normal. In a normal situation, when you bang your elbow, it hurts for a while, then disappears. With neuropathic pain, a small bang lingers. A peculiar feature of this pain is that it may first appear weeks or months after the injury, accident, or disease that brought it on. Why this happens is one of its many puzzles.

AT THE ONSET OF NERVE PAIN: A SURPRISE ATTACK OF SHINGLES

A couple of months ago, my friend Jake called complaining of a crashing headache and piercing, throbbing pain around his left eye. It had hit the morning after a big night celebrating, and at first he assumed that it was a hangover. But thirty-six hours later it kept pounding, and the usual drugstore remedies of aspirin, Tylenol, and Advil had not helped. The pain was unlike any Jake had ever felt. It wasn't exactly like pain, and he was hard-pressed to give the feeling a name, but everything set it off, including loud noises, bright lights, the feel of water from a shower, the sound of his kids crying, the touch of warmth against his skin. His entire body felt like a pain sensor. Worried that something serious was amiss, Jake had seen his primary-care physician, who found no clear problem. Since the pain was near Jake's eye and he complained of problems with reading, he was sent to an eye doctor, who, after a brief examination, told him his eye was fine and that he was possibly suffering from a migraine.

The pain did not disappear, and a day later, he felt a light burning sensation around his temple and eye. His doctor gave him a strong painkiller, but that only made him drowsy. He called me because he wasn't sure what was happening to him. By questioning him over the phone I found that gentle touch hurt his skin. This extreme sensitivity, called "allodynia," is common when there's inflammation from an injury, but that wasn't the case here. Jake's symptoms clearly declared that his nerves weren't working right, but I still couldn't be sure what had caused the problem. I put together the facts so far: He had nerve-type pain around the eye and the temple that came on suddenly after a rowdy night followed by a good hangover. One of the few disorders that present like this is shingles (herpes zoster), which is stirred up by an underlying virus. This was a long shot, particularly since he didn't have the telltale rash that almost always accompanies shingles. Still, Jake's symptoms were right over a nerve that this virus loves to attack.

Sure enough, later that day, a rash broke out over his eye and across the side of his forehead. The rash perfectly outlined where the top branch of the trigeminal nerve spread beneath the skin, providing a clear illustration of how the nervous system is mapped in all of us and how it can announce itself when disturbed.

Besides on the face, the rash of shingles also tends to occur around the ribs, the lower abdomen, and the legs. Even though Jake at age forty-four was on the young side for shingles, aging appears to make us more vulnerable, so shingles tends to erupt more in people over fifty. It had probably erupted because of a temporary letdown in his immune system from stress over work and family matters, coupled with the physical stress of lots of celebratory drinking and a whopping hangover. Using corticosteroid drugs can also compromise the immune system and invite a shingles attack.

Shingles arises from the chicken pox virus, a member of the herpes virus family but not the branch that causes other herpes infections such as genital herpes. If you've had chicken pox, you have the virus for life, even though it's dormant and inactive. The virus never leaves the body but lives quietly in your sensory nerves until some stress to the system brings it out of hiding.

For an acute attack of shingles, treatment is a two-front assault: deactivating the virus and quieting the overexcited nerves. Jake's doctor reassured him that the problem would soon pass. He gave him a prescription for acyclovir, a special antiviral drug that shortens the duration of symptoms as it weakens the reactivated virus. Jake also took gabapentin (Neurontin) which helped turn off the very busy nerves that caused the pain. And, he took analgesics like Tylenol or aspirin that helped smooth the rough edges of his discomfort.

Jake also found relief from an unexpected quarter. His pain eased up when he was distracted and lost in a high-pressure work project. When he obsessed over his pain, it worsened, but then it faded into the background as he shifted his attention to other thoughts. This regimen of acyclovir, gabapentin, other pain relievers, and distraction worked. He was soon on the mend, except for one strange thing. Although everything else had healed well, Jake was left with an itching on his forehead that, although not painful, was almost as bad as the initial pain. I suspected that the itch was probably from sickly nerves that had not fully healed and I suggested that he apply a cream called capsaicin on the itchy skin. This cream is made from hot peppers and halts pain by depleting the skin of the chemicals that fuel pain. Without these chemicals, the nerves in the skin can't transmit pain signals. Jake took care not to get any of the hot-pepper cream near his eye, and by the next day, he was no longer itching. A week later he was off medication and the whole episode was history.

DAMAGED NERVES THAT DON'T HEAL:
POSTHERAPETIC NEURALGIA

Jake was lucky that the shingles passed like a brief but violent summer storm. But the herpes zoster virus does not always fade and sometimes can linger for a painfully long period of time. It can transform into a most unpleasant entity called postherpetic neuralgia. A big variable in whether shingles evolves into postherpetic neuralgia is how aggressively it's treated, particularly how quickly the nerves are parked, or turned off. If the virus is allowed to develop into postherpetic neuralgia, the nature of the pain changes and the condition can become intractable. While shingles is localized burning and hypersensitivity, the chronic form can either be more of the same or vague sensations of discomfort that spread.

Most people who get shingles improve soon without lasting trouble. But not everyone. Doctors don't yet know exactly who will develop the more chronic form, but older people and those with other health problems have increased risk. Also, letting the initial episode of shingles go untreated for too long is probably risky. The experience of a patient at the Mass General Pain Center will show you how crucial it is to jump on the herpes zoster virus as soon as possible.

Perry Jones, a thirty-four-year-old computer executive and new father, was also seized by a sudden, unexpected attack of shingles, although the conditions were ripe for it. Right before Perry and his wife were to leave for a needed vacation, her mother was diagnosed with breast cancer. The family vacation was canceled, Janice Jones went to care for her sick mother, and Perry was left at home to look after their new baby. About a week after his wife left, Perry woke up with what looked like a bad sunburn around his hip, groin, and upper thigh.

Like Jake, he was mystified until the bubbling blisters propelled him to the doctor, who explained that what he had was shingles and prescribed an antiviral drug. However, unlike Jake's sores, Perry's did not fade. His whole body was hypersensitive to all sorts of sounds, lights, and touch. The blisters made wearing clothes impossible, so he stayed home from work and spent days on the couch watching TV, able to wear only boxer shorts. His doctor recommended that he see someone at the Pain Center, who after examining him, recommended a nerve block but also reassured him that even though his pain had lingered longer than that of most, he'd probably get better fairly soon. Perry rejected the idea of an injection, saying that it was too invasive for what seemed to be a harmless condition. In young people, shingles rarely persists. But several weeks later he was still hurting. Virtually housebound, irritable, and isolated, he seemed to be on the verge of acquiring the chronic form of shingles, postherpetic neuralgia. A rule of thumb is that if the pain of acute herpes zoster or shingles persists beyond a month, you're into the land of postherpetic neuralgia. Perry seemed to have arrived.

He returned to the Pain Center several weeks after talking with a family friend who had had a block for herpes zoster and quickly healed. It may have been just in time. Nerve blocks for this condition work best if done early. Those performed months after the infection has wreaked its havoc are often less successful. His symptoms were so severe, and had gone on so long, that a single temporary block was probably not going to be adequate.

The procedure delivered a local anesthetic, lidocaine, into his lower spine to quiet the nerves of the sympathetic nervous system that were involved in the flare-ups in his groin and upper thigh. Normally, this treatment is a single injection, a lumbar sympathetic block, but with Perry the duration of the block was stretched from a few hours to several days. This was done by placing a catheter in the epidural area near the spinal cord and giving him a steady solution of just enough local anesthetic to dull his sensory nerves but not his motor nerves. If Perry's pain had been in his head, neck, or upper arms, I might have given him a stellate ganglion block. It differs mainly by its route into the sympathetic nerves, which is through the base of the throat.

Perry dozed on the block room exam table during the procedure. Once the catheter was in place and tested to ensure that it was working well, a nurse wheeled him into the day surgery recovery room, where he rested for a few hours before being admitted to his hospital room. He could walk, but his lower body felt slightly numb. His pain was gone. The next day, hours after the catheter was removed from his back, he was no longer slightly numb and the pain was nowhere in sight. "I should have done the block sooner," he admits. "Next time, rather than wait to see if the pain will go away on its own, I won't waste a day."

Nerve blocks like Perry's are a powerful weapon against other kinds of nerve pain. Giving a break to a nervous system that's racing out of control with pain allows it to regain its normal function. Somehow, stopping the engine and letting the car sit quietly in park for a while allows it to run better when started next. This may be true with other forms of suffering, too.

One particular type of suffering, severe itching, is a cousin of pain, although most people with awful itching probably don't usually think about seeing a pain doctor. The nerves that control pain and those involved with itching are either the same or so closely related that doctors have not been able to tell them apart. And while it's not exactly pain, itching meets my criteria of sensation amplified to the point of discomfort.

John, a thirty-seven-year-old man with AIDS, was sent to me by his doctor after "trying everything." The man itched all over, probably because of his diseased liver. Despite all the known anti-itching medicines, like antihistamines and bile resins, even anticonvulsants and narcotics, the itching would not stop, and his entire body was scratched and scarred. "I'm at my wit's end," he declared, "I don't know how much more I can take."

As often happens, I was faced with suffering that wouldn't be occurring if the usual treatments had worked. Now I had to do something for sensations that were every bit as bad as pain. Since the symptoms were similar, I thought the treatments should be as well. I decided to treat his itch as if it were a burning sensation, like with neuropathic pain. I gave him a treatment called intravenous lidocaine, the same local anesthetic that calms the nerve fibers aggravated in neuropathic pain. The first treatment was a five-minute injection, after which we were both delighted to find his itching was completely gone. While the effect of the medicine would last for less than an hour or so, his relief persisted for weeks. He returned a few weeks later looking like a new man, the itching only a fraction of its original torment. I administered a quick intravenous injection, and again the treatment was successful. A few weeks later, the itching had crept back a little bit. Each time the lidocaine doused the symptoms for a number of weeks, but eventually, after the fourth block, the cycle of itching had been broken.

PAINFUL SOCKS AND GLOVES: DIABETIC NEUROPATHY

The most common forms of diabetes, juvenile and adult onset, which afflict more than fifteen million Americans with 800,000 new cases diagnosed yearly, can damage many organs and systems. As happens with kidney damage, diabetes can make it hard to digest food, cause heart disease, and destroy small blood vessels. In the face of this devastation, the nervous system often becomes an innocent injured bystander. The disease's most common pain syndrome is diabetic neuropathy.

William Rice was referred to the Pain Center with feet so sore he could barely walk. Mr. Rice, a middle-aged man who had been a diabetic since childhood, was insulin dependent and took care of himself. He seemed to have adjusted easily to this lifetime condition—his chart revealed a busy life with two teenage sons, a passion for sailing, and a successful career as a criminal lawyer. As I glanced through his initial evaluation, I wondered what had upset his seemingly even-keeled life.

When I walked into the block room where he was waiting, I took a quick inventory of his appearance. He wore a coat and tie and light-weight chinos, which surprised me a bit because it was February and twenty degrees outside. What really got my attention were his feet—he wore soft, heelless-type slip-ons and no socks. If it had been summer, I possibly wouldn't have noticed. But in the dead of winter, bare feet and ankles stood out like a Hawaiian shirt.

He was a man of few words, no nonsense but personable and engaging. The way he described it, diabetes was no more an inconvenience than shaving. I doubted it: Diabetes is such an intrusive disease that either he was taking heroic measures to manage it or he was minimizing the impact. As with any new patient, I tried to fill in the blanks of his personal history. Something had recently changed in his "it's-all-under-control" health. Since he said nothing out of the ordinary about his physical health, I looked for other possible points of stress. I couldn't help notice that his questionnaire was blank under the space for his wife's name, so I inquired about her.

Mr. Rice's lined, weathered face sagged. "She's dead," he said, point blank. "Died three years ago, January second, in the evening."

The sharp edge of his statement, with its distant tone, threw me off. It's moments like these when it seems that anything I could say would either be trivial or trite. All I could do was continue to be very interested in hearing what he had to say. After a pause, he picked up again. "Yup," he said looking away. "Hasn't been the same since."

It took about twenty minutes of back-and-forth before I pieced together that his wife's sudden death from a freak subway accident, a son's arrest for drinking and driving, and the loss of a big legal case had unraveled his neat life. As far as his physical health went, the biggest toll these personal crises were taking was in his alcohol consumption. He admitted that he drank daily, a couple of ounces of hard liquor before dinner and a glass of wine with his meal, and I mentally doubled his intake, figuring he was probably understating it.

I shifted our conversation to his painful feet. "Why no socks?" I began. "Wearing socks hurts," he explained. He hesitated to use the word "pain" and said that his feet felt like they were on fire with a constant burning sensation. The discomfort faded when he stopped walking and put his feet up, and occasionally the burning flared when something touched his feet, like a rough blanket in the middle of the night, or just socks. These were the symptoms of classic neuropathic pain.

I was struck by Mr. Rice's insistence that what he was feeling was not pain but an unusual, and uncomfortable, sensation. At what point does amplified sensation become pain? This may seem to be an irrelevant philosophical question, but it has real ramifications for devising treatments. The subjective nature of pain always makes treatment look beyond nerves firing "ouch" and raises the question of how much a patient's sensations are affected by attitude—either stoicism or hypersensitivity—and how much by neurophysiology. Trying to determine the most influential part is like trying to dissect the ingredients of a good broth. At some point it transcends its parts and it's just soup—or in my business, it's pain. But treating pain requires considering all the different influences on the final product.

Researchers have been trying for centuries to devise a comprehensive, objective, and accurate scale for measuring pain. A leading scientist in pain research is Gary Bennett, director of Pain Research in the Department of Neurology at Allegheny University in Philadelphia. His work in making models of neuropathic pain has shed enormous light on this disorder and helped develop treatments. The technique he created is widely known in pain medicine as the Bennett model, which other scientists speak of with the same enthusiasm as golfers describe titanium clubs.

Professor Bennett's lab, a windowless room with bright fluorescent lighting and stacks of small wire cages on workbenches, is inhabited largely by dozens of small white rats. Rats, being little mammals with nervous systems akin to our own, in fact, have much to teach us about pain. The Bennett model is a deceptively simple way of inducing and monitoring nerve pain. Dr. Bennett makes an incision on a rat's leg and finds the sciatic nerve, which he ties off with a suture. This soon produces neuropathic pain in that one nerve, the degree of which can be measured.

He pulled out a small leather case with instruments that looked like toothbrushes with only one bristle each, and each a different thickness. It was a von Frey hair, an instrument devised in the late nineteenth century as one of the first pain measurements and still used today. A strand of nylon of known thickness (von Frey used horse hair), which requires a known amount of force to bend, is pressed against the skin until it begins to bend. In this way, a doctor can go from strands that require less force to those that require more and find the exact amount of force that causes pain at a specific area of skin. Heat and cold also can cause pain and can be useful probes in measuring pain. To do this, Dr. Bennett uses a technique call thermal sensory testing. He places a metal disk, called a Peltier thermode, on a finger or animal paw and leaves it there as the disk precisely heats to the point when the subject pulls back. I pulled my finger away after thirteen seconds, which Dr. Bennett says is a predictable reaction.

Since neuropathic pain can crop up from an injury anywhere in the nervous system, doctors need an assortment of ways to test it. The autonomic nervous system controls involuntary functions such as blood pressure, heart rate, and blushing. It alters skin temperature by contracting the blood vessels in the skin. Dr. Bennett measures this with a device called a Doppler scanner. It scans a hand or foot, showing blood flow in bright colors, red being increased flow and blue decreased flow. If a subject hears a sudden loud noise or even takes and holds a deep breath during the imaging of their hand, Dr. Bennett can show in vivid pictures that the sympathetic nervous system reacts by changing blood flow. This makes for a novel way of following patients who have pain due to damage within the sympathetic nervous system.

"Five years ago, you might have asked a patient, 'How's your pain?'" Dr. Bennett says. "Today, that's the wrong question because we now know there are many kinds of pain sensations. This is especially an issue in drug trials. Some drugs eliminate pain and others do not. This doesn't mean the drug isn't working, just that it's not attacking the pain in question." He continues, "There are multiple kinds of spontaneous pain—burning, aching, electric shock pain, pain that occurs episodically. The mechanisms and the stimulus may be different for each—different pathways, different chemicals, and so different responses to drugs."

When he looks into his crystal ball, Dr. Bennett says, "In about fifteen years, there will be a standard battery of tests for everybody that measures and characterizes their pain. It will be a basic tool that won't require a pain clinic. It'll be as routine as getting your eyes checked when you get a license at the DMV. Better yet, we'll have a whole new bunch of treatments for neuropathic pain. We're already adding new classes of drugs, like NMDA regulators and calcium channel blockers, and there are still whole classes that we didn't know about. And the rate of discovery for drugs is escalating."

Although the kind of tools that Dr. Bennett uses are not yet standard tests, Mr. Rice allowed me to study his thermal sensitivity as well as his blood flow profile. Four days after his tests, Mr. Rice returned to go over his results, which bore the unmistakable stamp of diabetic peripheral neuropathy. He was hypersensitive to both heat and cold, and his blood flow was decreased. The confirming detail was that for both heat and blood flow, his feet were mirror images of each other. Only a systemwide disease, as opposed to injury to a specific nerve, could affect each side so equally. The symmetry of Mr. Rice's symptoms pointed straight to his diabetes.

We were in the block room again; Mr. Rice was sitting on the examination table, his legs and sockless feet dangling off the end. I wondered how many pairs of the flimsy, cloth half-shoes he went through every winter. I was feeling reasonably certain that I knew why his feet hurt and, even better, that I could offer a medicine chest of treatments to help control his damaged nerves.

We went into detail about the problem at hand, or more precisely, foot. "Your problem is not socks, or shoes, as such, but how the diabetes has altered sensation in your smallest nerves, which happen to lie at the end of the peripheral nervous system in your hands and feet. Diabetes essentially starves these tiny nerves, resulting in your nervous system becoming confused about what is and what isn't painful. Stockings, gloves—anything that touches skin served by these tiny, hypersensitive nerves is going to send signals to the spinal cord, where they will be mistaken for pain. It's like having a stereo with frayed wires in the speakers so that you can't hear normal volume. To adjust for the poor connection, you crank up the stereo to the highest volume—but while it may get louder, it doesn't necessarily get clearer."

I said that we needed to treat his nervous system, not his feet, and to calm the nerves that were misfiring. In essence, his nerves were acting as if they were having tiny seizures and I had to stop their abnormal signals.

The first step to getting Mr. Rice back into socks was to test his response to a five-minute infusion of the local anesthetic lidocaine. If the lidocaine took the pain away, I would give him similar drugs that could be taken orally. If not, I would look for different types of drugs. The odds that the lidocaine would halt his pain were high; and unknown to Mr. Rice, we were still on the winning side when his pain returned hours later. Understandably, his pain came back as the lidocaine wore off, but I now knew lidocaine-type drugs would help if taken regularly.

Because of his good response to lidocaine, I started with an oral version of an antiarrhythmic drug, a heart medication that smooths out irregular nerve activity and acts as an analgesic. I put him on mexilitine, an oral form of lidocaine. Later on, as symptoms eased up but did not completely disappear, I layered on an anticonvulsant that would similarly quiet the erratic nerve signals. Anticonvulsants—carbamazepine (Tegretol), clonazepam (Klonopin), gabapentin (Neurontin), phenytoin (Dilantin), valproic acid (Depakote), and others—are as fundamental to pain medicine as sutures are to surgery. I opted for gabapentin (Neurontin), but if any of the drugs I gave him didn't do their job, that did not mean that the approach was wrong, only that I had to try another drug from the group.

Much of the excitement over new neuropathic pain remedies is coming from chemicals that halt or slow down nerve seizures. Animal studies that test a class of drugs called calcium channel blockers are raising tantalizing results for easing pain. Scientists are beginning to learn more than ever about newly discovered calcium channels and their tendency to alter the flow of calcium, and electric signals, in and out of cell membranes. For years, drugs in this class such as verapamil, nifedipine, diltiazem, nicardipine, and nimodipine have been prescribed for hypertension and arrhythmia. Now, scientists are finding new calcium channel drugs that have special properties, one of which may be potent pain relief.

But as Dr. Bennett and other neuroscientists will tell you, it's a long leap from animal studies to humans. Translating from the rat's nervous system to your central nervous system is much more complicated than adjusting the dose from a small body to a large body. Tinkering with the way nerve cells emit and receive signals can generate seismic changes in your body. It's almost impossible to modify one chemical system in the body without upsetting others, and if I'm administering drugs, this means I may set off a barrage of side effects. When anyone promises a stronger drug, it may well be accompanied by sizable side effects.

Another new entry into pain medicine is a class of drugs called NMDA inhibitors. Scientists are fairly certain that NMDA receptors are major culprits in causing nervous system malfunctioning. Blocking this receptor may be one of the keys to halting the transformation of acute pain into chronic pain. Physicians have had access to several of these NMDA blockers for years, but they've either proven to be too weak or throw off too many side effects. So scientists are working hard at coming up with an NMDA blocker without the side effects. Presently, many pain centers are using a modest NMDA antagonist medicine called dextromethorphan (DM), which you may know as an ingredient in cough syrup (e.g., Robitussin DM). Its unclear how much punch DM has, but scientists are hopeful that it will help prevent a patient from developing tolerance to narcotics. Despite doctors' reservations about currently available NMDA drugs, they remain optimistic that it's a segment of pain medicine that is going to blossom and produce wondrous results.

Gradually Mr. Rice felt better, with symptoms arising only late at night when he tried to sleep. So I added a medication that does double duty for pain and sleep. To his surprise, and initial resistance, this was the antidepressant nortriptyline. He protested that he was not depressed, and I didn't argue, but I explained that antidepressant medications also work as analgesics. Some patients worry that being prescribed an antidepressant for pain means that the doctor doesn't believe their pain is real. So I carefully explained that these drugs are also antiarrhythmics in their own right and this is probably why they work for neuropathic pain. Patients frequently assume that antidepressants are good painkillers because depression can be intimately wrapped up in the pain experience, acting as a magnifier of physical discomfort. They do this, and much more.

When I have a patient with neuropathic pain who's depressed, I try to treat the two as separate conditions. Since the drugs' pain-relieving properties are probably different from their power over depression, a practical, sensible approach is to divide and conquer. Not all antidepressants disarm nerve pain. The proven pain relievers are tricyclics, such as amitriptyline (Elavil), nortriptyline (Pamelor), nortriptyline (Norpramin), and imipramine (Tofranil). The Prozac-type SSRI antidepressants, such as fluoxetine (Prozac), paroxetine (Paxil), and sertraline (Zoloft), don't seem to moonlight the same way as painkillers. This is probably because the Prozac-type drugs don't block seizures. However, since Prozac and its compatriots often have fewer side effects than tricyclic antidepressants, and depression can increase pain, they can be the best choice for a patient with depression and neuropathic pain.

TACKLING TRIGEMINAL NEURALGIA WITH NEW ARMAMENTS

Scientists like Gary Bennett are learning more every day about the electrical activity of nerves and scouring the world of known pharmacological treatments looking for new uses. There are lots of drugs patients take, to good effect, that scientists don't fully understand, like the antidepressants just mentioned. Another obvious example is aspirin. Researchers continue to find new uses for it beyond pain relief. As doctors now know, aspirin helps head off heart disease and may even prevent colon cancer. In the business of treating pain, science frequently finds new life in old drugs. Neuropathic pain, because of its wide impact on the body, is especially fertile ground for reapplying familiar nostrums.

A patient I treated for neuropathic pain involving the trigeminal nerve in his face needed repeated onslaughts of medication to bring it under control. Nick Ingersoll was a successful stockbroker. His work life was chaotic, packed with financial stress, and it took many months before I found the right pharmacological combination. His case was tough to crack, and unfortunately not that uncommon. Typically, a medication may bring relief for a few months, then gradually the ache and tenderness return.

The neurologist who first diagnosed Nick started him on the anticonvulsant Tegretol, and while it initially calmed the seizures in his facial nerve, its effects did not persist. As many chronic pain patients discover, arriving at the right drug is a tricky business. It requires more than just choosing the right category of drugs because even close relatives have different molecular structures and can produce different effects. Pain medicine is often a journey of trial and error, demanding persistence. The Tegretol was making Nick sleepy during the day and unable to sleep at night. So after talking with his psychiatrist to avoid unpleasant interactions with other drugs he was taking, I started him on another anticonvulsant, Klonopin (clonazepam)—the same drug I had added to Mr. Rice's regimen for his diabetic burning feet. Klonopin can have multiple benefits, quelling not only seizures but also insomnia and anxiety. Antianxiety medications often help with pain because anxiety has a tendency to magnify anything that is disturbing or uncomfortable.

The Klonopin worked wonders, completely eradicating Nick's facial pain and transforming him back into a high-powered financial broker who once again relished eating and could control his temper. However, a month after starting this anticonvulsant, he called up insisting on an immediate appointment. His buoyant mood had vanished; he was glum and irritable. Like floodwater that had been briefly contained behind a restraining wall, his pain had crept around the edges and returned in force. He was understandably discouraged, but I explained that my grand strategy was finding not a quick fix but a permanent one. Our progress might be slow, with some steps backwards, but we'd find the way and it would be a safe, sure route. If these drugs did not work, there were numerous others.

"It seems as if your body's developed a tolerance to the Klonopin." He slumped in a chair in the exam room as I delivered this verdict. His expression was downcast, and he fidgeted nervously with a ballpoint pen. I admitted that I wasn't completely surprised at this development. I knew that the delicate art of finding the right anticonvulsant at the right dosage demanded some degree of trial and error as well as gradual adjustments. I told him I wanted to keep cutting the Tegretol and upping the Klonopin dose. Since an earlier lidocaine test had shown that his pain also responded to this form of local anesthetic, I added the pill form of this pain reliever, mexiletine, hoping it would take a good bite out of his pain.

"Are you sure taking me off Tegretol is a good idea?" Anxiousness dripped from Nick's voice. He had read that Tegretol is the essential drug for trigeminal neuralgia and was afraid of abandoning it.

"What's keeping you from functioning," I explained, "is the sedation as much as the pain, and the Tegretol does that to many people. You are struggling to fire on all cylinders, to be alert, quick-thinking, not anxious. The Klonopin seems to still help with that, but we also need to look at what in your life is making you stressful and anxious."

It was time for me to address the anxiety that was a mainstay in his life. I tried to put myself in his place, and it wasn't hard. In a moment of frustration in trying to reconcile his pain and hard-driving life, I found myself sharing with him some of my own personal struggles as a Type A personality to lead a balanced life and adapt to stress. He seemed surprised to hear a doctor speak so personally about himself, but my intention was to help drive a message home. Nick and I had a common adversary in stress.

Before Nick left, we again negotiated to adjust the dose on the Klonopin and lowered the amount of Tegretol he was taking.

Unfortunately, Nick's story does not end with finding the right dose of the right anticonvulsant. Gradually, his body grew accustomed to the Klonopin, although I was able to bolster its defenses by having him take small doses of the mild opioid oxycodone before eating in order to head off any seizure that might be hovering. I was constantly watching out for toxic reactions, angling to keep doses as low as possible to minimize side effects. We talked regularly so I could gauge how he was doing with the various medications. Each drug worked well, but only for a short time. It was as if each time the nerve pain learned to get around the trap.

Like many patients, Nick was uncomfortable on a steady diet of narcotics, and his unease was accentuated by a family history of alcohol addiction. Dependence was an ugly word in his mind, despite my pointing out that dependence is a totally different animal than addiction, that dependence just meant that his body had become used to having that drug all the time. Nevertheless, he was a reluctant drug taker, and over the months, as the effects of the different medications waned, he asked about other treatments.

Under the Gamma Knife

When Nick came to the Pain Center for his next appointment, he brought his wife, Cathy, to ask tough questions about his treatment options. He expressed uneasiness about the drug regime, while she insisted that we aggressively pursue alternative therapies. I laid out the possibilities, and she asked most of the questions, which largely revolved around effectiveness and side effects. I gave her a brief sketch of noninvasive treatments that had shown good results with some patients, including hypnosis and acupuncture. I had to explain that unfortunately, there just aren't good studies to predict which will work. She was most curious about surgical procedures, including an open-skull operation and a less invasive operation called radio-frequency lesioning, which can leave one with numbness and other problems. Finally, we talked about a new high-tech instrument called a gamma knife.

The gamma knife is sometimes referred to as "cybersurgery"

because it employs invisible gamma radiation instead of cutting tools like a saw or knife. In fact, the gamma knife is leading a new era in surgery that has merged the latest computer technology with advances in knowledge about the structure of the brain and behavior of diseases. The gamma knife was developed by Swedish scientists in the 1970s as a bloodless way to demolish cancerous brain tumors. Gamma rays are a form of energy and can go much deeper into the brain than normal radiation or X rays. Scientists have known about gamma rays since the Curies identified them early in the century, and now medicine has the imaging technology that enables doctors to see through hundreds of layers of tissue and hit exquisitely small targets. In the last few years, technological refinements in MRI-guided techniques have provided three-dimensional pictures of the brain that now serve as a precise targeting mechanism.

MRI images can now identify a problematic trigeminal nerve that the gamma knife can possibly help repair. The gamma knife is a cutting instrument that concentrates more than two hundred beams of cobalt-60 gamma rays on a minute spot within the brain, be it a tumor or a malfunctioning nerve. And it does this without damaging the surrounding tissue. The knife works by emitting multiple gamma rays, each directed at a slightly different angle, and each too weak to cut tissue. But when the many rays converge on a specific point, the cumulative power can cut tissue at the spot of the convergence, but nowhere else.

Being methodical and accustomed to examining things from all angles before advancing, Nick investigated other surgeries. He talked with neurosurgeons and vascular surgeons about decompression surgery as well as radio-frequency lesioning. But the gamma knife held the most appeal because it had the least risk. With the gamma knife, no incisions are made, minimal tissue is cut, and there is almost no blood loss. The patient is conscious during the whole operation, which takes less than an hour, and can walk out of the hospital the same day.

With my referral in hand, Nick and his wife traveled to Presbyterian Hospital in Pittsburgh for the procedure. This was one of the few places where this technique had been perfected for trigeminal neuralgia. Nick was an ideal patient for the procedure because of the nature of his pain: It was flashing and electrical, not constant, and it hurt especially when he chewed or moved his jaw.

On the day of the operation, Nick was dressed in a hospital gown and wheeled into a windowless beige room surrounded by large metal machines. Before starting, the technician took one more magnetic resonance scan to ensure that the neurosurgeon had a good picture of Nick's trigeminal nerve. As Nick lay stretched out on a surgery table, the surgeon attached a metal cage to his head and gradually secured it to his skull with four screws. Its purpose was to hold Nick's head steady. Although it looked like a medieval torture contraption, Nick says he hardly felt anything, even though he was given only a light local anesthetic. Once the cage was in place, another shiny steel structure, which resembled a helmet of crisscrossed metal straps and bolts, was placed over his head. This was the computer-guided targeting device that, working from the latest images, would aim hundreds of individual gamma rays at a few centimeters of Nick's trigeminal nerve. Once the stabilizing and radiation machines were in place, the doctors and technicians left the lead-lined room. They would operate the instruments from an observation bay next door.

Nick lay on the surgery table in the stone-quiet room and waited. He wondered how Cathy, a veteran worrier, was doing in the waiting room. Although Nick was oblivious to anything happening, a few minutes after the doctors left the room, they launched a concentrated barrage of gamma radiation at his brain. The individual gamma rays passed largely unnoticed through his brain cells, but when all two-hundred-plus rays arrived at the same spot, like a magnifying glass pulling together thousands of beams of sunlight, the tissue was targeted and apprehended. Nick neither smelled, heard, saw, nor felt anything strange. He lay there, waiting for something to happen, and realized it was over only when the neurosurgeon returned to the operating room to tell him he was finished. As a precaution, Nick stayed in the hospital that night.

When he left the hospital the next morning, his face and jaw felt exactly as it did when he entered. For all he knew, this could have been a sham treatment, for there were no scars, no side effects, no changes in how he felt. Then, over days, he detected the pain slipping away. Ten days after he left Presbyterian Hospital, Nick was pain free. He was so astonished by the absence of pain that he almost hesitated to cut back on the truckload of medications he had been taking. Nevertheless, he slowly tapered off his daily intake of Tegretol,

Klonopin and methadone, and for the first time in years, Nick's face stopped seizing.

The gamma knife is no silver bullet. While it's a wonderful advance using the latest computerized imaging technology, it ventures into forests of tissue and nerve cells that do not always respond the way scientists expect. The only way to confirm that nerves have been deadened is by how they do or don't respond. Equally difficult is guaranteeing that the nerve has been disarmed in the right place. And, there's always that nagging possibility of nerve rejuvenation, making the gamma knife a promising but not foolproof treatment.

Two months after Nick left Pittsburgh, he felt a twitch on the left side of his face. Alerted, he braced for the pain to return, which it did. A call to his Pittsburgh surgeon confirmed what he suspected. "Oh, that's typical and to be expected," he was told, and the surgeon advised him to wait six months to see whether the pain progressed or receded. Nick is now in a waiting mode and back on a partial dose of the analgesics and anticonvulsants that had been keeping the pain in check. The next rung in Nick's treatment ladder is possibly a repeat of the gamma knife surgery.

If this doesn't work, he may choose to undertake a riskier surgical option: vascular decompression surgery, which would physically relieve or free up his trigeminal nerve from the blood vessel that may be squeezing it and making it misfire. Like a minority of patients with trigeminal neuralgia, Nick may need decompression surgery to disengage blood vessels, scars, or anything else that might cause undue pressure on a nerve. In the meantime, he is now on a new anticonvulsant, lamotrigine, with good results.

THE ENEMY WITHIN: CRPS, RSD, AND OTHER MYSTERIOUS PAINS

There's a certain kind of patient who remembers the exact day and time when they were hurt and their life was forever changed. The trauma might have been a major accident, like a car crash or a mishap at work that put them in the hospital; it might have been a minor incident, like a sprain or a broken bone; or it might have been a routine surgical procedure like repairing a herniated disk. With many patients, the trauma seemed minor, a familiar injury they assumed would heal and pass, and they almost forgot about it. Then, sometime weeks or even months later, the pain returned.

Mathew Green's accident happened on May 2, at 5:35 P.M., as he was driving some teenagers to a prom dinner. He was at a four-way stop, trying to locate a certain Holiday Inn, when a sedan loaded with high school kids late for a football game barreled through the crossing and hit his car head-on. Matt's head crashed through the windshield (this was before airbags were standard) as the car's engine was rammed into the front seat and the steering column collapsed into a pretzel. Remarkably, none of the teenagers in the backseat were injured. But Matt's right hand was crushed between the steering wheel and dashboard. When the mass of crumbled steel stopped moving, Matt was bleeding profusely but conscious enough to know that he was alive and hurt all over.

Matt was taken to the closest emergency room, where he received X rays of almost every part of his body. His mangled hand ballooned to boxing-glove proportions, and the ER doctor told him that he needed to see a specialist at Mass General immediately or risk losing it. Still alert and a little calmer, Matt agreed to be rushed to MGH. His hand looked awful and had a numb, throbbing sensation, but he figured it was not fatal and would heal.

The doctors at Mass General regarded his hand with more gravity and whisked him into the operating room, where they tended to a smashed median nerve and attempted to rebuild surrounding damaged structures. Matt was in the hospital for a week, then started physical therapy to regain use and sensation in his hand. Black and blue and all cut up, his hand was barely useable, but Matt struggled daily through fine-motor and strengthening exercises. For the next three months, Matt religiously did hand exercises and made all of his physical therapy appointments at Spaulding Rehabilitation Hospital. He had to relearn simple activities like how to dress himself and cook, and the doctors told him that he might not ever regain full use of his hand. The pain mostly subsided, erupting only suddenly, as if he'd hit his funny bone and unleashed an excruciating electric shock.

Almost a year after the accident, Matt's doctor referred him to the Pain Center. By that time, he had had two surgeries on his hand, and the surgeon said he could do no more for the burning, throbbing pain that was making him miserable. He even went as far as to say that he just didn't understand why Matt had such strange symptoms of pain and swelling. Matt was skeptical about the prognosis for his hand

and, at first, listened halfheartedly to me. I explained that this mysterious pain that had planted itself in his hand was most likely from damaged nerve paths. He looked relieved when I named his tormentor—complex regional pain syndrome (CRPS)—and could describe how it felt. This disorder goes by many other names, most commonly reflex sympathetic dystrophy (RSD).

Because this type of pain is often misdiagnosed, for instance, as a repetitive soft-tissue strain, a hairline fracture, an infection, a trapped nerve, fascitis, or bone spurs, doctors can only guess at its prevalence. It seems to appear in up to 15 percent of people with traumatic injuries. However, it can occur without any known trauma, just out of the blue. It crosses all ages but peaks in people in their fifties and strikes almost three times as many women as men. Matt's CRPS was classic: His hand was red and swollen, it would suddenly change color and temperature from hot red to cool blue, and it hurt even with light touch. His pain was almost constantly burning and sometimes accompanied by a jolt of electricity.

The picture of CRPS is not always crystal clear, particularly since the pain can appear without any preceding traumatic event. I've had patients who had what looked like CRPS but could recall no accident, no trauma, no operation to set it off. To tease out the culprit, I often try a diagnostic procedure that attempts to unmask whether sympathetic nerves are involved. Similar to the lidocaine infusion, a preliminary injection with a drug called phentolamine may temporarily immobilize the sympathetic nerves and the patient may instantly feel relief.

Soothing the Sympathetic Nerves

The first line of treatment for CRPS is to try to turn off the alarm that is stuck in the ringing position. Since many of the characteristic symptoms of CRPS are under the control of the sympathetic nerves, doctors have long thought that the sympathetic nervous system may be at fault, although it is also possible that this nerve network is an innocent bystander. The sympathetic system carries out automatic reactions like heart rate, blood pressure, and sweating and probably causes such CRPS symptoms as sporadic swelling, asymmetrical sweating, and either warm reddened skin or occasionally cold and white-bluish skin. Consequently, treatment first focuses on deactivating the sympathetic system in the hope it will reset to normal. A rare treatment is to surgically cut sympathetic nerves or kill them with alcohol or other chemicals. Called a sympathectomy, this surgery can provide temporary pain relief, though lasting relief is not as assured.

There are several types of nerve blocks that shut down the sympathetic system. The block I deploy depends on the location of the pain. There are certain blocks for the face, neck, and arms, and others for the legs. Some blocks affect only a certain part of a limb. For Matt's hand, I first did a stellate ganglion block that turned off the sympathetic nervous system in his arm. These helped greatly, but only temporarily. This block, which goes through the neck, is straightforward and relatively safe. Since Matt's pain was controllable for about a month at a time, I chose an easier path to the same result. I delivered an intravenous regional block, a Bier block, named for the German doctor who first used an injection of anesthesia to deaden a limb. This block, which corrals the numbing agent in the lower arm and hand, can give some patients long-term pain relief.

For the Bier block, I first wrapped Matt's upper arm in a device that looks like a blood pressure cuff and injected a squirt of Novocain in the skin so he didn't feel the placement of the IV catheter. Then, right through the IV catheter, I infused lidocaine as well as another drug, bretylium, that would quiet the sympathetic nerves. For a few minutes, Matt felt a burning sensation, which is normal. Afterwards, his arm was almost completely numb for a short while. I removed the cuff after about forty minutes, and Matt's arm started to feel less numb but with much less pain than before. The Bier block not only quieted the pain but also gave him back some motion. One of the best features of the block, Matt said, was that it gave him enough freedom from pain to be able to exercise and even try driving again. So we scheduled this block for right before his physical therapy sessions.

Bier blocks are usually not permanent, and the pain generally seeps back within days, weeks, or months. For some patients, they last a month or two; for others they can last even longer. Matt's pain vanished for one or two months, and so he now comes into the Pain Center monthly for a Bier block.

CRPS can be a chameleon, quickly flaring up and dying down, revealing only one or two of its characteristic symptoms rather than the full spectrum. In some patients the disease causes hair loss along the limb; in others it stimulates hair growth. Similarly, a patient's skin may be warmer than normal, or cooler.

Complex regional pain can invade almost any part of the body, and when it storms through the chest or trunk area, the best way to block these sympathetic nerves may be to go through the epidural space near the spinal cord. The pain of CRPS that lodges in the head or face may call for a stellate ganglion block. The stellate ganglion is a knot of nerves at the base of the neck, and an injection here prevents select nerve activity from traveling upward.

A lumbar sympathetic block is the injection of choice for CRPS that lodges in the hips or legs. This injection is given at a specific area of the back where the sympathetic nerves congregate just in front of the spinal bones. It is occasionally used to quell the fire of chronic shingles (postherpetic neuralgia) in the lower extremities, and it's a common treatment for CRPS.

Early treatment has the best chance for success with CRPS. When the problem has lingered, it's rare that a single block can defeat it. Often, treatment entails a series of injections, and even with this approach, I am never surprised if the pain returns. This pain syndrome is a tough customer, a shape-shifter with many origins, some known and some not. It usually demands an arsenal of treatments. Nerve blocks are my initial barrage, but if they fail, lose their impact, or miss their mark, I storm the sympathetic nervous system with drugs as well as nonpharmacological treatments.

The sympathetic nervous system can be calmed with drugs that are often used to treat other conditions that involve these special nerves. The most common are drugs for high blood pressure. If you take medication for high blood pressure, you will recognize the names of many of the drugs given to manage CRPS. Clonidine is one of the common drugs used, as are oral forms of phenoxybenzamine and propranolol as well as many other drugs used for hypertension. But such drugs raise pros and cons that patients have to weigh: They circulate throughout the body, cooling pain wherever it flares, while also producing such side effects as low blood pressure, slowing or racing heart, stuffiness, sexual dysfunction, and diarrhea.

A Blitzkrieg of Drugs

If I find that turning off the sympathetic nervous system isn't winning the battle against the burning, swelling, and electric shocks, I look elsewhere for vulnerable spots. I treat the pain like any other form of neuropathic pain. Since neuropathic pain arises from convulsions or seizures somewhere along nerve pathways, the best weapons are anticonvulsant or antiseizure medications. There is no clear science yet to guide me as to which drug to choose first, so I usually start with the safest. Neurontin (gabapentin), a relatively new epilepsy drug, is one of the first medications I reach for when I'm expanding pharmacological treatment. Another anticonvulsant that has a regular role is the well-known anticonvulsant carbamazepine (Tegretol). Many other anticonvulsants and antiarrhythmics can be used with equal benefit, including mexiletine (Mexitil), Dilantin, topiramate (Topomax), lamotrigine (Lamictal) as well as tricyclic antidepressants (Elavil, Tofranil, nortriptyline, Desipramine) and others. They help slow down nerve signals and weaken pain signals.

Complex regional pain, as you may have surmised by now, does not play by the rules. Treating it is like trying to lasso an angry bull—it keeps changing directions, charging and retreating, motionless at one moment and running and darting at another. So when it does not act like neuropathic pain and seems immune to its remedies, I look for any other way to corral it. I treat it as idiopathic pain—pain that defies rhyme or reason—and consider using other analgesics, from over-the-counter remedies like ibuprofen to a strong narcotic.

The Ups and Downs of Narcotics

Susan Susman had been through the CRPS war zone. Following a minor automobile accident, which jammed her arm into the steering wheel, the arm ballooned into an angry red bulb that was hypersensitive to heat and cold and unusable. In the six years since the accident, she had had surgery, extensive physical therapy, psychological counseling, and enough drugs to overwhelm any medicine chest. When she came to the Pain Center, she had been gobbling Percocet, and her primary physician, suspecting she was abusing the drug, was questioning her requests for refills. A perky, active woman in her thirties, Susan's distress during our first appointment was visible. Her eyes watered as she described her uncontrollable pain, and she shifted uneasily in her chair as we talked about her medication and her doctor's latest cutback in her dose.

Percocet is a combination of acetaminophen (Tylenol) and the narcotic oxycodone that works for about three to four hours. If you've ever had an operation, like a ligament repair or hysterectomy, chances are good that you were given Percocet or a close relative for the post-operation pain. Percocet and other short-acting pain relievers often contain two ingredients, a narcotic like oxycodone, a derivative of codeine, and an analgesic like acetaminophen, aspirin, or ibuprofen. The narcotic content is usually much smaller than the other analgesic, which boosts the potency of the opioid. The double ingredients usually make these painkillers the wrong drug for the long haul.

As Susan took Percocet over many months, she naturally developed a tolerance to the drug's narcotic, oxycodone, and needed increasingly larger doses for effective pain relief. But as her Percocet doses got higher, so did the amount of the drug's second ingredient, acetaminophen (Tylenol), to which people do not develop tolerance. Its impact on her liver and kidneys also rose and would eventually reach toxic levels. Ironically, her body could handle gradually higher doses of opioids but not larger quantities of the supposedly more benign acetaminophen (Tylenol).

This double-edged sword is a problem with any of the pain relievers that combine a narcotic and another analgesic. One of the ingredients can literally poison a patient. The upshot is that these drugs are best used for no more than a couple of weeks, not for pain that lasts for months and years. These are well-known medications, and include Darvocet N-100 (100 mg. propoxyphene and 650 mg. acetaminophen), Darvon Compound (32 mg. propoxyphene, 389 mg. acetylsalicylic acid, and 32 mg. caffeine), Percodan (5 mg. oxycodone and 325 mg. acetylsalicylic acid), Tylenol #3 (300 mg. acetaminophen and 30 mg. codeine), Tylenol #4 (300 mg. acetaminophen and 60 mg. codeine), and Vicodin (7.5 mg. hydrocodone and 750 mg. acetaminophen). Two new narcotics, Vicoprophen (hydrocodone and ibuprofen) and Norco (hydrocodine and acetaminophen), offer slightly different combinations but similar risks. This is why I don't prescribe Percocet or any of these combined medications for chronic pain. Instead, I use the single opioids alone and if necessary add the other drug separately.

Susan was on a pain roller coaster. Since the oxycodone in the Percocet only worked for a short time, she was constantly reaching for pain medicine. This was exactly counter to the goal of prescribing opioids for chronic pain to improve a person's normal functioning. Also, the rising level of acetaminophen was very risky. So I immediately changed the Percocet to the active ingredient, oxycodone, alone.

Then I changed the opioid to a time-release formula so that, once the right dose was reached, she would need only a few doses a day. In most patients I can get this to one or two doses per day or once every three days (with the fentanyl patch, Duragesic). Susan settled down on a few daily doses of methadone, which, for unknown reasons, worked best for her.

All narcotics have side effects, and no one can predict which patients will feel which side effects. Constipation, nausea and vomiting, sleepiness, itching, slower breathing, and tolerance can be companions to opioids but usually are not. Some patients feel sleepy when they're taking methadone but feel fine when taking morphine. Others feel exactly the opposite. While I can't anticipate all side effects, the one experience that everyone has is constipation. And unlike other side effects, which often fade after a while, the constipation never does. Constipation is such a consistent outcome that if a patient's not constipated, I wonder whether her dose is sufficient. Although annoying, constipation is controllable, and every patient on chronic opioids is also on a laxative.

In trying to find the right drug for a patient, I watch not only for which side effects crop up but also how he or she tolerates the drug. Some patients may acquire a tolerance for opioids, but despite public belief, growing need is not a bottomless slide into addiction. It simply means that a drug's effect at a certain dose is wearing off and a larger dose may be needed for the same effect. Some patients can need higher doses as they are starting their medications but within months arrive at a plateau dose that they can live with for a very long time. If a patient's tolerance shoots up, I may modulate the patient's reaction by switching drugs. I also have to keep in the back of my mind that the medicine may be wearing off because the disease is getting worse.

There is a whole new class of drugs that I call opioid stabilizers because they look like they actually decrease tolerance. These drugs are called NMDA antagonists, blocking a certain receptor involved in pain becoming chronic as well as the development of tolerance. So far, the most useful one is an over-the-counter cough medication called dextromethorphan (the DM in Robitussin DM), although I prescribe DM in much higher dosages for pain than for cough suppression. Many other NMDA blockers for pain are being studied and readied for use.

Occasionally a patient asks for one drug over another because he or she believes it's more potent. While it's true that some opioids pack more punch, this does not necessarily make them more effective. Patients frequently confuse potency with effectiveness. Much more vital is the dosing. The opioid fentanyl is sixty to eighty times more potent than morphine, while codeine is less potent than morphine, but what they do for a person depends on how much they take. For instance, a patient who needs five milligrams of morphine can get the same effect from about thirty-five milligrams of codeine. Potency is always moderated by the dose, and I can achieve the same effectiveness with fentanyl or the weaker cousin meperidine (Demerol) by adjusting the dose. However, I rarely use meperidine because it has more serious possible side effects than almost any other commonly used narcotic.

Whenever I lecture on treating chronic pain with narcotics, I find that the subject is not only heated and controversial but greatly misunderstood by doctors and patients alike. The discussion is always about more than medicine, crossing over to social and legal issues as well. The subject is loaded with misconceptions and myths, fears and fallacies. Most physicians and patients know opioids as the primary treatment for acute pain or pain at the end of life, and many of their assumptions about these drugs do not hold up when they are given for chronic pain.

The Cost of Addiction Phobia

Perhaps one of the most widespread notions about using opioids is that they are always addictive. Doctors fear addiction, patients fear addiction, indeed, our entire society is terrified of the possibility. When doctors prescribe narcotics, which they do not always do even in the face of awful discomfort, the type of drug and dosage are greatly influenced by the specter of addiction. Doses tend to be too low, the right narcotic preparation tends to be avoided, and the prescribing period is often too short. Medicine's reluctance to use appropriate doses of opioid drugs gives patients the wrong message—their pain isn't that important, they are not trustworthy, they may be addicts, they are bad people if they take the drugs even if they are prescribed. It's a vicious cycle. Every now and then patients refuse my prescription for an opioid that I know they need because they're convinced it's "wrong."

Exacerbating doctors' reluctance to prescribe narcotics is the enormous scrutiny and regulation they face every day. Most narcotics are what the government calls Schedule Two or Schedule Three drugs, which means that unlike other prescribed drugs, their prescription is restricted and closely monitored. In many states, doctors have to write opioid prescriptions in triplicate, with the original going to the patient, the doctor keeping the second, and the third sent to the state regulatory agency. Individual states and the federal Drug Enforcement Agency (DEA) keep a close watch on the kinds and amounts of narcotics doctors prescribe and fine the doctor or revoke a license if they suspect abuse. Legitimate pain doctors have been fined and lost their licenses for perceived overprescribing, and this has had a chilling effect across the board. Doctors are also acutely aware of an added layer of scrutiny from media and medical watchdogs poised to jump on any physician suspected of overprescribing narcotics. While certainly some doctors and patients abuse these substances, the hysteria surrounding this problem has deprived many patients of the most effective pain relievers available.

Doctors are not the only people reluctant to venture into the opioid jungle. Patients also have been led to believe that all narcotics are addictive and if they need or want their pills too much, they're just one step away from becoming a junkie. Patients worried about getting hooked on their drugs either downplay their pain and say they don't need opioids, take only part of the prescribed dose, or stop taking them altogether.

As I explained to Susan, there are sensible ways to prescribe opioids for chronic pain that minimize the chances of addiction and increase the chance that addiction will be noticed if it occurs. For starters, the long-acting opioids that I use for chronic pain are much less likely to produce the euphoria that everyone believes is a basic feature of narcotic abuse. Opioids for chronic pain are time-released or long-acting drugs that are taken in pill or patch form, not injected, and slip into the bloodstream gradually, then circulate at a steady level without large peaks and valleys. There's not the rush or high that comes when short-acting drugs speed to the brain.

When you receive your pain relief in steady levels, the pain isn't completely abolished but diminished enough so you can return to normal activity. Instead of euphoria or addiction, you feel pain slide from unbearable to bearable, freeing you to rejoin your family, return to work, do favorite activities, and enjoy being alive. The opioids mute your pain enough to help you function better; they don't eliminate it. Restoring function is so central to using opioids for chronic pain that it clearly defines the critical line between addiction and effective treatment. So simple is this distinction that it sometimes even takes physicians by surprise.

Opioid addiction and effective treatment of chronic pain with opioids are diametrically opposite when it comes to function. A person who is addicted to opioids has a disease that makes it impossible to function optimally and drives him to compulsively use a drug, despite the negative consequences. Everything this person does revolves around getting more drugs, not living life. However, the pain patient who is dependent on opioids finds life restored. With the pain muted through a stable and steady, controlled use of long-acting opioids, they reclaim their lives, go back to work, return to family life, and purse favorite pastimes. The difference between a patient with opioid addiction and a patient who is on opioids for chronic pain is simple: The pain patient does better and the addicted patient does worse.

Pain doctors have known for years that taking opioids for medical reasons over a long time does not have to lead to addiction. More than a decade ago, neurologist Russell Portenoy, who is presently president of the American Pain Society, reviewed studies of almost twenty-five thousand cancer patients, most of whom had been on opioid therapy for many years. Of the whole group, only seven showed any signs of drug abuse, drug craving, or drug-seeking behavior.

Every one of these cancer patients was dependent. However, their physical needs were worlds away from what medicine, and the government, consider addiction. Addiction is a psychological condition that compels a person to satisfy that need, and keep satisfying it, no matter what. It's compulsive behavior that demands more and more drugs, regardless of the consequences that lead to dysfunction. Dependence is a physical state that occurs when the lack of a drug causes the body to have a reaction. This can occur with almost any kind of drug. A good example is caffeine. If you are used to several cups of coffee each day, you soon learn about physical dependence when you miss a day or two. This doesn't mean you are addicted. It only means your body is surprised not to see what it has become used to. In the case of opioids, a certain amount every day fills the glass, and no more is needed or asked for. If the medication is removed, the consequences are physical, like sweating, racing heart, or nausea, not psychological. As any diabetic will testify about insulin, or any heart patient will testify about blood pressure medication, dependence on regular medication is not necessarily addictive or abusive—in fact, it may be essential for good health.

Like many patients, Susan was terrified that she had become addicted to her medication, and the conflict between the insistent pain that cried for relief and her agonizing over addiction made her even more miserable. She withdrew from family and friends, hiding out in the family room watching television, shut off from the shopping, daily aerobics, and a job that once shaped her days. To her doctor, her husband, even herself, she seemed to be addicted to Percocet because she kept needing larger doses and, despite taking more medicine, was able to do less and less. As I listened to her describe what had been happening, I suspected that her real problem was "pseudoaddiction." Her behavior showed signs of inadequate pain treatment—she was on the pain/analgesic roller coaster and the Percocet was not doing the job. Her problem wasn't psychological craving or drug seeking. When the drug delivered its relief a few hours a day, she was able to do essential grocery shopping or talk with friends. She didn't go out looking for more drugs. Then the narcotic wore off and the pain came roaring back, making her even more uncomfortable and more desperate for relief. Rather than freeing herself from her pain, she became conditioned to watching her pain every moment.

Once I shifted Susan from the short-acting Percocet to opioids that lasted longer and only required a few dosages per day, she was off the roller coaster of temporary relief. Her pain receded enough for her to get on with her life. She happily stayed at the same dose for over a year as she recaptured the small pleasures in her life that had slipped away. She no longer had to plan shopping and household chores around a certain dose of a pill. She was able to reconnect with her family and enjoy a social life, and even have regular exercise that she so enjoyed before that fateful auto mishap.

ELECTRONIC STIMULATION

One of the first things Steve Matthews said to me when he came into the Pain Center was, "I don't want to leave here with a drug problem." I soon learned why he was so concerned: He had been taking Percocet for three years and was also consuming upwards of fifteen

Tylenol a day, anticonvulsants, tricyclic antidepressants, and sleep medication. He wasn't on just any roller coaster of pain and relief, he was on the Big Dipper.

Steve's chronic regional pain was the result of a construction acci-dent when a ton of concrete blocks slipped from a forklift and crushed his foot. The foot was so swollen and damaged that the ER physician called in others to see it. Bones were broken or badly bruised and flexed, and since then, Steve had not been off crutches, back to work, or barely out of the house he shared with his parents. From the start, his experience with pain medication had been troubled. He left the emergency room with instructions to wait for the swelling to go down before his foot could be casted and twelve Percocet to last him two weeks.

The casting proved a disaster—his foot became infected and he had to be hospitalized. Even after it apparently healed and he had com-pleted months of physical therapy, it was still black and blue and stone cold. He had to quit all the sports he loved—playing in two ice hockey leagues, pickup basketball and baseball—and his usual sixty-hour work week was now filled by time on the couch, waiting for delivery of daily newspapers and trying to lose himself in novels about adventure travel.

I explained that he had CRPS, a version of neuropathic pain, and that there were more options for him than just drug therapy. My immediate recommendation was a lumbar sympathetic block, and though this is a routine pain procedure, I had to repeatedly reassure him that it would not hurt or cause any further damage. "What hap-pens if I sneeze during this—will I end up in a wheelchair?" he asked. He had been badly burned by the medical establishment with his pre-vious treatments and was understandably leery.

Although he was nervous during the first block and indeed jerked his head to say something during the middle of it, the local anesthetic diminished his pain by about 70 percent. Over the next year, he had seven lumbar sympathetic blocks that toned down his pain, though a little less each time. I suggested we shift to a Bier block, which would stop the pain from marching up his leg. But like the other block, this too did not shut down the entire syndrome. He was still bedeviled by his painful foot, its burning and hypersensitivity so intense that wear-ing shoes was akin to stepping into a torture device.

Like most neuropathic pain, Steve's had its own patterns and style, and like a willful child it was incredibly stubborn to the remedies that usually subdued it. When he came in to renew his prescriptions for the pain and sleep medications he was using to supplement the regular blocks, I told him about another option. "Look, Steve, I know you are reluctant to venture into anything new, and I don't blame you. But as your doctor, really your consultant, I have to be sure you know all your options. There is another way to attack this pain, and although it may seem more drastic, more medically intrusive than what you're doing now, it may offer relief. It's a surgery and a device called a spinal cord stimulator that has few, if any side effects, unlike the drugs you're taking now, and might free you from the short tether you're on with the Pain Center."

Spinal cord stimulators are the technological offspring of the gate control theory of pain. As you may remember, that theory explained how pain is transmitted from damaged nerve and tissue through the dorsal column to a "gate" in the brain that regulates what is and is not felt as pain. The gate control theory has come under skeptical review in the past decade, but it has spawned technological devices designed to change the nature of the signal that gets to the gate. In the 1970s, scientists began designing electric devices that altered nerve signals; at first they used them for all sorts of chronic pain, with mixed results. Many of the early complications are attributed to poor patient screening—they were given to the wrong people—and equipment failures.

Those bugs have been worked out, and today spinal cord stimulators have become a safe option for patients for whom other treatments have not worked. Recent research suggests that they are especially welcome by patients suffering from neuropathic pain, particularly CRPS. Steve was a good candidate for a spinal stimulator and met all the patient criteria: He had tried all conventional therapies, further surgery or other drugs were not likely to improve his pain, he had no psychological complications, and he had no potential medical complications, such as needing a pacemaker.

The theory behind spinal cord stimulators is easy to understand. It generates constant electrical stimulation that feels like tingling, essentially counteracting the pain signals so that the sensation at the spinal cord is not perceived as pain. This is the theory, but in truth doctors don't really understand how spinal stimulation alters the perception of pain. We think it works in the same way as rubbing your elbow after you've jarred the funny bone—that is, by producing an alternate or masking sensation so that the pain signal can't get through.

The surgery and device are fairly uncomplicated. The surgery takes place in a sterile operating room, and the patient is given a numbing agent and sedative but is awake throughout. An electronic lead or thin plastic cable containing electrodes is gently passed into the spine exactly where the nerves from the painful limb enter the spinal column. In this phase of the operation, the doctor tests the placement of the lead by activating it with an external transmitter and asking the patient where he feels the sensation to make sure it's connected to the pain area. The lead is then connected to a battery/transmitter device that is about the size of a deck of cards, which is tunneled around the patient's trunk to the abdomen. A transmitter determines the strength of the signal that produces the electric pulse. It can be adjusted by the patient or, with an internal device, by the doctor, and the patient can turn it on or off by passing a special magnet over the area.

Spinal cord stimulators use electric signals to distract the brain from feeling pain. Many patients turn them on only when they expect pain to surface or while they're sleeping so they won't be awakened by pain. In some, just knowing it is there makes a huge difference.

Of course, I explained to Steve that spinal stimulators are not perfect or risk-free. Sometimes there are complications from the surgery or afterwards, like bleeding, infection, allergic reactions, failure to stop the pain, and, very rarely, paralysis. But compared with other pain therapies, the odds of bad side effects for spinal cord stimulators are small. For many people, they become the lifesaver that at last enables them to reclaim what neuropathic pain had stolen from them.

At the UC Davis Pain Management Center, we have found that spinal stimulators are sometimes the miracle cure that triumphs when all else has failed. Dr. Karen Pantazis has implanted many of these devices in patients with pain following back surgery as well as neuropathic and complex regional pain, and she has watched patients routinely experience substantial improvement.

Dr. Pantazis implanted a spinal stimulator into an athletic young woman who had been sidelined for years with painful knees. The twenty-seven-year-old mother and basketball player had had arthroscopic surgery on both knees, followed by repeated pain therapies, such as blocks and medication. Almost crippled by complex regional pain, she was likely to never again lace up a pair of high-top sneakers.

Dr. Pantazis implanted a stimulator with two leads in the epidural space where the nerves for each knee meet the spinal cord and positioned the electrical generator just above the belt line in her abdomen. The pain was not completely removed but reduced so much that she was able to play basketball again. All she has to worry about now is setting off airport metal detectors. (She carries a card that explains her implanted medical device.)

9

MEETING HEADACHES HEAD-ON

Tension Headaches, Migraines, and Other Monsters

> If migraine patients have a common and legitimate second complaint besides their migraines, it is that they have not been listened to by physicians. Looked at, investigated, drugged, charged, but not listened to.
>
> —DR. OLIVER SACKS,
> *Newsweek*

Given the millions of people who suffer from headaches and especially migraines, it's no wonder that treating headaches has become a medical specialty unto itself. As a result, people with severe headaches often seek help from a specialized clinic rather than a pain center. The headache patients I see have pain that has resisted a barrage of remedies and defied the best efforts of other doctors. With the pervasiveness of headaches, it's become a fertile field for discovery with better treatments than ever before.

While many people blame stress for the modern plague of headaches, this special form of torture is as old as mankind. Ancient Egyptians described a "sickness of half the head," Mesopotamians declared, "Headache roameth over the desert, blowing like the wind," and around 460 B.C. Hippocrates told of "a violent pain supervened in the right temple." Despite its timeless history, much about the headache still baffles doctors, and only in the past ten years has medicine begun to make headway in treating it.

As you may know, headaches can be a symptom of a serious disease or a condition in itself that's not fatal but severe enough to make you miserable. The headache that indicates to a neurologist that a patient has some other health problem is usually not the same creature that attacks the forty-five million American chronic headache pain sufferers. Doctors distinguish between these two categories of headaches by asking a patient about how the headache started and accompanying symptoms, and by a clinical examination. Although you may at some time have wondered whether your headache is really a brain tumor, only about 1 percent of headaches point to another ailment. Headaches that are a harbinger of a more severe malady often come on quickly and severely, sometimes following a blow to the head or head injury, or are accompanied by convulsions, confusion, loss of consciousness, fever, stiff neck, loss of balance, slurred speech, weakness, or tingling in the body. Fortunately, this variety of head pain is rare. The other type spares few of us.

WHY HEADACHES HURT AND OTHER PUZZLES

For years, scientists and researchers ignored headaches as a legitimate subject of study. They were dismissed as a "woman's problem"— women suffer them much more than men—and so they were relegated to the realm of psychological disturbance. Scientists were further discouraged because headaches do not reveal any organic causes and cannot be "seen" with normal diagnostic techniques. Researchers have also been limited because they can't use animals in their studies, since there's no way to know if a rat or cat has a headache. However, with the advent of high-tech scanning devices that opened a window into the human brain, headache knowledge has advanced significantly. Applying sophisticated technology that can measure electrical activity and chemical processes in the head and brain, scientists have now started to piece together the mechanisms that bring on headaches.

The science and treatment of headaches received a tremendous boost in the early 1990s with the development of a new class of drugs, triptans, that are remarkably effective for treating certain types of headaches. Dr. Elizabeth Loder, director of the Headache Management Program at Spaulding Rehabilitation Hospital in Boston, is a leader in this new specialty and has treated thousands of headache patients. "The new drug sumatriptan changed the ways doctors think about migraines," she says. "They became a real medical condition that could be treated, not just a woman's problem."

A substantial number of migraines run in families and point to a genetic origin. But genetics are only part of the puzzle. Headaches arise from a complicated, sometimes perplexing stew of chemical and neurological activity. Although scientists have not figured out all the deep-seated causes of headaches, doctors do know why they hurt. The pounding, throbbing, stabbing, and aching are so painful because of the dense web of sensory nerves around the head. The pain is not generated in the brain, which has no sensory nerves, but in the nerves of the scalp, face, mouth, and throat, as well as in the muscles of the head and blood vessels at the base of the brain. This generous supply of pain nerves is crucial to your protection and survival. Stress, muscle tension, dilated blood vessels, and other triggers launch a chemical reaction that stimulate these pain nerves, which send the awful message of headache to the brain.

One source of aggravation, though surely not the sole one, is dilated blood vessels pressing on sensory nerves. For many years, doctors believed that the expansion, and quick contraction, of blood vessels in the head were the chief sources of pain. They now know that a lot more is going on, too. "The problem is not blood vessels alone," insists Dr. Loder. She believes that many other causes are probably also common. These may include the trigeminal nervous system and release of brain chemicals such as prostaglandin and serotonin.

THE WORLD OF HEADACHES: FROM ICE CREAM TO TENSION

Doctors have identified about a dozen major varieties of headache and at least sixty subtypes. If this sounds like a lot, consider all the variations that you may have suffered from yourself: tension headache, an "ice cream" headache, sinus headache, hangover headache, eyestrain headache, menstrual headache, hunger headache, temporomandibular joint (TMJ) headache, caffeine withdrawal headache—the list goes on. Although there is no such thing as a "headache personality," headaches do afflict women three times more than men, possibly because of hormones. The headaches that most often come to the attention of doctors are migraine, tension, rebound, cluster, and post-trauma. Not infrequently, patients suffer unknowingly from more than one kind.

The Headband Headache

This headache has gone by an assortment of names, including muscle-contraction headache, chronic daily headache, and tension headache. But by any name, it's the headache that you know as a gradual pressure or tightness around the head, like a hat that's too small, that advances into a dull ache or intense pressure. As the headband image suggests, this headache attacks both sides of the head and in this way can differ from migraines or cluster headaches. Other than the tight headband sensation, tension headaches don't follow a pattern. Some last for hours, others for days; some occur daily, others weekly; and some come with feelings of fatigue and, at their worst, loss of appetite. A caffeine-withdrawal headache can resemble a tension headache, though the latter is caused when blood vessels in the head, accustomed to constriction from a daily dose of caffeine, dilate in its absence. You may think that a sure way to tell if a headache comes from caffeine withdrawal is to see what a cup of coffee does for the pain. But caffeine is a well-known pain reliever that works for almost any headache.

Tension-type headache, which is the term doctors use today, was once thought to be caused by muscle spasms of the many muscles of the head and neck. However, scientists suspect that the underlying causes of tension headaches probably have more to do with blood vessels around the brain and disruptions in the normal flow of the brain chemical serotonin.

The infamous triggers that you hear about, like alcohol or chocolate, are probably much less to blame for tension headaches than emotional stress or depression. When depression is fueling a headache, the pain often appears soon after waking. "The science behind studies of food triggers is very poor. Most of the evidence is anecdotal—it's hard to double-blind red wine," says Dr. Loder, referring to the standard study protocol in which both the patient and doctor are in the dark about who's getting the substance being tested and who's getting the placebo. "Some patients do have food triggers, but they're very individual. Alcohol is definitely a vasodilator, but the evidence on dairy products is uncertain. Same with fruits. I resist giving patients lists of foods to avoid because they can become neurotic about their eating and lose an important pleasure. I suggest that patients eliminate one food at a time for a week or two, then slowly reintroduce them and notice any effects."

Migraine Misery

Migraine sufferers say that the migraine is as close to hell on earth as they'll ever come, and I believe it. Although there are variations of migraines, most share telltale characteristics that let the sufferers know that they are in store for more than routine discomfort. Migraines generally hit on one side of the head with a pain that throbs and is made worse by any activity or motion, even sneezing. The pain is often accompanied by nausea, vomiting, and difficulty in thinking, and you may become acutely sensitive to light and sound. People who suffer from migraines may feel them as often as every few days or as occasionally as once or twice a year.

The search for the cause of migraines has gained momentum in recent years as doctors and patients have become frustrated with weak or ineffective treatments. Driving much of the research has been the knowledge that once an organic cause is identified, scientists can then devise drugs that have an impact. For many years, doctors believed that migraines were caused largely by dilated blood vessels pushing on nerves. Until recently, the leading drugs to fight these headaches were ergotamines (trade names Cafergot, Wigraine) or an injectable form, dihydroergotamine mesylate (DHE), which causes blood vessels to constrict. But as scientists have refined scanning and imaging tools and delved into genetic research, they have downgraded the "vascular theory" from main culprit to an accomplice and have identified other sources. While vascular dilation surely plays a role, it may well be the result of something else going on, such as unusual chemical activity.

One theory suggests there is an electrical or chemical disruption in the brain stem, which then discharges signals to nerves in the head and face. Something sets off a chemical or electrical chain reaction that affects blood vessels and head muscles as well as the flow of powerful neurochemicals, like the inflammation moderator prostaglandin. What doctors call "sterile inflammation"—meaning that inflammation occurs for no reason—is thought to be a possible cause. When researchers confirmed that the neurotransmitter serotonin was mixed up in the migraine stew, pharmacologists created a drug to interact with serotonin and hinder the migraine chemistry. The first of this class of drugs, sumatriptan (trade name Imitrex), has proven to be wonderfully powerful in suppressing migraines. Scientists looking at causes could also not help but notice that migraines frequently arise in families, and so they are actively hunting for the gene(s) at fault. Locating this gene could lead to a test to diagnosis who's likely to get these headaches and help doctors distinguish between a migraine and serious neurological disorders.

Migraines fall into two categories, depending on how the pain develops and the accompanying symptoms. Migraines that are preceded by an aura (visual auras are the most common), a warning sensation like sensitivity to light, were once dubbed a classic migraine and known to occur in fewer than 20 percent of people who get migraines. Aura migraines may include other temporary sensitivities as well, such as numbness and tingling, and can impair a person's ability to speak and move. Most doctors apply the criteria of the International Headache Society when judging whether a headache comes under the "migraine with aura" class. You must have had at least two headaches with three of these four characteristics: pain associated with aura symptoms; auras developing gradually over minutes or two or more in succession; no aura lasting more than an hour; and headache appearing within an hour or less of the aura or at the same time. Furthermore, say headache experts, your migraine with aura also has to possess the qualities of a nonaura migraine.

This other version of migraine, without an aura, was once called a common migraine and is much more prevalent. While harboring no distinct aura, these migraines may also bring a sensitivity to light and last for hours or sometimes days. This is why most migraine sufferers find a dark, quiet room when they're stricken. Most migraines crop up early in the morning, and occasionally awaken someone from nighttime sleep. Generally speaking, for your headache to be a migraine without aura, you must have had at least five bouts that lasted four to seventy-two hours with at least two of these qualities: pain on one side of the head, pulsating feeling, moderate or severe pain, and pain that intensifies from routine physical movement. Also, your headache has to be accompanied by nausea, vomiting, sensitivity to light and/or sound (photophobia or phonophobia), and not be related to any other physical problem.

Individual triggers—foods, stimuli, environmental changes, and personal chemistry—are a central cog in the migraine machinery. Researchers are certain that triggers can launch a migraine and suspect they can be influential in starting other types of headaches, too. Scientists at the government research agency, the National Institute of

Neurological Disorders and Stroke, which is investigating migraines, say about triggers, "It's like a cocked gun with a hair trigger. A person is born with a potential for migraine and the headache is triggered by things that are really not so terrible." Triggers vary from person to person, and there are literally dozens of suspect substances and events, so each headache patient has to discover on her own what sets off the pain. Lists of likely triggers often start with foods or drinks, and the most often mentioned are alcoholic drinks, chocolate, aged cheese, the flavor-enhancer monosodium glutamate, the artificial sweetener aspartame, caffeine, nuts, and nitrites and nitrates, chemical preservatives found in meats like baloney and salami. A change in your habits or environment can set off a migraine. Fluctuations in weather, seasons, altitude, sleeping habits, physical activity, mealtimes, time zones, and personal schedules have all been implicated. Personal habits or patterns, for instance intense activity, or a quick drop-off in activity, moving, a dramatic change in your job, or a personal crisis can set off a migraine. And changing levels of hormones, especially among women, may precipitate an attack.

More unusual forms of migraine include the hemiplegic migraine, which temporarily paralyzes a person on one side of the body for ten minutes to more than an hour before the head pain starts. An ophthalamoplegic migraine centers pain around the eye and usually comes with a droopy eyelid, double vision, and other sight problems. The basilar artery migraine stems from a disturbance of a major brain artery and produces such early signs as vertigo, double vision, and poor muscle coordination. This type, which generally strikes adolescents and young women, is connected to a menstrual cycle. The benign exertion headache is a version stirred up by running, lifting, coughing, sneezing, or bending, and though the pain starts with activity, it doesn't last more than a few minutes. Status migrainosus is a rare form of headache that lasts for days with pain so intense that a person may need to be hospitalized and treated with a combination of medications. Perhaps the most unusual species is the headache-free migraine, which is a collection of migraine symptoms, namely visual problems, nausea, vomiting, and diarrhea, but no head pain.

A Cluster Attack

The cluster headache is one of the fiercest types of head pain and fortunately much rarer th migraine. This headache besets mainly men between the ages of twenty-five and fifty, beginning quickly and stimulating excruciating pain around or behind one eye, often during the night. Though the pain is usually deep and constant, it can also throb, and some men say that sometimes there's the sensation of ice-pick-like pain around the eye. The pain usually stays on one side of the head during a cluster period, although it may switch from one cluster headache to the next. Companion symptoms include runny eyes and stuffy nose, sweating, and paleness. The pain lasts between thirty minutes and three hours, and for most sufferers the pain always comes at the same time of day and frequently happens two or three times a day, hence the tag "cluster." The episodic cluster arises a couple of times a day for a month or two, then usually vanishes for months and occasionally even years. The chronic cluster, on the other hand, doesn't have long periods of remission—it's relentlessly regular.

Although blood vessels are dilated during a cluster headache and feed the pain, vasodilatation is probably the result of some other malfunction and not the root cause. Researchers have noted that cluster headaches disturb circadian rhythms, and so they think that a person's biologic clock may be involved in generating the pain. They also have theorized that the symptoms of a cluster attack could stem from a lesion on one of the main vascular channels of the brain. As with most headaches, clusters may be stimulated by triggers, particularly alcoholic drinks and heavy smoking.

The Rebound Headache

It's a cruel twist of fate that one of the worst sorts of headaches is the direct result of taking too much headache medication. This headache is the offspring of painkillers, like barbiturates, opioids, or over-the-counter analgesics, to which a patient becomes physically dependent. Another common ingredient in these headaches is some form of caffeine, whether it's multiple cups of coffee a day or sipping a soft drink loaded with caffeine all afternoon, every afternoon. Often, rebound headaches afflict someone who's taking regular medication for migraine or tension headache. The headache sufferer becomes trapped in a cycle of daily pain pills for headache; after a few weeks or months of steady consumption, the body grows dependent on the physiological effects. In just three weeks, you can become dependent enough on medication to feel a rebound headache when you stop the medication.

Thus, when the pain reliever wears off, headache returns and more medication is needed to quiet it. Any pain reliever taken more than once a week, whether it's generic aspirin or heavy-duty opioids, can bring on a rebound headache.

THE BIRTH OF THE HEADACHE CLINIC

Given the prevalence of headaches—epidemiologists say that 95 percent of the population has them, and government researchers report that forty-five million Americans experience a chronic variety—it's not surprising that clinics that specialize in treating them have sprouted across the land. Headaches have always attracted their own brand of medicine and unique treatments. Remnants from Stone Age settlements indicate that ancient medicine men used flint tools to cut away part of the skull to relieve pain. Sixth-century Christians cured headaches by pressing their brow against the rail of a saint's tomb. Settlers in the British Isles around A.D. 800 drank concoctions of cow's brain, goat dung, and the juice of elderseed to relieve head pain.

Modern medical professionals first recognized the need for specialized treatment of headaches around the end of World War II as soldiers arrived home with head injuries. In 1945, the first headache clinic was established at the Montefiore Medical Center in the Bronx, New York, but it wasn't until almost twenty years later that the first private headache clinic was created. This treatment center, the Diamond Headache Clinic in Chicago, tilled fertile ground, and since its creation in 1964, hundreds of headache clinics have followed. Headache treatment has become so specialized that often patients are referred from a primary-care doctor, or even a general pain center, to a neurologist or internist specializing in headache management, or to a comprehensive headache center. When I was at Mass General in Boston, I occasionally treated headache patients, particularly unusual cases that hadn't responded to standard remedies. I directed more complex headache cases to my friend Dr. Zahid Bajwa, director of the Headache Center at the Beth Israel Deaconess Hospital on the other side of town.

A neat, precise man born and educated in Pakistan, Dr. Bajwa's medical training is in neurology, with a specialty in headaches and pain management. He completed a residency in neurology at the Montefiore Medical Center, a hospital with one of the premier headache centers. Dr. Bajwa and I first met when we did our fellow-ship in pain medicine together at Mass General. From that time on, he was my first stop whenever I had a patient with difficult headaches. Once we finished our fellowship program and became bona fide pain specialists, I stayed on at Mass General and Dr. Bajwa moved across town to Beth Israel, joining a prestigious group of pain special-ists. "Headaches are fascinating, especially migraines," he declares. "And they're very treatable, although patients tend to be poorly man-aged because most doctors don't know much about them."

Let me take you into his clinic for a behind-the-scenes look at the latest treatments for a wide assortment of headaches. As you read through these cases, you will see how Dr. Bajwa, like the best practi-tioners working today, address the full complexity of headaches, teas-ing out symptoms that mean little harm to the patient from those that may be much more serious.

Every Wednesday, Dr. Bajwa walks from his office to the headache office in the hospital's neurology department, where for six plus hours he sees a steady stream of diverse patients. Generally, patients at the Headache Center have already been seen by a primary physician, a neurologist, and perhaps even a headache or pain specialist, and usu-ally organic causes of their head pain have been eliminated. But with all of his new patients, Dr. Bajwa extracts a full medical history, plus a physical and neurological exam, making few assumptions about what might be causing their pain.

Migraine Without Aura

Dr. Bajwa's first patient of the afternoon is Deborah, a thirty-year-old woman who says that she's been plagued by headaches that began soon after she graduated from college. Healthy in every other way and taking only Excedrin and birth control pills, Deborah describes her head pain as a severe throbbing in both temples, with stabbing pain behind one eye and pain darting down the back of her neck. Dr. Bajwa asks about her family, and she says that neither of her parents have headaches or migraines. She explains that her family life is chaotic and hectic because she is working as a paralegal while going to school at night, and that she and her husband are working extra hard to save money for a house and toward a time when they can afford a child. She extracts from her purse a small diary of the details surrounding her headaches. The record shows that they have become worse in the past two years, coinciding with her going on birth control pills and starting school.

"There's not necessarily a direct relationship between stress and migraines," Dr. Bajwa informs her. "Only about a third of people get migraines when stressed, and some get them at the end of a stressful period. So far, I don't see a clear pattern, here."

Dr. Bajwa gives the Deborah a brief physical and neurological exam, taking her pulse and blood pressure, feeling around her head, neck, and shoulders, examining spine and neck muscles, and checking head and neck arteries. He asks her to walk heel-to-toe, touch her nose with her eyes closed, walk on tiptoe, and walk on her heels. A headache has many possible causes, so he is on the lookout for danger signs indicating a problem with her brain such as a brain mass, a problem with the brain's blood vessels, infection, or a metabolic or systemic problem. Also, he wants to eliminate the possibility that her head pain stems from another condition, such as sinusitis, glaucoma, a compressed optic pathway or mass on the pituitary gland, hemorrhage, some other vascular abnormality or inflammation of an artery, or optic neuritis (inflammation of a nerve).

Deborah tells Dr. Bajwa that the headaches are impinging on much of her life; she hesitates to socialize with friends, knowing one beer can bring on the throbbing, and is afraid of making weekend plans, worrying that a headache could force her to cancel everything. When the headache comes, she's sensitive to light but sees no stars or sparkles. She does feel numbness or tingling, and occasionally throws up. She says that the headache builds for an hour or two, then stays for hours, sometimes days. They appear erratically, sometimes like a painful parade, one after the other, and at other times, only every few months. She tried treating her headache with caffeine and Motrin, but they did little, and though the Excedrin takes off the edge, it does not eradicate the pain.

Fairly soon, Dr. Bajwa feels comfortable in making a diagnosis and tells the young woman that she has a common migraine, without the aura, and that it doesn't seem to be directly related to hormones. However, he cautions that the migraine frequency and severity may well be influenced by stress and environmental triggers. Because her headaches are so frequent, he first suggests a preventative medication. His rule of thumb is that when a patient has more than four headaches a month, some type of medication is needed to halt them before they start. Preventative or prophylactic drugs represent close to half of today's treatment approaches. Doctors and pharmacologists have discovered numerous chemicals that effectively block migraines, even though most of these medications are not typical painkillers. Through clinical studies and trial and error, doctors have found that drugs used for hypertension (beta blockers and calcium channel blockers), nonsteroidal anti-inflammatory drugs, antidepressants, anticonvulsants, and a serotonin inhibitor that is a derivative of ergot help block migraines. Scientists don't know why most of these drugs prevent migraines, and so in deciding which to use, they consider any other conditions a patient may have or other medications she may be taking, then opt for the safest with the fewest side effects.

Dr. Bajwa is partial to calcium channel blockers, like verapamil, nifedipine, and diltiazem, and explains to the woman, "These work for sixty to seventy percent of my patients, and they may be particularly helpful for patients with hormonal or menstrual migraine." He adds that they can cause constipation and warns her to drink lots of fluids to avoid dehydration.

For breakthrough pain, they discuss the relatively new drug that has revolutionized migraine treatment by bringing relief to patients for whom nothing had worked. This drug, from the triptan family, was developed by an English pharmaceutical firm in 1993 and first sold only in an injectable form under the name sumatriptan (Imitrex). The triptans, which effect serotonin activity, are not only fast-acting, halting migraine pain within twenty minutes, but also combat accompanying symptoms like nausea, vomiting, and light sensitivity. And the side effects are usually minimal, mainly dizziness, tingling, a warm sensation, and a light feeling of pressure in the chest (which may be why it isn't advised for people with heart problems or high blood pressure). Since Imitrex came out, other varieties of triptans have come on the market, and manufacturers have devised a pill and nasal form. Three other triptans, zolmitriptan (Zomig), naratriptan (Amerge), and rizatriptan (Maxalt), are also now available in the United States. Although these come only in tablets, their effects last longer than sumatriptan. In prescribing a triptan medication, Dr. Bajwa also advises the patient to combine it with an anti-inflammatory (NSAID) if she finds that the relief does not last. "The problem," he explains, "is that triptans, particularly sumatriptan, have a short half-life, and your headaches last for a long time, so the NSAID may help prolong the relief."

Dr. Bajwa adds one more element to the young woman's treatment program—exercise. "It's a good treatment for migraine," he insists. "It alters your physiology and helps stabilize brain chemicals that may be fueling your attacks. And it boosts your resistance." Any exercise will do, he says, as long as it takes enough effort to break a sweat and produce heavy breathing, and is sustained for twenty minutes or so. "It's *regular* exercise that helps—at least three or four times a week." He also emphasizes that regular daily habits for healthy eating and sleeping can reduce headache frequency.

A Hormonal Migraine

The next patient has been taken into the examination room, and Dr. Bajwa reviews her chart before seeing her. Patricia is a long-standing patient who came to him after years of headaches and failed treatments. In her mid-forties and a single mother, she vividly remembers her first migraine attack around age five as she was sledding behind her home in Michigan. Every bump sent pain crashing into her head. Her physician father fed her a steady diet of analgesics throughout her teen years, which helped contain the severe episodes to two a year. She discovered her personal headache triggers—bright sun, loud noise, exercise, and aged cheese—and arranged her life accordingly. She also found that hers was a family affliction among the women. Her grandmother, mother, and aunt all suffered the same kind of headache, which gained momentum during their twenties, thirties, and early forties, then disappeared with menopause.

Patricia tells Dr. Bajwa that she cannot remember a time when her headaches did not dictate her life. She chuckles over all the money she has spent on sunglasses, which she wears year round. Less amusing is how the headaches have circumscribed her daily activities. In college and throughout her twenties, fear of a headache attack limited her social life. She didn't go to outdoor sporting events because the sun might be bright, and she avoided consuming alcohol or going to bars or restaurants that could be noisy. After college, she wisely chose a profession where the surroundings would be quiet and away from direct sunlight: She became a librarian. As she moved into her thirties, the migraines gained momentum, coming three or four times a month, then accelerating to three or four a week as she turned forty.

Over the years, Patricia experimented with any treatment that hinted at relief. She checked into a world-renowned headache clinic that focused on intensive group-therapy sessions. But it had little impact on her headaches, and she left after three weeks. She learned biofeedback and for a year diligently regulated her skin temperature; yet again, the headaches persisted. She visited an acupuncturist, a chiropractor, and a stress reduction clinic, all without success. Open to any possible remedy, no matter how unconventional and unproven, she took regular doses of the herb feverfew. It helped for a short while, then its effect faded. She consulted with a hypnotist who told her that she was not a good candidate because she had a hard time focusing her thoughts.

In Dr. Bajwa she found a headache specialist willing to reach into a varied and complex bag of medication options and readily switch when one loses its effectiveness. He is also comfortable with encouraging his patients to seek out other therapies he cannot deliver. Since her first visit, Dr. Bajwa's treatment plan for the librarian has been two-pronged: prevention and cutting the headaches off when they flare up. He started her on an antidepressant, amitriptyline (Elavil), not because he thought she was depressed but because the drug alters the activity of brain chemicals that play a part in migraines. For two years, the drug worked well, although Dr. Bajwa had to gradually increase the dose to hold off the migraines.

This afternoon's visit is relatively short as Patricia and Dr. Bajwa talk about fine-tuning doses. They discuss the preventative drug that she's now taking, another antidepressant, doxepin (Sinequan), and notching up the dosage. The medication she's using for breakthrough pain, Tylenol with codeine, is barely keeping the pain in check, and, although sumatriptan did little for her, she wonders whether the new generation of triptans coming out will help. She tried Maxalt tablets, which worked better than the Imitrex and lasted longer. Although she and Dr. Bajwa acknowledge that the best solution may come with age and menopause, they agree that it may help to consult a neuroendocrinologist knowledgeable about migraines and possible hormone therapies.

Tension-Type Headache

Most people do not seek out medical help for tension headaches, preferring over-the-counter remedies, which work remarkably well. But occasionally, a patient's tension headaches are more complicated and more persistent than the predictable head pain that precedes a crash deadline or follows a stressful meeting. Dr. Bajwa's next patient is Bill, a man in his forties, a police detective whose headache is written across his face. His left eye droops, and his mouth and eyes tighten as he talks. This is his monthly visit to Dr. Bajwa, and he says his head hurts worse than ever. The first thing the headache doctor notices is the asymmetry in the detective's face. He suggests that Bill dig up an old photo of himself and compare it with his present image to see how dramatic the change might be. Although Dr. Bajwa has not found any neurological abnormalities, he advises the detective to call him or go to an emergency room if his face changes dramatically or he develops any neurological symptoms.

The policeman's headaches started after his retina was damaged in a fight during an arrest. The eye pain after that fight prompted his primary doctor to do an MRI scan, which revealed a tumor. Since the diagnosis, he's been off work with head and eye pain and embroiled in a lawsuit with the police department over who's responsible for his disability pay.

"This week is not going well," Bill tells Dr. Bajwa. "I've had a bad couple of days—my son is sick and I've got this strange feeling in my head. It's not quite pain but feels like a really tight police hat." When the pain strikes, he takes Percocet and a serotonin-modifying antidepressant and escapes to a dark, quiet room. Dr. Bajwa asks whether the physical therapy he recommended has had any effect. He had suggested that the officer do structured exercise at least three times a week, not only as a way to relieve the anxiety over returning to work but also to help him shed a few pounds. Dressed in baggy sweat pants and sweatshirt, Bill says that he has gained weight, which has added to his stress. He admits that he exercised for a few weeks, but stopped when he started to feel better.

Dr. Bajwa asks more questions about the medications the detective is taking. From other patients with tension headaches, he's deduced that the rebound effect, particularly from acetaminophen, is a large part of the pain. His suspicion gains ground when Bill says that he's been on a steady diet of Percocet, which is a combination of an opioid and acetaminophen. Dr. Bajwa explains rebound headaches, particularly the role of acetaminophen hidden in other medications. The policeman agrees to taper off his Percocet consumption, especially when Dr. Bajwa assures him that there are other equal potent drugs available that don't contain acetaminophen. Yet he cautions Bill that regardless of which pain reliever he takes, he'll have to pare back the frequency.

They work out a schedule for reducing his medications, while Dr. Bajwa also tells him that he believes his headaches will improve when his job situation is resolved and his daily stresses, like feeling over-weight and worrying about his family, ease up. And the doctor impresses on him the need to keep up the physical therapy workouts and suggests a biofeedback program for relaxation and stress management.

Rebound and Tension Headaches

Dr. Bajwa has not seen the next patient for six months and is eager to hear how she is doing. Cece originally came to him with a mixture of headaches that appeared a couple of times a week and sent her to bed with severe fatigue and nausea. Her body language on this visit tells him that not much has improved. She sits clutching her purse in her lap, almost doubled over, and looks pale and haggard. Since she last saw him, she relates, her life has taken a turn for the worse. Both her parents have died, and she has been saddled with the complicated job of executing their estate. Furthermore, she has left her live-in boyfriend, who had become abusive, and is camping out on a friend's couch. And, she has quit her job.

Cece's first complaint is about sleep. "I'm not sleeping very well, though I'm in bed a lot, reading novels or watching videos," she says. "Maybe I'm depressed," she adds. The doctor suggests that perhaps her problem is too much sleep or taking medications at the wrong time of day. She reports that her headaches move around her head, sometimes encircling it and sometimes lodging around one temple. Knowing that she is seeing other doctors, Dr. Bajwa asks what med-ications she is taking, and she recites a long list, beginning with blood pressure medication, asthma medication, an antidepressant (Paxil), estrogen, Tylenol with codeine, Fioricet, and Saint-John's-wort. Some of these drugs, she tells him, help relax her.

Dr. Bajwa asks her to stand up so he can exam her head and neck. He gently feels around her shoulders and neck, probing for tight mus-cles. He explains what he thinks is happening to her and offers a treat-ment plan. "We need to sort out the issues here—your sleep problems, the depression, and the muscle tension," he announces, implying that each requires separate attention. "Some of your sleep difficulty may be because you're taking the Paxil at night, which in some patients can cause insomnia. This change alone could make a difference." For tension, he strongly recommends physical therapy and stress reduction, and he refers her to a physical therapist and psychologist, key members of the doctor's comprehensive headache team. He pointedly does not add to her medications but declares the he would like to reduce the number of drugs she is taking. "Pills won't solve all our problems," he concludes.

He believes that her headaches may be getting worse because of a rebound effect. Over the months, Cece has gradually taken more and more Fioricet with codeine, which is a combination of a barbiturate, caffeine, acetaminophen, and an opioid. He explains how over time her body has become tolerant and that as the drugs wear off, a headache returns and demands a larger dose to quell it. Her problem is probably compounded by multiple medications that overlap in their effects. Almost any analgesic, including most over-the-counter medications, can produce this rebound effect, and the solution is to lower the dose gradually, reduce the number of drugs she's taking, and find longer-acting drugs. Furthermore, he recommends that she should consolidate her doctors and let just one prescribe her medications. By the end of the appointment, the tense woman is sitting more relaxed and occasionally smiling. She wants to be on fewer medications, and Dr. Bajwa's non-drug suggestions clearly fit with her aims.

The Awful Cluster Headache

Toward the end of the afternoon, Robert, a middle-aged construction worker who has combated cluster headaches for twenty years, steps into Dr. Bajwa's office. Like many chronic headache sufferers, he vividly remembers the first attack. It was summertime, he was thirty-five years old, and he had left work early with a headache, for which he took aspirin. "It might as well have been a sugar pill for all the good it did." The headache stayed with him not only for that day but the entire week, the pain stretching from his right eyebrow to his jaw and into his teeth and neck. He became hypersensitive to light as well as touch or sound—even a brush against his hair hurt.

His wife, a nurse, urged him to see a doctor immediately, and the physician quickly diagnosed the awful cluster headache. He and his pain fit the classic profile: male and a heavy smoker, with the headache appearing suddenly at night on one side of his head and coming in bunches or clusters, generally during the warm, summer months. His headaches were frequently triggered by alcohol, especially red wine—"That was like throwing fuel on a pilot light," Robert says—as well as Chinese food laced with monosodium glutamate. For a year or so, the headaches came like clockwork, hitting him every week or so at almost exactly 10:55 P.M. Although his doctor knew full well what was happening to Robert, he could offer no truly effective treatment, and the suffering construction worker was left with home remedies.

Each time a headache came on, Robert got out of bed, put a cold facecloth over the most painful part of his head, made a pot of hot coffee and dry toast, took a Sudafed for his clogged sinuses, which always played a part in the headache, and went outside, coffee and toast in hand, to pace around the yard. The pain was often so bad he yelled and screamed, and he still marvels that the neighbors never complained about the barefooted man raging in the middle of the night in the backyard.

His wife urged him to experiment with painkillers. He tried an assortment of opioids—Demerol, Dilaudid, morphine, Percocet, Fioricet, Tylenol with codeine, and Stadol nasal spray—and found that they affected him about as much as drinking a Coca-Cola. The opioids just made the pain worse because they raised his expectations, then failed. Other medications that came and went with little impact, or intolerable side effects, included anti-inflammatories, both nonsteroidal and steroids, anticonvulsants, and hypertension medication.

Until two years ago, Robert floated from doctor to doctor, trying their remedies, feeling no relief, and seeking out yet another treatment. The first drug that halted his headache pain was an injection of sumatriptan. Within ten to fifteen minutes of a shot of Imitrex, the pain faded, although it did not completely disappear. Robert at last had a drug for breakthrough headache pain, but he needed more. When he sought out Dr. Bajwa, who was recommended by a friend, Robert desperately wanted to find a drug to complement the sumatriptan that would prevent the clusters from occurring.

In his first visit with Dr. Bajwa, they talked about the drugs Robert had been taking and the adjustments he had made to his daily life—

particularly the foods he avoided—in order to forestall a headache. He pulled from his jacket a two-page list his wife had prepared of all the drugs and doses he had taken over the years. One of his first questions to the headache doctor was, "Why me?" Dr. Bajwa had no answers to that one. Cluster headaches do not run in families or appear more frequently with any particular ethnic group or beset people who are highly stressed. The only qualifier seems to be middle age and male. Dr. Bajwa put Robert on two medications to help prevent the clusters: a calcium channel blocker (verapamil) and lithium (Eskalith), a drug prescribed mainly for manic depression that has a twenty-year track record in clinical trials of preventing chronic clusters.

On this visit, Robert is in good spirits. It has been almost seven months since his last headache, and though he's afraid of tempting fate and announcing that he's cured, he's very hopeful that he will make it through the coming summer months without a headache attack. In truth, this visit is mainly a quick checkup and an opportunity for Robert to renew his prescriptions. Dr. Bajwa considers Robert to be one of his great successes and an example of what experienced headache doctors can accomplish.

HOPE FOR HEADACHE SUFFERERS

The pharmacology of headache treatments has been gaining steady momentum since the development of triptans. Second-generation triptans are already producing even more wondrous results. What's special about these drugs is that they're like a bouncer in a rough bar—when a fight, or headache, breaks out, they're on the spot to halt any further hostilities. Unlike many migraine medications that work only if they're taken when early signs appear, these drugs can stop a fully launched headache cold. And the new generation of drugs help reduce nausea and a patient's sensitivity to light and sound, all without sedation. They don't work for everyone, but for some they are a miracle. One newcomer to the triptan family, rizatriptan (Maxalt) has an ingenious delivery system. It's available in wafer form and dissolves on the tongue within seconds. This is particularly helpful to migraine sufferers who may not like having to need a glass of water to take their medication.

Lately, patients have been asking me about the herb feverfew, which has been shown to be of some help. The problem with herbs is usually twofold: There are few, if any, controlled studies of these substances, and what few studies exist are not well designed. Doctors at the University of Exeter in the United Kingdom recently reviewed all the studies of feverfew they could locate and concluded that while feverfew appears to work better than a placebo, its effectiveness for treating migraine remains in doubt.

Herbal remedies in general are potentially strong medicines. Most strong remedies that come from plants and herbs are just crude forms of drugs. And yet, I never automatically reject a treatment simply because there's no hard data backing it up. There are many treatments that work wonders even though scientists do not understand why. As you'll read in the next chapter, many so-called alternative treatments may work in mysterious ways and yet can be powerful pain relievers.

10

THERAPIES THAT CHALLENGE
THE LIMITS OF SCIENCE

*Acupuncture, Trigger Point Injections,
Hypnosis, and Behavioral Therapies*

> Take care of the sense, and the sounds will take care of
> themselves.
>
> —LEWIS CARROLL

Because I am a physician grounded in the scientific tradition, believing things that I can't prove doesn't come easily. So convincing myself of the power of the mind has sometimes been an uphill climb. But in a world where we understand only a fraction of the mystery of life, we are all faced with a universal dilemma of what to believe. Believing only what is completely proven leaves a limited perspective on a vastly complex world. Believing everything on faith is not much better. In medicine, gray is far more common than black or white, and distinguishing what is real from what is bogus is one of the great challenges for patients and physicians.

If medicine were perfect, there would not be "alternative" treatments—conventional therapies would suffice. But medicine is not perfect, and its success often relies on supporting the body's own healing powers. Any treatment that boosts our ability to heal ourselves can help overcome an illness. That is why I have adopted a pragmatic approach of harnessing any treatment that is safe and effective. I try to be critical of what I do not know, but also careful to avoid judgment until I'm certain. In my business, I'm rarely certain. So I have learned to suspend disbelief. While I'd *like* to know exactly why something works, I don't *need* to know. If I did, I'd be left with a very limited arsenal.

My first lesson in the power of alternative treatments for pain was when I was in college and traveling through Europe for the summer. Being on a student's allowance, I lugged around a heavy backpack and spent my days sitting on the hard seats of third-class railway cars and nights sleeping on saggy, lumpy beds. It probably was inevitable that one morning I would wake up with back pain. Despite being young and healthy, one day my low back went into painful spasm, hunching me over like an old man. I could barely dress myself, and walking any distance was impossible. In the middle of Switzerland and desperate for relief, I visited the local pharmacy and consumed large amounts of aspirin, acetaminophen, and all other over-the-counter remedies that I thought might help. But nothing brought me relief.

Like millions of other pain sufferers, my desperation made me more open than usual to experimentation. I readily accepted the advice of a local resident whose back pain had been successfully treated with acupuncture. She gave me the name of a Chinese immigrant who practiced in his home, and I appeared at his small apartment shuffling slowly and unable to stand up straight. It was a secretive place. At that time, acupuncture wasn't a legal treatment in Switzerland, and the practitioner was careful to explain that he was not charging for this work but would accept a cash gift. The treatment consisted of his placing thin needles on various points of my body including my back, legs, feet, and ears. He explained that this would stimulate and correct my personal energy field, my "chi." It took about forty-five minutes, and after he removed the needles, I lay on his couch for a few minutes recovering. When I was ready to leave, I stood up straight for the first time in days, and I left his place a little sore but upright and mobile. My pain was not cured as much as diminished, but all I knew was that I could get on with my travels. This was my introduction to alternative medicine. As I suspect is true of many pain sufferers, I was willing to try a treatment I did not understand, even one that reputedly reorganized mysterious, intangible "energy fields."

"Alternative" medicine encompasses more than unconventional or non-Western therapies. It's the realm of medicine that ventures beyond double-blind controlled studies into areas of human health that appear to defy rigorous, scientific investigation. Given that chronic pain is such an elusive and all-encompassing ailment, understanding how every treatment works is not possible. Many standard therapies in the pain arsenal are far from proven.

The therapies you'll read about here have shown success with easing chronic pain and repairing its collateral damage—even though we can't always explain why or how they work. Most of these are well-established treatments that offer either physical remedies for pain-induced disabilities or psychological approaches to reducing the impact of suffering and improving daily function. Unfortunately, many of these effective techniques are often applied only after more standard therapies have failed and much time has passed.

LOOSENING TRIGGER POINTS: MYOFASCIAL PAIN

Nancy Chang is a woman in her fifties who came into the Pain Center racked by muscle aches, fatigue, and depression so bleak that it had turned her life upside down. She had a constellation of disorders, many of which sprang from the extreme physical discomfort of the musculoskeletal syndrome known as myofascial pain. Although cause and effect are often impossible to untangle, her fatigue, achiness, and extreme muscle tenderness had forced her to stop work as a school-bus driver and plunged her into depression, hallmarks of a pain syndrome that has become a modern epidemic.

The exact number of patients with myofascial pain is hard to come by for a variety of reasons, especially because of the countless undiagnosed and misdiagnosed cases. One group of physicians has reported that about 30 percent of their pain patients showed symptoms and that myofascial pain was the most common reason patients came to them for treatment. For reasons doctors do not understand, myofascial pain attacks many more women than men and is concentrated in women ages twenty to sixty.

For years, controversy has swirled around this syndrome. This is largely because it is really a hodgepodge of symptoms characterized by mild to extreme discomfort emanating from skeletal muscles and soft tissue almost anywhere in the body. Although sometimes called myofascial pain or fibromyalgia, the condition also encompasses other disorders, including temporomandibular joint pain (TMJ). Historically, the condition has been given various medical labels: muscle hardening, muscular rheumatism, fibrositis, myofascitis, myogelosis, and interstitial myofibroitis. Some of Hippocrates' writings describe what sounds like myofascial pain, but only in the past hundred years or so have doctors identified this condition as a distinct entity. The terms myofascial pain and fibromyalgia are often used interchangeably, but they are not identical twins. Myofascial pain is the umbrella term, and fibromyalgia is a specific variety that encompasses widespread symptoms in muscles throughout the body.

The centerpiece of myofascial pain is trigger points—small areas of muscle that cause pain in a distant area when pressed. They are often associated with tender, hard knots within muscle tissue but are not always tender. Trigger points and tender points are often confused, but they are not the same thing.

As with many pain conditions, there are no laboratory tests to diagnose myofascial pain. For years, patients have been complaining to doctors about achy pain in their muscles that comes and goes, moves around their bodies, and produces fatigue. Yet the shifting character, seemingly vague symptoms that come and go, and undetectable causes have confounded successful treatment.

In 1990, doctors took a great step toward quieting the debate. For the first time, the American College of Rheumatology set forth specific diagnostic criteria for myofascial's enigmatic offspring, fibromyalgia. To be diagnosed with fibromyalgia, a patient must have widespread pain and clear signs of muscle tenderness at eleven of eighteen specifically identified spots on the body. The scientist who first identified these clumps within muscle described them as feeling like "rubbery Rice Krispies." Lodged within a taut band of muscle or neighboring tissue, they are tight knots. When pressed, they're usually tender, and when pressed hard, they may cause the whole muscle to twitch or a person to flinch, which is known as a jump sign. They frequently congregate in one area of the body, such as in a neck, shoulder, or back, and radiate discomfort to neighboring muscles. If you have had occasional knots in your muscles, like a kink in the neck, you may have had what's considered latent trigger points because they can radiate pain but quickly disappear.

The underlying cause of trigger points is frequently a mystery. They can crop up after an injury or disease, or from repetitive motion, like lots of lifting or a repeated sports motion. Or, for no apparent reason, areas in muscle or connective tissues or at the junction of bone and tendon suddenly or slowly become sensitive to pressure. This is what happened to Nancy. She could not recollect what, if anything, had stirred the first pains, but she had discernible tender areas. These spots clustered in her upper body, not in the eighteen places identified by the rheumatologists. She had myofascial pain, and I swiftly referred her to Dr. Joseph Audette, a specialist in physical medicine and rehabilitation (physiatry) who treats myofascial pain with a technique known as trigger point injections.

Dr. Audette's primary bases of operations are Spaulding Rehabilitation Hospital and an outpatient program outside Boston where he serves as medical director. Like Nancy, more than half of his patients have suffered from myofascial pain for at least six months. Many have been on a merry-go-round of doctors and treatments such as nerve blocks, massages, electrical stimulation, and ultrasound, to no avail. Dr. Audette offers a procedure called dry needling. "I'm confident that I can make a difference with just one treatment," he declares, and his track record bears this out.

Finding and feeling the trigger points of myofascial pain requires experienced, sensitive hands. The source of pain in a muscle can be hard to pinpoint. Tender spots resonate when pressed on but do not radiate pain down muscles or limit motion. At some time, each of us can find such spots in tired or sore muscles. However, trigger points, which are not only tender but also radiate pain to distant muscles, are much harder to detect. Doctors unaccustomed to this kind of pain may well lack the touch. But during both a cursory physical exam and later a thorough, time-consuming scrutiny, Dr. Audette readily sorted the trigger points from the tender spots. In his initial exam of Nancy, he traced her pain to her shoulders, neck, and upper back, and gently pressed muscles, asking her how it felt. Among other things, he was looking to see whether the discomfort was on one side or both, knowing that myofascial trigger points are often one-sided.

Nancy was in a hospital gown for the next part of the exam. Although fifteen minutes had passed since Dr. Audette first located and pressed on her trigger points, he noticed that the areas were still red, yet another sign that pain nerves had been abnormally activated. Now he focused on individual points, quickly releasing his fingers across the muscle and causing it to twitch. Dr. Audette considers the twitch response, which results from a single motor unit and is impossible for an individual to voluntarily control, definitive for trigger points.

During my initial evaluation, I decided that Nancy was a good candidate for Dr. Audette's treatment because she met two basic criteria: She had myofascial pain, and the trigger points were clearly radiating pain outward. She also could tolerate being examined, which meant she could likely bear the trigger point injections. Some patients suffering from myofascial pain can barely stand to be touched; for these people, the needling technique inflicts too much distress.

During the treatment Nancy lay facedown on an examination bed. Dr. Audette wanted her muscles as relaxed as possible; otherwise he would have a difficult time penetrating their tense fibers. He identified five or six trigger points and swabbed each area with alcohol. With fingers poised on each side of a spot, he pinched a small fold of skin and inserted a fine needle. The needles he uses are very thin, but not especially long, acupuncture needles. His technique, dry needling, means that he does not inject anything such as the local anesthetic agent that many other practitioners use. He uses the needle as a tool instead of a delivery system.

Soon after the needle broke the skin in Nancy's shoulder, the muscle twitched, confirming he was in the right place. He slowly pressed the needle, knowing by feel when it reached the muscle's fibrous coating. Once he was on the mark, he gently tapped the needle with a pecking motion. As the muscles twitched and he manipulated the needle, Nancy lay quiet, except for an occasional gasp or brief moan. Dr. Audette offered soothing reassurance as he proceeded, keeping in constant communication with Nancy, telling her each time he found a trigger point.

For Nancy, this was the best and worst part of the treatment. The good part came from the muscle, which went into uncontrollable convulsions, then gradually became exhausted and finally relaxed. Dr. Audette could feel through the needle when the muscle had spent itself and become quiet and supple. The trigger point had been dissolved temporarily, if not permanently. At this point in the treatment, it's not unusual for a patient to feel such an emotional release with the relaxation of a tormenting muscle that she cries. The downside of the process was that it hurt. The rapid muscle contractions along with the release of chemicals in the muscle produced pain that lasted throughout the procedure. Nancy said that the pain felt like a knuckle pressed into a muscle knot to break it up, but much worse. Dr. Audette asked her how she was doing and whether she could bear more needles. She nodded, and Dr. Audette slid another needle into a new trigger point and began the procedure again. Nancy received the full treatment, which consisted of placing and manipulating needles in six places. After they were inserted and the muscles spent themselves by contracting and relaxing, he left the needles in place for fifteen minutes while Nancy dozed and tried to relax.

The pain relief from this procedure was not instant. Nancy's muscles felt sore, as if she had just completed a strenuous workout at the gym. As the soreness receded over the next three or four hours, the pain relief was profound. Soreness and tension vanished, and for perhaps the first time in many months, Nancy could move, sit, and sleep pain free. However, Dr. Audette advised her to take it easy for a few days and keep her muscles relaxed. The twitching had exhausted them, so strenuous exercise, like working out with weights or heavy lifting, as well as massage, could send her muscles into spasm.

Dr. Audette's dry-needling treatment usually involves six to ten sessions. Patients are strongly advised to combine his treatment with physical therapy to improve body mechanics that can contribute to or result from the problem. Although many of his patients suffered an injury or trauma that precipitated their pain, a good portion developed the pain from some repetitive motion.

A complementary treatment to Dr. Audette's procedure is known as spray-and-stretch. Instead of a needle, this treatment employs a coolant sprayed on the muscle to relax a trigger point. After applying the coolant, the doctor gradually elongates the muscle in order to pull out the knots and, slowly, extend the muscle over its full, normal range of motion. Another new development in treating myofascial pain is injections of the chemical botulinum toxin, also known as Botox. Botox has been receiving attention lately because it's an extremely safe neuromuscular relaxant used by plastic surgeons to smooth facial wrinkles. In theory, Botox may help relieve myofascial pain and has the advantage over injections of local anesthetics of providing long-lasting pain relief of up to three months. Although Botox is a promising treatment, its not yet been fully studied for myofascial pain.

THE WONDERS OF NEEDLING

If Dr. Audette's dry needling reminds you of acupuncture, you're not far off the mark. He's the first to acknowledge that his technique belongs in the same universe as the ancient Chinese healing practice and believes that acupuncture may have originally aimed at eradicating trigger points. While acupuncture is a long-standing member of the alternative medicine clan, it has become widely accepted by conventional practitioners. The U.S. Food and Drug Administration has approved and now regulates acupuncture needles, as it does all medical devices. The National Institutes of Health has deemed the procedure to be effective for various types of pain and discomfort. The ultimate sign of acceptance for this treatment comes from the private sector: Some insurance companies and health maintenance organizations now reimburse for acupuncture. So it should come as no surprise that many of the country's leading pain centers, including my former pain center at Massachusetts General Hospital, now offer acupuncture treatment.

As a treatment, acupuncture occupies the hazy ground between time-tested, well-documented medical practices and poorly understood, almost magical ancient powers. The prospect of combining modern empirical medicine and a traditional healing art is what appeals to Mass General's acupuncturist, Dr. May Pian-Smith. She is a thoughtful, soft-spoken anesthesiologist who seems to glide between the formal medical specialty of anesthesiology and the vaguer boundaries of acupuncture therapy. While anchored in the hospital's obstetrics unit, where she delivers anesthesia for childbirth, Dr. Pian-Smith ventures to the Pain Center at least once a week to apply acupuncture to patients with all sorts of conditions.

Patients who come to the Pain Center for acupuncture may have a solitary problem or a host of complaints, and frequently they have a long history of treatments and procedures. Many are well acquainted with chronic pain and hope acupuncture can achieve what other therapies have not, while also freeing them from medication. And they know that it has very little downside. It's minimally invasive, quite safe, and produces no side effects other than a tired feeling. (Dr. Pian-Smith says it feels like jet lag.) If acupuncture has any drawbacks, it's that patients often decide that they don't want to mix it with other treatments or drugs. So, they may inadvertently deprive themselves of other effective treatments and suffer more in order to give acupuncture a fair trial.

Acupuncture is not a panacea, and Dr. Pian-Smith applies her needles mostly to particular types of chronic pain, namely musculoskeletal pain like arthritis, backache, myofascial pain, some neuropathic pain, and cancer pain and chemotherapy symptoms, especially nausea. She devotes a considerable amount of time to patients before treatment, familiarizing herself with their personality as well as their medical profile. Each patient completes a detailed questionnaire, covering symptoms and conditions plus a variety of personal traits spanning food preferences and temperament. The answers sketch a mosaic of specific symptoms and individual traits, what Eastern practitioners refer to as "yin" and "yang" qualities.

During this first session, Dr. Pian-Smith answers patient questions, one of which is inevitably about how acupuncture works. Despite her training in China, as well as her position on the faculty of Harvard Medical School, Dr. Pian-Smith freely acknowledges the uncertainties and skepticism surrounding this treatment. Scientists do not know the secret of acupuncture. So far, they have only a partial, disjointed picture of how it works. The theories include stimulating endorphins; prodding the hypothalamus and pituitary glands into action; altering immune activity; changing the flow of neurotransmitters, neurohormones, and blood; inducing distraction; and the placebo response. As all these theories suggest, inserting and manipulating tiny needles generates some kind of biological changes, but the full picture remains obscure.

Nevertheless, Dr. Pian-Smith has seen acupuncture ease pain time and again. She estimates that about 75 percent of her patients get some form of relief. Even patients whose pain is only slightly diminished say that they move more easily, need less medication, and sleep and feel better. Her usual course of treatment consists of five or six needling sessions, although patients who improve generally do so around the second or third visit. Occasionally, there's a lag between the needling and relief.

Dr. Pian-Smith's treatment of Ms. Babb, a forty-year-old woman whose knee was crippled in a car accident, illustrates both the potential and limits of acupuncture. This college teacher came to Dr. Pian-Smith after physical therapy and home remedies were unsuccessful at returning her to pain-free walking and swimming. An active woman who once enjoyed long hikes and daily laps at the Y, Ms. Babb decided on her own to veer away from conventional treatments and seek out acupuncture. The fact that her HMO would cover part of the cost was an added inducement.

Acupuncture treatments at the Pain Center are administered in the block rooms. Like all patients going through some type of invasive therapy, Ms. Babb slipped into a hospital gown and was prepped for a sterile procedure. Dr. Pian-Smith asked her to lie on her side, with her back exposed, so that she could insert tiny needles into her lower back, the back of her knee, and in her ankle—that is, along what the Chinese call meridians. Meridians are thought to be the highways of energy traffic that acupuncture redirects. They indicate where needles should be inserted in order to alter specific bodily systems.

Once the needles are in place, some type of energy must be applied to them. They can be rotated by hand, stimulated with electricity, or activated by burning a substance called moxibustion. The Chinese emperor who devised acupuncture thousands of years ago believed that a unique energy force—called "qi" and pronounced "chee"—travels along channels in the body and regulates its health and activity. They are like nerve pathways, although they do not follow the same paths. The body's energy, acupuncturists believe, can be stimulated by inserting needles along these meridians. The Chinese identified 365 points as pivotal, and over the ages, practitioners in Korea, Japan, and elsewhere have found other acupoints, which now total around 1,500. However, there is no agreement among acupuncturists as to the best points to change specific bodily processes, making comparisons and studies of various practices almost impossible. Similarly, techniques used in inserting needles and stimulating qi have been refined and modified, so there is no standard method. As a result, acupuncture is not a single, codified science—rather, it is a healing art that each practitioner administers differently.

In treating Ms. Babb, Dr. Pian-Smith used a combination of techniques, applying the needles to Chinese acupoints and employing a French technique of using mild electric current to stimulate the needles. After inserting the needles, she attached an electrode to each, emitting a slight tingle. Once the needles and electrodes were in place, Dr. Pian-Smith asked Ms. Babb to lie still for twenty minutes. She turned down the lights and left the room.

At the end of the treatment, Dr. Pian-Smith detached the electrodes, removed the needles, then rubbed the insertion points. "The theory is that we've added energy," she explained, "and we don't want it to escape so I rub the hole." Ms. Babb dozed throughout most of the therapy, and afterward felt relaxed. As she walked down the hospital stairs, she noticed that her knee moved more easily. She says that after her first treatment, she was able to walk to work for the first time in a almost a year. Ms. Babb is firmly convinced that her acupuncture treatments have restored some of her mobility and have warded off the stiff encroachment of osteoarthritis.

While Western scientists do not understand how acupuncture can reduce pain and make the body feel better, they acknowledge its power by investing substantial time and money in trying to find out how it works. Although some continue to believe that all or part of acupuncture's therapeutic benefits are due to the placebo effect, the fact that acupuncture can be effective with certain animals, notably dogs with hip dysplasia, appears to belie the placebo explanation. One of the theories for why acupuncture diminishes pain is the notion of distraction. The needles may be creating sensations that compete with, and triumph over, pain signals. While I don't think this is the major reason for acupuncture's effects, distraction as a form of treatment has a firm place in the pain medicine arsenal. Shifting a patient's focus away from the source of suffering can help alleviate it—athletes, such as marathon runners who "psych" themselves out of pain, do this all the time. Reducing the magnification of pain by redirecting focus away from it can have potent beneficial effects and is part of the rationale for a number of treatments.

The Power of Concentration: Hypnosis

Ever since Anton Mesmer, the eighteenth-century Swiss doctor, asked patients to hold a metal bar anchored in a tub filled with iron filings to treat nervous disorders and physical ailments, scientists have been fascinated by hypnotism. Originally regarded as a parlor trick and entertainment, hypnotism today is the subject of constant scientific scrutiny and gradual acceptance by the medical establishment and public. As with acupuncture, the absence of firm scientific understanding of how it mutes or halts pain sensation has relegated it to the realm of an alternative therapy. Yet its efficacy has been appreciated for much longer than many newer treatments.

Even though medicine does not have a clear picture of what a hypnotic trance does to pain signals, it has abundant evidence of its power to subdue pain. It can be particularly effective with an assortment of acute and post-op pains, and there are countless cases of it being used as the sole anesthesia during surgery, including brain surgery, tooth removal, thyroid removal, heart surgery, appendix removal, and Cesarean section, as well as to soothe burn patients as dressings are changed.

There are numerous reports of hypnotism saving the day after conventional treatment has been futile. A dramatic case involved the patient of my colleague, Dr. Anna Holmgren, a psychiatrist who was treating a woman named Barbara for severe depression and anxiety. Barbara's serious medical problems, including blindness and neuropathic pain from diabetes, frequently landed her in the hospital. She was well known to all of the nurses on the inpatient floor, and her many problems resulted in her taking multiple medications, all of which helped, but at the price of debilitating side effects. Her fragile health required constant medical attention and frequent adjustments in her medications. This time, she was hospitalized for a flare-up of abdominal pain. While in the hospital, she deteriorated. Diabetes not only caused her pain but also injured the nerves in her gut, slowing down the normal digestive action, a disorder called diabetic gastroparesis. This condition, plus narcotic pain medication, had caused so much constipation that her bowels became distended. She was in grave danger. Changing her pain medication and a constant infusion of laxatives had no effect. Her bowels were shut down. Barbara believed she was dying, and all of her doctors were walking a tightrope; cutting back on pain medication helped the bowel obstruction but left Barbara in agony. They tried every conceivable pain reliever, but either her bowels or her fragile kidneys would rebel. She hadn't slept in days and was a picture of misery.

Dr. Holmgren knew Barbara well, and they shared a degree of trust that allowed another option. She asked Barbara if she was willing to try hypnosis. As she explained, "It's like taking a familiar drive, during which you get lost in thoughts far removed from driving, but still arrive safe and sound at your destination." Barbara's extreme distress surely made it tough to focus away from her pain, so Dr. Holmgren was not optimistic that she could be hypnotized. She started by asking Barbara to close her eyes, even though she was blind, and picture her favorite place. Dr. Holmgren figured that, at best, this soothing exercise would help the exhausted woman relax. She told her to imagine this favorite place, which for Barbara was a beach, and to sense everything about it—the wind on her face, the sand between her toes, the briny smell of salt water.

Dr. Holmgren watched as her breathing slowed and became deeper, and her facial muscles, which had been twisted into a grimace, smoothed. Throughout, Dr. Holmgren asked the patient how she was feeling, and although she made no suggestions about a trance or dropping into a deep sleep, Barbara's head gradually drooped and she fell asleep. Dr. Holmgren stayed for a while, relieved that for the first time in many days, Barbara was able to sleep.

The next morning, Dr. Holmgren checked in with Barbara's nurse. The nurse reported that Barbara slept through the night, and like a triumphant sign from the heavens, awoke in the morning and had a bowel movement. Her pain was decreased, her bowel functioned, and she was out of danger.

Studies of people in hypnotic trances reveal altered brain waves. According to one theory, trance states activate regions of the brain that impede pain. Another notion is that it "disconnects" pain sensations from the mind's "receiving antennae." We simply do not know how hypnosis works, and such theories are far from proven. Despite the uncertainties about how it works, doctors who use hypnotism to treat pain have particular ideas about how it's best set in motion.

Not everyone is susceptible to being hypnotized. Dr. Maxwell Shapiro, a prominent psychologist and hypnotherapist at Massachusetts General Hospital, has found that people with higher intelligence and active imaginations that enable them to become absorbed in a movie, book, or activity are the most receptive. When treating someone with chronic pain, Dr. Shapiro looks for two other traits: their ability to form an alliance with him and their motivation. By alliance, he means their willingness to trust his skill and experience to guide them toward a hypnotic state and even to suspend any disbelief they may have about the treatment. Motivation is a patient's desire to break out of his pattern of pain. For instance, Dr. Shapiro is less optimistic if a patient is involved in litigation over his condition because any change in his condition has consequences outside his health. Someone suffering from an awful burn may be eager for relief and so becomes highly motivated. When treating someone with chronic pain, he asks about any previous success with overcoming a physical challenge, since the patient may be able to transfer such skills to the problem at hand.

Putting a patient into a trance is not complicated. Dr. Shapiro uses only his voice—no whirling gadgets, beams of light, or shiny objects. One reason he works gadget free is that he wants patients to ultimately be able to drop into a trance on their own without his cues. When a person is in a trance, he or she feels psychologically and physically different, and Dr. Shapiro repeatedly asks patients to be aware of what their trance feels like. "Hypnosis changes the way you experience the world and your body," he declares. He wants them to be able to recognize when their mind slips into a trance so that, ultimately, they will be able to induce one without him. This skill is like being able to recognize when you're hungry or full, warm or cold. It involves turning a mirror on your thoughts and sensations, knowing what is normal for you and when that has shifted. "All hypnosis is self-hypnosis," he says, emphasizing that the ultimate success of hypnosis for pain depends on an individual's ability to turn his mind away from thoughts of pain.

BIOFEEDBACK

Hypnotism and biofeedback both use the mind to control chronic pain. With hypnotism, a patient learns to develop alternative images in order to crowd out thoughts of pain. Biofeedback, on the other hand, teaches you how to use information about the state of the body to gain similar control.

Biofeedback broke into the medical world in the 1970s after scientists observed that rats could change their heart rate and blood pressure for rewards of food. To see whether people had any control over their physiology, psychologists attached electronic monitoring equipment to subjects' heads and chests to see if they could alter brain waves or heart rate. Once scientists saw that people could manipulate certain body functions, they applied biofeedback to conditions that were especially affected by blood flow and heart rate—in particular, migraine headache, hypertension, and Raynaud's disease, a disease that causes blood vessels in the hands to constrict painfully at the slightest drop in temperature.

Biofeedback persuasively shows that we have much more control over our body than we might believe. With a modest amount of instruction, you can learn to slow your heart rate and change your blood pressure—functions previously believed to be unconscious. From these basic functions, it has been a logical progression to apply the control we have over these basic functions to the control of pain and suffering.

Biofeedback can be performed by simply monitoring your pulse with your finger. But highly sensitive machines have helped patients go farther. Modern biofeedback machines can track changes in muscle tension, brain waves, electric signals across the skin (galvanic skin response), blood flow across the skin, heart rate, blood pressure, and the actions of some internal organs. Most pain centers tend to concentrate on muscle contractions using an electromyogram (EMG), skin temperature, and/or galvanic skin response. It's not unusual to combine several techniques. Back pain, headaches, and painful conditions that are aggravated by stress or tension, which can include almost any form of chronic pain, are prime candidates for biofeedback sessions.

Biofeedback is deceptively simple. The equipment and instruments are compact and easy to read, and the interaction between patient and machine is quick and unequivocal. Depending on the type of measurement applied, electric wires with tiny monitors are taped to a patient's forehead, neck, back, or finger. The patient watches some type of monitor that emits a beep, picture, or graph line to indicate what changes are taking place in the system being monitored.

My colleague, Dr. Daniel Rockers, the administrative director of the Pain Clinic at UC Davis and a psychologist, regularly treats pain with biofeedback. He declares, "This stuff is pretty fundamental, but surprisingly it's not well known. Relaxed deep breathing can raise the temperature of an extremity, like a finger, ten or fifteen degrees. When the body is physiologically aroused, capillaries constrict and blood rushes to the muscles. When you're relaxed, capillaries dilate and blood goes to the hands, feet, and internal organs. Cold hands can mean you're stressed and tense. So, raising hand temperature reduces that."

Electromyographic (EMG) feedback measures the electrical activity of select muscles, indicating whether they are relaxed or contracted. Muscles almost always hurt more when they're tensed than when they're not. Frequently, pain patients discover tight muscles they never knew about. EMG feedback does not always bring relief; for instance, pain from distant tense muscles—what's known as referred pain—may not ease up even when the source muscles are relaxed. And sometimes there is a lag time between when the muscle goes soft and the pain eases up, which can lead people to conclude that the biofeedback isn't working.

Depending on what body function is under fire, a psychologist shows a patient how to manipulate body reactions by tapping into visual images, relaxing selective muscle groups, altering rates and types of breathing, or concentrating on music or a taped voice. With clear instructions, most people can generate a marked change in skin temperature. For biofeedback to have a lasting effect, a patient has to learn to master certain functions, which means being able to assert control whenever it's needed. This takes practice and regular use. Most patients require several sessions in biofeedback therapy before they are reasonably adept at warming their hands, slowing their heart rate, or untensing muscles. The next step is exercising their newfound skills on their own, applying them in different situations and at different times of the day, figuring out what helps most and lasts the longest.

Learning biofeedback to cope with chronic pain is not like swallowing a pill or getting a nerve block. Instead of passively waiting for a medicine or medical technique to relieve pain, you become an active participant in the process. As you learn to master various facets of your physiology, you discover how particular physical habits or ways of thinking have been adding to your pain. Better yet, you learn how to significantly reduce your suffering.

OTHER BEHAVIORAL TREATMENTS

At the UC Davis Pain Center and the Mass General Pain Center, as with many medical centers, biofeedback is one of a wide range of behavioral therapies. As you may have figured out by now, chronic pain is usually much too complicated to yield to a single blow. This is why many pain centers pull together various brands of medicine and specialists to launch a coordinated assault. Behavioral medicine assesses the impact of pain on our lives and devises solutions that restore function and support healing. Chronic pain frequently consumes a person's entire life, so behavioral specialists help patients learn to cope with chronic pain and separate living from hurting.

Dr. Rockers treats many patients whose daily existence has become intertwined with chronic pain, and he starts off by dispelling the myth that the mind and body operate separately. While careful to point out to patients that acknowledging the psychological dimension of their pain does not mean that "it's all in their head" or that their trouble is psychiatric, he stresses that facets of their behavior and thinking can be fueling their pain, especially stress and tension. These conditions not only worsen pain but generate new ones, and the most direct way to counteract them is with relaxation techniques. Dr. Rockers states, "Relaxation and pain are opposing states and they usually don't coexist. Good centering or balancing mechanisms applied during daily frictions can help lower tension." Relaxation is one such balancing mechanism, and Dr. Rockers shows patients how to find it. He often uses breathing exercises as a means to finding deep relaxation.

The simple act of breathing has been the subject of increasing attention in medical circles as people have discovered that it represents a remarkably effective therapy. Breathing is closely connected to the body's panic alarm, which rings loudly when there is any hint of suffocation. At some level, perhaps deep within consciousness, you are aware of breathing, and whenever your intake of air decreases, you quickly become anxious. Hold your breathe for a minute and you'll see what I mean. This alarm is the same system that stirs up anxiety, agitation, high blood pressure, and the racing heart when you get frightened and sets off panic attacks. Since lack of breathing can trigger stress, control over breathing can relieve stress. Taking in and expelling a controlled, slow, easy breath of air soothes both the body and the psyche. Seemingly as basic as human functions get, deep, relaxed breathing is a mind-body event that stimulates the autonomic nervous system with feelings of calm and relaxation.

You draw air from one of two areas of your lungs. When you are under stress or anxious, you tend to breathe in short gulps, pulling air from the relatively shallow chest or thoracic region. These quick gulps of air trigger parts of the autonomic nervous system that prepare the body for fight or flight. The nervous system prompts the release of adrenaline, which speeds up the heart and breathing rate, raises blood pressure, and shifts blood flow away from organs to muscles. Your body braces to flee or defend itself. And like dry logs on a raging fire, more short bites of air and shallow breathing fuel the flames of anxiety. An inevitable accompaniment to this heightened state of alertness is an acute, even consuming awareness of physical discomfort.

The antidote to the tension that comes with your body's preparations to fight is slower, deeper breathing. This is called abdominal breathing, and it pulls air from deep within the diaphragm, avoiding the fight-or-flight alarm. This system counterbalances anxiety and stress by slowing the heart and lowering the blood pressure. To teach deep breathing, Dr. Rockers asks patients to lie on their backs and place their hands over their chest and abdomen as they breathe. In this position, they can feel how a large breath extracts air from much further down than a small sip of air. At the same time, they can feel the deep breathing relaxing their muscles and mind.

Of course, deep breathing is not the only path to relaxation, and Dr. Rockers combines his instruction and behavioral therapy sessions with other strategies. He has found that visualization and introspection improve physical awareness so that patients can divert pain sensations away from parts of their body and replace them with warm, relaxed sensations. With autogenic relaxation, Dr. Rockers asks a patient to close his eyes and focus on a part of the body, for instance arms, and to tune in to how they feel—their weight and how warm or cool they feel. As the patient explores the feeling of his limbs, Dr. Rockers offers a soothing phrase to repeat, like "I feel quite quiet." During this process, he may monitor and record the temperature of the patient's hands and ask what images he is visualizing. By heightening a patient's awareness of his body and generating warmth in a limb, Dr. Rockers gives him a tool to relax and a method that eventually he can take with him and perform anytime, anywhere he needs it.

Relaxation training is one element of Dr. Rocker's treatment, which varies depending on the patient. For instance, he offers busy patients who can't stop in the middle of their day to do deep breathing or autogenic exercises an abbreviated route to relaxation called a Quieting Response. And he may well fold into pain management therapy directions for biofeedback, hypnosis, very brief cognitive psychotherapy, and writing therapy. A patient's attitude toward their pain, and how it fits or doesn't fit into their life, is crucial for the success of behavioral therapy. For Dr. Rockers, attitude encompasses how motivated a patient is to get better and replace pain with something else in their life, and how open he is to working at it—doing the exercises, making all the appointments, initially pushing toward small goals that build into substantial results.

Attitude is also at the heart of the matter for Dr. Margaret Caudill, a leading behavioral medicine specialist, codirector of pain medicine at the Dartmouth Hitchcock Clinic in Manchester, New Hampshire, and author of *Managing Pain Before It Manages You*. With her pain patients, she looks for acceptance. "I often see patients who've been in pain for years, and their attitude may be, 'I don't want to manage my pain, I just don't want it.' Acceptance is the crux—they have to accept their pain and that there's no cure. They have a choice—they can continue to be oblivious, and hang their identity on their pain, refusing to act as if they have no pain, or they can take control." She explains that acceptance is like going through the grieving process. It requires coming to terms with there being no cure and saying good-bye to a dysfunctional way of looking at the world. It requires reframing the meaning of healing and adopting behaviors and activities that account for pain and diminish it. It hinges on seeing the difference between being cured and being better.

The greatest obstacle to acceptance is denial, what she calls "Push, Crash and Burn." She explains: "Patients aren't flexible, they don't adjust for their pain. They continue to do activities in the normal way, as if they have no pain. They'll work all day, exercise, do leisure activities, then collapse in pain. They don't pace themselves. For example, a patient will spend hours on her feet cleaning the kitchen instead of breaking it into pieces, and sitting for a bit to do something else, like paying bills."

Dr. Caudill's behavioral therapies revolve around the tripod of relaxation skills, techniques for altering thought patterns, and learning better ways of relating to others. Patients must be active participants in the process, learning and practicing direct pain control, distracting themselves when necessary, and developing a feeling of peace and calm.

Learning what doctors call "coping behavior" is a central theme of behavioral medicine. Early in my career, Dr. David Ahern, director of the Behavioral Medicine Unit at Massachusetts General Hospital, first showed how patients in chronic pain lose crucial parts of their lives, cease important activities, become absorbed in their painful condition, and abdicate control of their lives to pain. "I tell patients that they can put their lives on hold waiting for a cure that will probably never come, or learn various coping behaviors." The coping behaviors are familiar to all pain doctors and are neither difficult nor complicated. Undoubtedly, most chronic pain patients have heard of them, too. They're relaxation and distraction techniques, pacing, suitable exercise and conditioning activities, and elimination of destructive habits like heavy alcohol consumption or watching television all day. The key is to avoid doing too little or too much. Either extreme will defeat the goal of getting on with life and taking back control from the pain.

LIFE MANAGEMENT: INSIDE A PAIN UNIT

Occasionally, a chronic pain patient is overwhelmed by his situation. The weekly visit with a behavioral therapist or acupuncturist doesn't dent their pain. While most chronic pain patients do not need to be hospitalized, some need more intensive attention. Chronic pain can derail a person, throwing a life into such turmoil that restoring it has to start with focusing on regaining simple daily functions like getting out of bed and dressed every morning. Or the situation at home requires that the initial work of recovery be done in a hospital. Such is the case with patients admitted to the Chronic Pain Inpatient Unit at Spaulding Rehabilitation Hospital in Boston. What's special about the Spaulding Pain Unit is that it intensively encourages patients to fold the skills learned for managing pain into all aspects of daily living. Inpatient therapy is more about learning how to live with pain than learning how to conquer it. It is a brief respite from the real world with every goal geared to making the real world a far less painful place to live.

Patients who check into the twenty-one-bed unit, which spreads across the tenth floor of the hospital, are generally veterans of the chronic pain wars. They've been wrestling with intractable pain for an extended period and have usually been through an assortment of treatments, all without success. The exact nature of their conditions varies, although common maladies include migraine headaches, low back pain, and myofascial pain. Regardless of their ailment, the usual length of stay is twenty-eight days, although it's entirely voluntary and some opt to leave early.

Many patients at first struggle to accept the unit's basic philosophy, which affects everything from how they spend their days to their treatments and medication. "The focus here is on function, not pain," explains the unit's medical director and prominent headache specialist, Dr. Elizabeth Loder. "Reasonable pain management has not worked for them, even narcotics haven't worked." The program is designed to repair the damage from the fallout of chronic pain, which usually encompasses some type of disability. A patient may have stopped working, withdrawn from social activities, and even ceased leaving their home. And physical disability may have spawned emotional disability, like depression or anxiety disorders. The program also aims to give patients sufficient resources and skills so that they stop shopping for a cure or bolting for the nearest emergency room when they can't tolerate their pain.

Each patient in the unit follows the Master Schedule, an almost hour-by-hour timetable beginning with 7:30 A.M. breakfast—in the common room and fully dressed—and ending with 9:00 P.M. medication dispensing. While this may sound like a military boot camp, the reason for a regimented schedule is persuasive. "Patients often lack a model for learning how to keep going and how to schedule themselves," explains Dr. Loder. "They're used to staying at home and quitting work because they hurt. We help them to regain order and learn how to keep functioning." All members of the inpatient community are in pain, and hurting does not provide an exemption from getting on with the day. Dr. Loder underscores that patients are not allowed to miss scheduled activities—which include meals, education groups, physical therapy, occupational therapy, and meetings—because of their pain.

The daily timetable also helps patients pace themselves, often a significant issue for someone in chronic pain. Patients often get caught in a downward spiral of exhausting themselves when they feel OK, then collapsing in even worse pain when their condition flares up. Pain medication is also dispensed on a strict schedule rather than on demand. This dissuades patients from depending on drugs to bail them out of uncomfortable times—they must do it themselves through other means. And the unit teaches a wide variety of nondrug treatment techniques called modalities, such as heat and ice massage, transcutaneous nerve stimulation (TENS), stretching, and hot-cold baths. Many patients come to the program after trying escalating doses of drugs and finding that they haven't helped. These drugs need to be decreased carefully, so while some medications may be continued, most patients are put on a medication-reduction program, and the doses are diminished over the weeks of their stay.

A cornerstone of the Spaulding pain treatment is physical therapy, which is tailored to each patient's abilities. A staff physical therapist evaluates every patient, looking for how mobility and function have been compromised, then devises a plan for improvement. The critical part of the physical therapy is education. Through individual and group sessions, therapists show patients exercises that can ease their pain, protect against flares, and get them moving again. For all patients, the day starts with stretching exercises. Then they pursue their individualized regimen, which may include aerobic or endurance exercises, working out in the unit's small gym, or even slight postural changes.

Many patients opt for treatment with a transcutaneous electrical nerve stimulation device—a TENS unit. This small device, which contains a battery pack and looks like a pager, has wires and electrodes that attach to the skin over any part of the body and that emits a steady electrical impulse that feels like a slight tingling. A patient may wear it for hours or all day for conditions including low back or neck pain, neuropathic pain, complex regional pain, abdominal pain, the itching of shingles, and phantom limb pain.

TENS units are a controversial part of the pain management arsenal because science doesn't understand how they mute pain and studies of their effectiveness conflict. It's nearly impossible to do a blind study because patients can immediately distinguish between a real and a sham unit. One theory suggests that they create a diversion, distracting patients from their pain. Another theory suggests that they alter neurophysiology and block the pain gate, closing off the path pain takes to get into the brain. And there's always the placebo possibility. Also, therapists disagree over where to place the electrodes, either directly on the painful region or at a distant site. For many patients, the scale tips in favor of using TENS because it's remarkably safe, produces almost no side effects, and often makes them feel better. Penny Herbert, clinical supervisor for physical therapy for the pain unit, finds that TENS helps soothe dull, achy pain but that it's best applied as an adjunct to treatment rather than as the primary modality.

Occupational therapy (OT) is another key ingredient of life on the Spaulding pain unit. While physical therapy centers on ways to foster moving with less pain, OT shows patients how to function better in various parts of their lives and eliminate behavior that aggravates pain. For instance, OT instruction sessions cover ways to reduce stress, improve tolerance for sitting or walking, cook a meal with a minimum amount of pain, conserve energy while doing a single task, pace oneself at work, and find better ways of talking, or not talking, about pain. Occupational therapy also helps patients plan outings away from the hospital while applying techniques they've learned about managing their pain and the mechanics of normal functioning. For patients who have jobs, a vocational rehabilitation counselor can help devise a realistic strategy for returning to the workplace while keeping their pain in check.

Occupational therapy also reinforces independent self-treatment. Between the OT and PT interventions, patients are coached in the basics of applying heat or ice for reducing specific kinds of pain, like tense or stiff muscles, or nerve sensitivity. They learn relaxation techniques like progressive muscle relaxation, deep breathing, visualization, and meditation. And they learn how to use a gadget that looks like a short hard rubber cane, called a theracane, for massaging sore back muscles.

Inpatient centers or hospital units like Spaulding's are unusual for practical and medical reasons. Insurance companies are reticent to pick up the tab for a lengthy stay not requiring urgent daily medical attention. And being in a hospital can have its own set of negative effects—particularly when the goal of treatment is increased function and greater autonomy. So living in a hospital for almost a month is a last resort and suggested only for people who have tried everything else and whose entire lives have been capsized by their condition. This is because almost everything that can be done in the hospital can be done as an outpatient. As a result, outpatient chronic pain programs are growing in number and offer many advantages.

THE BOGUS, THE HARMLESS, AND THE POSSIBLE

Over the ages, the mysteries of chronic pain have spawned a profusion of therapies, some grounded in solid science and others more the product of the imagination. Since ancient times, unorthodox treatments for pain have flourished. Medical history is replete with tales of magic potions, gadgets, and bizarre procedures that miraculously purge pain and heal the sufferer.

But in all fairness to primitive miracle cures, there are also modern, conventional treatments that squelch pain but that scientists do not fully understand. While there may be clues and theories, the complete underlying science and logic is still elusive. Being unproven does not make a treatment worthless or bogus. More than once, yesterday's quack cure has developed into today's almost mainstream alternative treatment. Hypnosis surely fits into this category.

As I write this book, one of the hot new therapies is magnets. Magnets as medical treatment have been around at least since Anton Mesmer. Magnets continue to captivate people's attention, even though there's only limited hard evidence of their efficacy.

So, as is the case with unproven treatments, until the evidence is firm, I wait and see. I accept their use as long as such treatments are safe and do not preclude another, better-substantiated intervention for someone in dire need. What makes me suspicious of magnets, as well as copper bracelets, electric zappers, homeopathy, and the whole panoply of either unproven or yet-to-be proven pain treatment is the nature of pain itself. History and practice have demonstrated that it's easy to concoct a treatment that works. But because of pain's inherent complexities and all the mind-body influences that are a natural part of any treatment, it's extremely difficult to prove that a single treatment inherently reduces pain.

By the time this book is published, very likely a new, untested pain remedy will be the subject of late-night infomercials and Web site chat rooms. Our wish to invest new treatments with miraculous healing powers is changeless and an enduring testament to our hopefulness in the face of chronic disease.

11

PAIN AT THE END OF LIFE

Untangling the Threads of
Physical and Psychic Suffering

> We all must die. But pain is a more terrible lord of man
> than death.
>
> —ALBERT SCHWEITZER

I only began to understand why "pain is a more terrible lord of man than death" during my final years of medical training. I spent time working in a hospice program and witnessed people confronting one of life's most unkind challenges: facing pain and death simultaneously. This is when I first realized that standard pain therapies aren't always enough. Pain at the end of life is unlike any other kind of pain—it is a medical and emotional emergency that demands extraordinary measures. It transforms the traditional rules of pain management in clinical settings, as doctors strive to address the extreme demands on patients and their loved ones.

At first, it seemed ironic that treating and caring for a dying patient's pain could make a monumental difference in his quality of life. But then I came to realize that treating pain during a terminal illness is so urgent because pain can drain the humanity from the precious time remaining. Pain at the end of life is inescapably interwoven with—and often amplified by—multiple levels of emotional and spiritual angst as the inevitability of death looms. Fear, a potent pain magnifier, is the dominant emotion—fear of pain, fear of death, fear of the unknown. Studies have shown that people at the end of life fear pain even more than they fear death. Sadly, for many dying patients, pain is the ultimate torment and death is the cure. It does not have to be this way, and if you or a loved one are facing death, you have every right to demand that your final days not be consumed by pain.

Fear is just one of the powerful emotions in the mix. Dying patients are often prey to a host of anxieties—about the state of their affairs, about the fate of those who will grieve their loss, about how their behavior will be seen, and possibly judged, during their final hours. And of course, there are usually deep spiritual and religious questions to address. Did my life have meaning? Will my soul survive my body? Am I at peace with myself, my family, my friends?

And not least of all, people at the end of life worry about how their pain will be managed. Will they be undermedicated and have to ask, or even beg, for relief? Will they be overmedicated and lose consciousness during their precious waning days and hours? They may even be afraid to complain. If they do, will they be seen as whiners or quitters? If they ask for narcotics, will they be judged by their doctors as drug seeking, or even cowardly? Or will their medical care be relegated to comfort measures only, while all efforts to cure their illness are suspended?

For doctors, ameliorating a dying patient's pain and suffering poses both professional and personal challenges. Physical pain at the end of life, regardless of whether it comes from cancer, AIDS, end-stage heart disease, end-stage diabetes, pulmonary disease, or any other disease, is usually fed by a constellation of complications that demand an all-encompassing treatment strategy. Even diagnosis of the source of pain is tricky, because pain may be caused by the disease as well as by diagnostic procedures, side effects from drugs, or from something else like a broken bone due to a malignancy. Tissue damage, inflammation, pressure on nerves, or damaged nerve pathways or nerve systems hurt the same whether or not someone has a terminal illness.

Pain has to be addressed, and so, too, do such accompanying difficulties as nausea, vomiting, constipation, fatigue, infections, shortness of breath, and anorexia. The array of weapons I use to fight pain at the end of life are the same as those I apply to other types of acute and chronic suffering. But instead of systematically directing a succession of therapies, I often don't have the luxury of time and have to choose a more aggressive approach, applying a simultaneous barrage of medications, procedural therapies like a nerve block, psychological and social interventions, or some other extraordinary treatment.

One of the challenges of pain management at the end of life is to ensure that the patient's needs are met and their wishes are respected. Doctors are used to searching for cures or definitive diagnoses and treatments. Sometimes, the compassionate zest for resolving the cancer or other medical problem can overshadow the patient's immediate needs for physical, emotional, psychological, and spiritual comfort. It's up to the patient to decide how much pain relief they need and want at the end of life. No doctor can reliably intuit how much pain a dying patient might be in without asking and watching closely. Offering pain relief neither excludes simultaneous curative treatment nor does it generally require extraordinary measures—the treatments usually consist of the same medications, procedures, and therapies applied for other types of pain. However, many dying patients may need these treatments applied with much greater force.

Whether from a feeling of helplessness or aversion, caregivers may spend less time with someone who is dying or neglect to offer simple human comfort, like holding someone's hand or sitting with them for a moment. Dying patients who sense reluctance and avoidance feel abandoned and rejected. Loved ones may need to bring this to the attention of everyone involved, including the treating physicians and even other family members. One of the most universal human fears is of dying alone or being emotionally abandoned. The cloud of imminent death casts a shadow of abandonment at the time when a person most needs to feel connected and loved.

Rabbi Harold Kushner, in a talk to pain medicine professionals that I attended, explained that abandoning dying patients is especially cruel because a caregiver's simple presence can provide comfort. "People going through hard times want consolation, not explanation. Yes, they want to be told the name of their disease, and yes they want to be told the prognosis. But what they want to be told more than anything else is that you care about them as a person. You're sorry that they're hurting. You want to do whatever you can to make the pain go away. And before you give them a single pill and before you prescribe any medication, just telling them, 'I am here to make you feel better, I am going to do something to ease the pain,' that eases the pain."

Treating the whole patient at end of life means bringing together meaningful support from many different directions. This may mean going beyond tradition medical issues. For instance, I always inquire whether a dying person is religious, and I never hesitate to enlist pastoral care as part of my team. An agnostic patient may still have deep feelings that he or she may need to confide to a nonfamily member. I can be that confidant, or I can find a counselor who may be a better fit.

IMPROVING QUALITY OF LIFE AT END OF LIFE

When someone is dying, time is a luxury and wait-and-see is not an option. As a person's days and weeks grow shorter, time becomes more precious. What matters most in the final days is that patients are free of crippling pain and unbearable suffering so that they can finish their lives in ways that bring comfort, peace, and completion. Concerns about lasting side effects from months of using a drug or diminished physical capacity become secondary to making a patient comfortable. When I weigh relative risks and benefits, the urgency of end of life always moves me to intervene aggressively to maximize benefits.

Another common belief among both medical professionals and people close to someone who is dying is that suffering, either physical or emotional, is to be expected and is somehow inevitable. I reject this view categorically. *No one has to die in pain. I believe that all suffering is treatable.* Sometimes, I can "magically" make it go away—if not, I can subdue it to the point where a patient's last days can be ones of connection and closure rather than pain, loneliness, and despair.

Anyone who argues for assisted suicide as the answer to persistent suffering needs to understand that a comprehensive treatment approach can restore the will to live. An overlooked aspect of Dr. Kevorkian's assisted suicides is that the vast majority of the people who want to kill themselves are almost always suffering from extreme physical and emotional pain. If only the physical pain is treated and the emotional dimension is ignored, the patient will continue to suffer. Likewise, if treatment misses the physical component, no amount of spiritual or emotional care will yield significant pain relief. No one needs to die in pain, or even in despair, but many people will continue to do so until all end-of-life care becomes comprehensive.

Being terminally ill carries a different personal meaning for every individual—and that meaning affects how, and how much, he or she suffers. A woman with breast cancer may be as tormented by threats to her sexuality as the specter of death, or a lifetime smoker who is dying of lung disease may be consumed with guilt over abandoning his family. Cultural or ethnic background can also play a role in the degree and nature of someone's suffering. Researchers at the New England Medical Center have been conducting a cancer pain education program called "Taking Control of Your Pain." They have found that some groups of people refuse to talk about their disease, even with family members, and so suffer in silence. People of Latino origin, they found, hold medical professionals in such high regard that they rarely complain about ineffective pain remedies, and so they too endure more discomfort than necessary. You may find yourself or loved ones falling into similar patterns that may reflect family or cultural traits. If they are only making matters worse, the first step to improvement is recognition of the situation.

Most people do not die in isolation—there are usually friends, family, or medical people tending to a dying patient, and their suffering is often palpable. It may be hidden beneath anger or denial or distancing, but few people can fail to be anguished by the passing of another. An attentive doctor incorporates the suffering of close family into his treatment approach. Everyone in the company of suffering is at risk, and ministering to them is an important part of comprehensive end-of-life care. A few months ago I was asked to visit a man who was dying of prostate cancer. Mr. Briland was in his final hours, apparently comfortable with the aid of morphine. However, he had persistent hiccups, and while he did not complain, his wife was heartsick, believing that her husband was in distress. The hiccups made him briefly writhe and thrash in bed, which was a disturbing sight. My treatment was not a pain medication but a drug to halt Mr. Briland's hiccups and, not incidentally, relieve his wife's agony over what she imagined her husband was going through. In essence, I treated his symptom and her suffering.

Treating someone who is terminally ill is as much about addressing suffering as it is about subduing physical pain. Physical and emotional suffering are usually tightly intertwined at the end of life. The doctor's job is to untangle that knot and diagnose and treat the strands of affliction individually. As you'll see from the patient stories that follow, a doctor can be of most use to a dying patient when he listens attentively—with his ears, his eyes, and his heart—and responds with all his professional and human faculties.

PAIN AS A SYMPTOM OF TERMINAL ILLNESS

Mike Benjamin looked like the soul of New England—a full head of white hair, ramrod-straight posture, a soft accent, and dressed in the East Coast, foul-weather uniform of corduroy pants, crewneck sweater, and duck boots. When I first met him in the Mass General Pain Center, he seemed to possess another well-known New England quality: stoicism. From his awkward way of walking and sitting, I suspected that he came in for chest pain. But he betrayed no grimacing, no verbal or body language to describe his discomfort. He was very matter-of-fact about what he needed and wanted. As we sat in a block room, surrounded by posters of diagrams of human anatomy and coding sheets for different procedures, he pointed to the wall next to him and said, "See number 730245—I want one of those." Number 730245 is an intercostal block, which his primary doctor had told him might help his chest pain. "Look," he said, "Saturday is my seventy-fifth birthday. I'm having a party with friends on the golf course and I want to be able to swing my clubs again."

I nodded in astonishment; no one had ever asked me for a block by its billing code before. "That's certainly a good block," I said, "and that's part of our medicine. But can you tell me why you're sure this is what you need?"

Mr. Benjamin's pain had begun over a year earlier as an ache that shifted around the left side of his chest, and which he thought was a strained muscle. He visited his internist, who prescribed drugs for muscle ache, but the pain kept up. When it didn't improve, he had a complete battery of tests including a CAT scan of his chest, ultrasound, and blood workups. The doctor detected only a small buildup of fluid outside his lungs, suggested it might be an infection, and told him to wait and see if it cleared. Several months later, another CAT scan of the area still showed a small amount of fluid, and again, his doctor advised a wait-and-see strategy. Months dragged by, and by the time Mr. Benjamin reached me he had a medical file as thick as a phone book and was still in pain. The pain itself wasn't as bothersome to him as what it was doing to his most treasured activity, golf. He couldn't carry his bags anymore and barely had enough energy to play nine holes.

He gave me a brief history from his time as a young man and as a welder in a navy shipyard, through family life and two children, and his recent retirement from his job as a traveling salesman for a textile company. I listened to his lungs breathing, and they sounded like sandpaper. I don't like to treat symptoms when I don't know the cause, and I suspected more was happening inside Mr. Benjamin than a pinched nerve. He had lost weight, was obviously fatigued, and his lungs did not sound healthy. Although I wished I didn't have to face my suspicions, I had to wonder about a rare cause of such a problem. Mesothelioma is a cancer associated with asbestos that grows very slowly, appearing many years after exposure. Navy shipyards were full of asbestos! I couldn't fully treat his pain without eliminating this possibility.

"I tell you what, Mr. Benjamin. Let's make a deal—I will give you the intercostal block if we can first take one more CAT scan. I know you had one several months ago, but I'd still like to see recent pictures. If everything comes back OK, I'll do the block first thing tomorrow morning." Although not the type of person to question a doctor, Mr. Benjamin hesitated. He was tired of hospitals and procedures, and more to the point, previous doctors had assured him that they had seen nothing to indicate that his lung pain was connected with anything serious. His earlier scans had even appeared to rule out cancer. Understandably, he did not want to reopen that possibility.

In the morning, I had the scan results, and Mr. Benjamin returned to the Pain Center, this time with his wife, Sally. When we made the appointment, I had suggested that he bring his wife of fifty years. She had been an active partner in his earlier treatments and surely would want to be part of this. There is no easy way to tell someone that you think he needs an immediate biopsy, and while Mr. Benjamin reacted calmly, a dark cloud settled over his wife. She was as frightened of the word "biopsy" as most people are of "cancer" and quizzed me on the reasons for my recommendation. She later told me that she was convinced that previous doctors had been holding back the truth. Although probably not the case, her feeling of being deceived, or even lied to, added yet another layer to her anguish over her husband's health.

Mr. Benjamin's biopsy did indeed indicate mesothelioma cancer, and soon afterward he underwent surgery to have most of the lining surrounding his lungs removed. He then underwent a complete course of radiation to stem the cancer's spread. Although his oncologist was in charge of his care, I had promised Mr. Benjamin that I would be an active member of his treatment team. I assured him that I would not let him live in pain, and if a treatment lost its impact or did not help, I'd have a replacement ready to take its place.

As usually happens with cancer, there was no cure for his disease and little I could do for the underlying cause of his pain. While the surgery and radiation had slowed its progress, it soon became clear that the disease had metastasized, spreading to other organs and parts of his body. The pain in his chest had crept into his abdomen, spine, and hips, a clear indicator that the disease was attacking his skeletal system and generating one of the worst and most universal types of fallout from cancer—bone pain.

TREATING BONE PAIN

Many cancer patients experience bone pain—upwards of 85 percent, according to experts, regardless of where the disease first strikes. It's the result of a tumor invading bone either close to the original cancer or in a distant part of the body. Cancer that has spread (metastasized) frequently lodges in vertebrae, the pelvis, and/or long bones. Patients say bony pain is a constant dull or deep ache that often gets worse at night or when the patient moves or carries heavy objects. A bone scan may confirm my suspicions—but not always. In past decades, doctors struggled mightily with trying to control this almost omnipresent cancer pain and usually failed, which medical historians believe may have contributed to the coining of the expression "intractable pain." Fortunately, pain medicine has made great advances in mastering cancer pain, and the word "intractable" has faded as bone pain has been blunted.

Cancer's complex chemistry and mechanisms make bone pain obstinate. The pain may be the result of many possibilities including tiny fractures from weakened, disintegrating bones or bones that are forced to accommodate an intruding tumor. One of my first interventions may be to refer a patient to radiation therapy to stem the tumor invasion and slow the painful bone disintegration. While radiation can halt cancer growth, even in patients whose tumors cannot be contained it can shrink them enough to relieve pain. An alternative to radiation is a radioactive drug, strontium 89, which helps retard bone breakdown and may help prevent more deterioration. And it's shown good results in easing pain from the bone metastasis of prostate cancer. It generally has a more widespread effect than radiation but also has the drawback of needing three or four weeks to take effect.

Drugs can be powerful adversaries of bone pain, particularly anti-inflammatories like corticosteroids and NSAIDs. Surprisingly, NSAIDs, even over-the-counter NSAIDs such as ibuprofen, can have extremely potent effects—sometimes even greater than morphine. Steroids have the added advantage for some patients of stimulating appetite and elevating mood. Although NSAIDs also combat bone pain, patients may not want to put up with their side effects, which pose serious limitations. There is hope, though, that the new family of NSAIDs, the COX-2 inhibitor drugs, may also work for bone pain.

Normally steroids are not my first choice for an anti-inflammatory because they can suppress immune function and produce osteoporosis, infections, and ulcers. But when I am treating pain from a terminal illness, a steroid's long-term side effects are often outweighed by its strength and how it helps boost the effects of other drugs. Both steroids and NSAIDs notch up the impact of opioids, which cancer patients often take for accompanying pain.

Clinicians have recently discovered that a group of drugs called bis-phosphates (pamidronate is the most commonly used) halt bone corrosion and in some cases reverse bone loss. And it's shown potency in controlling pain. In rare cases when nothing else works, miraculous results have sometimes come from a surgical procedure whose effectiveness cannot be explained. Doctors have discovered that, for unknown reasons, removing part of a patient's pituitary gland has a remarkable deadening effect on the pain of bony metastasis. They theorize that it may have something to do with altering hormone activity, but they have no solid explanations. Nevertheless, in some, it has produced immediate pain relief. However, doctors have seen less convincing long-term results, and the surgery remains controversial because it hasn't been thoroughly studied. Yet another unusual method of attack that's shown good results, especially for bony metastasis, is percutaneous electrical nerve stimulation (PENS), which delivers a mild electrical current to the painful region. Using needles similar to those in acupuncture, doctors deliver about thirty minutes of stimulation and may repeat the treatments depending on how the patient feels.

HEALING WHAT WE CAN'T CURE

As is so often the case with cancer, bony pain was not Mr. Benjamin's only complaint—he had internal, or visceral pain, and equally crucial, his joy of life was slipping away. The pain and fatigue continued to curtail his beloved golf, he worried about being a burden to Sally and, alternately, despaired about leaving her. His emotional turmoil became the focus of my attention.

So often, worry and anguish about the toll one's dying is taking on loved ones adds another element of suffering. On top of wrestling with physical pain and grieving over one's own demise, a patient may be consumed by concerns about strained or unfinished relationships, finances, and the desire for closure in their personal and worldly affairs. To help Mr. Benjamin, I had to minister to an entire life that had been turned upside down. I had to consider not only his physical discomfort but also the many things that were a source of meaning to him and his vision of how he wanted to spend the remainder of his life. Together, we needed to fix the little things as well as manage the larger problems. Rabbi Kushner's words were never far from my mind: "There are things we can heal that we can't cure. We can heal things by making people feel better about what is unfixable."

Having seen Mr. Benjamin and his wife together at our second meeting, and hearing him speak of her, I knew they were worried more about each other than themselves. They instinctively tried to shield each other from unpleasantness and pain. They were spending much of their energy protecting each other from the terrifying eventuality of death—each too afraid to directly confront the situation because they believed the other couldn't handle it. Our sessions together, although veiled as visits for pain management, became time to talk about their stressful experience that was robbing them of quality in their last days together. By acknowledging that Mike was dying, and by talking about how to make him as comfortable as possible, they were able to turn the time into an occasion of togetherness and love. They got Mike's worldly affairs in order and tended to his personal relationships through reminiscing and saying good-bye to loved ones. I knew we had made progress when Mike told me he knew it was time to use the many frequent-flyer miles he had accrued from all his business travels to take his bride of fifty years on the trip they had always talked about.

In one of our early meetings, I explained that on top of the discomfort of the encroaching illness, Mike might feel unpleasant side effects from some of his treatments. "These drugs harm both normal cells and cancer cells—with the hope that more cancer cells are debilitated than are the normal ones. With this kind of strategy, it's no wonder that there are side effects." The good news, I told him, was that they were manageable. He just had to tell me what was hurting, and we would find a way to alleviate it.

After we got past his reluctance to complain because he thought it would disturb Sally, he let me know that taking his medication was difficult because it hurt to swallow. This was due to an infection that resulted from his chemotherapy, so I prescribed an antifungal drug to eradicate it. Being unable to swallow medicines can be a significant problem. The question of the best route for delivering medication to someone terminally ill comes up early and regularly, and it's an issue I constantly keep my eye on. Pain relief is not going to work if a patient cannot tolerate its path into the body. But the pain reliever shouldn't also cause pain. For this reason, I rarely give a patient with severe pain an intermuscular injection—these are usually painful and there are almost always other less painful ways into the body that are just as direct, such as intravenous infusions, infusion under the skin, suppositories, or patches that deliver medicines through the skin directly into the bloodstream.

Another seemingly minor problem was fatigue, and Mike only mentioned it when I asked about how he was spending his days. He said he could not do much, and even grocery shopping exhausted him. He described severe fatigue that Sally characterized as "a loss of spark." Again, I reached into my bag of medications and gave him a stimulant, methylphenidate (Ritalin). There are several forms of stimulants such as amphetamine, each working well to counteract sedation and fatigue. While best known as a drug for attention-deficit disorder in children, stimulants are also the only antidepressant drug that begins to work almost immediately. Ritalin's relatively safe, and as I told Mike Benjamin, it would not cause insomnia if he took it in the morning.

Mike never used the word "depressed," but he confessed to being afraid and so glum about his future that he would feign sleep to stay in bed in the mornings. The previous small pleasures in his day, like doing the crossword puzzle or talking to friends, were no longer of interest. Depression and dying are an odd couple, and not as wedded to each other as many people assume. Most people think that it's natural to be depressed at the end of life—*a life is ending,* they reason. Of course it's natural to feel sad about dying and to grieve over the loss of one's life. And it's often helpful, even therapeutic, for someone who is dying to be able to talk about these feelings and not have to hide them for fear of upsetting loved ones. But persistent feelings of fear and helplessness—clinical depression—are not normal, even when someone is dying. While depression may be understandable, it is never appropriate and always needs treatment.

I started Mike on an antidepressant and told him we would try other types if this one didn't work. On many occasions during the last months of his life, I reassured Mike and Sally that I would not tolerate his pain. At one point, when I was just about to reassure him one more time, he stopped me with a wink and the bright spirit that was still inside, saying "I know, you're going to attack the pain." He came to the pain clinic at least once per month, and our visits seemed more social than medical. Sally came with him, except for the times that he wanted to talk about how much she was suffering. His greatest fear seemed to be that his pain would cause suffering for Sally, and he desperately needed to maintain his emotional and physical composure. Sally later told me that our visits helped Mike feel reassured that I was still on board in case pain returned. Fortunately, small adjustments in his regimen were enough to maintain comfort.

Sally and Mike were able to take care of good-byes, particularly to each other. His death was expected and yet still hit me like a shock. He, and patients like him, are the reason I feel so privileged to do my job. By allowing me to participate in his last months, Mike Benjamin poignantly showed me the value of life. At his funeral, I finally met all the people he and Sally had told me about—his daughters, grandchildren, and special friends. As I left Mike's funeral feeling like I had lost a good friend, his daughter came over to say thanks. I accepted her gratitude, and for a few moments we talked about some of his special qualities. In truth, her gratitude was hard to take because I felt that anything I gave Mike was returned and more. Benevolence seemed so selfish.

SAME DRUGS, DIFFERENT EQUATIONS

The drugs I prescribed for Michael Benjamin were the same compounds I apply to garden-variety pain. Good pain management is good pain management, as long as it is delivered with regard to the individual context of a patient's life. At the end of life, the risk of slowly dosing a medication to avoid side effects can result in missing the window of opportunity for relieving suffering. This is why pain at the end of life is an emergency. Such was the case for Gabriella

Carlucci, a woman in her late forties whom I met several hours after surgery to remove her pancreas.

Pancreatic cancer can be one of the most virulent and painful tumors, and it can sneak up on a person with the force of a tornado. Gabriella Carlucci's pain began as an innocuous backache that wouldn't go away and defied the diagnoses and treatments of her primary doctor. As you might recall from an earlier chapter, cancer pain often deceives people because usually its symptoms erupt long after the disease has burrowed into the body. Gabriella trudged between her primary doctor and specialists for months as they tried to find the source of the achiness that shifted between her ribs and back. Finally, a gastroenterologist ran yet another scan of her abdomen and detected a spot on her pancreas, which is tucked behind the stomach and secretes digestive juices and hormones—and her life went into fast-forward. He scheduled her for immediate surgery to remove part of her pancreas and intestine.

I was asked to meet Gabriella just after her surgery to help control her pain. She had done well with postoperative pain, mainly because of an epidural catheter. After several days, the epidural was routinely removed and she was transitioned to oxycodone, an oral opioid for the surgical pain and for the persistent ache in her back. Her back pain, caused by a group of nerves just behind the pancreas called the celiac plexus, was of most concern to me, since it was a common feature of pancreatic cancer. I suggested a celiac plexus block, an injection that would permanently numb these nerves within her abdomen. I discussed this in detail with her and her husband, John, who had taken a six-month leave of absence from his job as a newspaper editor to care for Gabriella. He visited her twice daily in the hospital and tended to their home and ran errands when he wasn't at her bedside.

Cancer pain often stems from growing tumors and injured tissue, so an effective block for it is frequently neurolytic, meaning a treatment to deaden or destroy nerves. Neurolytic blocks are appropriate only when the pain is clearly identified as coming from specific nerves. For instance, it made sense for Gabriella's pancreatic pain but would not have for Mike's all-over bone pain. The chemical used to kill nerves is either alcohol or phenol, and clinical studies report major pain relief from neurolytic blocks in 50 to 90 percent of cancer patients. The downside of damaging nerves is that, as you know by now, the effect is not permanent and may last only months. But for someone with a terminal illness, that can be a lifetime.

Neurolytic blocks can halt pain stemming from various regions of the body as well as from internal organs. Intercostal blocks help quell pain in the chest or abdominal wall, while peripheral blocks halt sensations coming from an arm or leg. These blocks, as with other cancer treatments, involve potential trade-offs. For instance, a peripheral block for severe leg pain runs the risk of causing paralysis. But if a patient has only a short time to live and is in so much pain that he cannot move, stopping that agony by deadening nerves may be a welcome trade-off. Neurolytic injections in the spinal cord are a viable option when they offer a patient the best chance for dying without pain.

Gabriella and John were hesitant to undergo yet another invasive procedure, and their surgeon believed that the worst of her pain had passed. While my recommendation was that she have a block, I also told the couple that there is no single right way, but a variety of workable approaches, and in truth, her doctor was more familiar with her case than I. She decided not to undergo the block, so for the short term, I continued to tailor an effective regimen of oral analgesic. Mrs. Carlucci was discharged with a prescription for pain medication, and I heard nothing about the case for months until her name appeared on my roster of patients in my weekly rounds of the cancer pain clinic.

She, John, and their grown daughter, Julia, were waiting for me in an examination room, a small beige box barely large enough for an exam bed and a couple of plastic molded side chairs. John did most of the talking while Gabriella sat beside him and Julia leaned against a wall. Gabriella was a shadow of the woman I had met months earlier. She had lost so much weight her clothes were half empty. She sat rigid and unmoving, like a stage prop, and spoke in monosyllables. Her eyes were almost shut, as if she was dozing.

John described how Gabriella had gone into a free fall several months after her discharge. Her pain had never abated—it gnawed at her—and she spent more and more time in bed or on the living-room couch. Her medication made her drowsy during the day, but she slept little at night. Julia volunteered that she often found her mother in the middle of the night on the living-room recliner, staring into space and muttering about putting John "through this misery." Not only was her sleep-wake cycle a jumble but she had lost any interest in food. When a patient no longer enjoys eating, I automatically think of depression. Gabriella's flat appearance was probably the result not just of paralyzing pain but of loss of the desire to live.

"My wife's not a complainer," John said, "so I know something's wrong." He gave her hand a soft pat.

"And how are you doing?" I ventured. He, too, looked as if he had lost weight.

"So-so. The doctor gave me some pills to help me relax and sleep, but I don't like to take them. And it's kind of hard to keep my mind on work." He added as an afterthought, "I just want our life back."

As it so often does, the cancer was cutting a broad swath through this family. Gabriella had a terrible constellation of problems orbiting around her cancer, and it was no wonder she wanted to die. And she was not the only family member who was suffering. Nevertheless, I felt reasonably confident that if we could get her troubles under control, then John and Julia would also brighten.

This family's misery represented a genuine medical emergency. The first step was to separate Gabriella's physical pain from the family's emotional suffering. My first goal was to reset Gabriella's sleep-wake cycle to its natural course, which would lift her mood. Pain control would come next. Since her daytime naps and drowsiness coupled with nighttime insomnia were making her tired all the time, I took her off sedating drugs during the day and gave them back to her at night. She needed to be awake and alert during the day if she was going to sleep well, so I added a stimulant, an amphetamine, to her morning medications.

What kept Gabriella awake at night was not just the absence of sleepiness. As she lay in bed, worrying about her family and feeling guilty about what her illness was doing to them, Gabriella's mind was too wrapped up in fear to drift into sleep. Fear is rooted in irrational thinking that magnifies pain and suffering. I prescribed the psychotropic medication Trilifon to calm her agonizing thoughts and allow some conflict-free space in which to get some sleep.

Since she was on so many medications, I tried to simplify the drugs and the different dosing intervals—choosing drugs that could do double duty and eliminate unnecessary ones. I asked about her diet and Julia interjected, "Mom's been living on chicken broth and Jell-O because there's always some test coming up." We all agreed that was no way to live, and I suggested she make an appointment with the hospital nutritionist to investigate dietary supplements to add to her calorie intake. While neither she nor anyone in her family acknowledged that she was dying, I suspected that that reality was gnawing at her. The real source of her lack of interest in food was her depression, so I put her on an antidepressant. Although antidepressant medication takes a couple of weeks to kick in, I knew that the stimulant would immediately improve her spirits, and perhaps her appetite.

A further drag on Gabriella's peace of mind was her discomfort over being constipated—which may also have eroded her desire to eat. Opioids almost always cause constipation, and she had a bad case, so I gave her a drug to block the effect of the morphine on her gastrointestinal tract for a day or so, then started her on a strong laxative. The bulk of Gabriella's pain medication was quick-acting opioids for breakthrough pain. Although they usually kept a lid on the worst pain, such fast-acting opioids only added to her sleepiness and constipation and did little for dull, achy background pain. She needed something that would last all day, but she didn't want to take any more pills. So we decided to try an opioid patch that would deliver a constant amount of the narcotic medication fentanyl right through her skin and into her bloodstream.

Opioids like morphine are the centerpiece of pain management for a terminal illness because they remain our most potent and reliable painkillers. And they can be administered in a variety of ways. With the right dose and the most appropriate delivery method, opioids can contain virtually any pain. Nevertheless, surveys of hospitals and doctors reveal that medical practitioners continue to undermedicate cancer pain, even for someone terminally ill like Gabriella. Hesitant because of social and legal concerns, as well as medical misconceptions, many doctors avoid applying the full might of these ancient and modern wonder drugs.

Both doctors and patients worry about addiction, overdoses, and decreased breathing. But with weeks or months to live, addiction is rarely a significant concern. I answer concerns about overdosing and repressed breathing by explaining that when a medication is gradually increased with an eye on the patient's breathing rate, the body adjusts. Despite what many people believe, there is no ceiling or single maximum amount of opioids a person can take or a dose that is automatically fatal. An effective dose for stifling pain can always be found. Dr. Ira Byock, in his book *Dying Well,* tells the story of a woman with kidney cancer whose pain exhausted the entire supply of injectable Dilaudid (hydromorphone) in all of Missoula, Montana's pharmacies and two hospitals; at her worst, she needed nine grams of morphine an hour (one-tenth of a gram will knock out most healthy adults). It all depends on the individual, and the pain. And sometimes the pain accelerates not only because of increasing tolerance but because the disease has worsened.

I use opioids more liberally for end-of-life pain, but rather than considering a person's ability to function as my gauge for choosing a specific drug and dose, I aim to maintain or improve the quality of their daily life. For instance, if a pain reliever is making someone drowsy and the patient wants to be alert, I add a stimulant to the drug regimen rather than backing off the opioid. The same is true if a drug brings on nausea and vomiting—I add an antinausea medication to the mix rather than cut back on the pain reliever.

The delivery route of opioids into the body—orally, by injection, through a skin patch, through mucus membranes, or via an implanted tube or pump—can have a significant impact on pain relief and side effects. Pills or liquid by mouth take a circuitous path to the pain site, first filtering through the gastrointestinal tract and liver, which detoxifies and metabolizes the opioid. As a result, taking opioid medication orally delivers only a fraction of its punch. Furthermore, as the opioid passes through the stomach, intestines, and bloodstream, it can cause constipation along with nausea and vomiting. However, taking medications by mouth is still the most common and usually the most convenient method of treatment. Other routes are usually used only if oral medication is not possible.

Gabriella's oxycodone pills were not quieting her pain yet were stirring up lots of side effects. We settled on a skin patch that releases a steady flow of the opioid fentanyl (trade named Duragesic). Fentanyl, a synthetic opioid 75 to 125 times stronger than morphine, is the most fat soluble of narcotics, so it quickly speeds through skin and into the brain. Although available in an injectable short-acting liquid, fentanyl through a patch offers a steady, sustained-release infusion. The patch is composed of four layers of material that keep it glued to the skin and full of enough time-release medication to last for days. The drug needs about twelve hours before it reaches its optimum dose and usually needs to be changed every two or three days.

A PCA device (patient-controlled analgesia), which patients recovering from surgery regularly use, can also be fitted for portable use by someone with cancer or a terminal illness. This lets the patient control the flow of pain medication and is an especially effective weapon against the breakthrough pain that besets many cancer patients. As its name suggests, breakthrough pain comes hard and fast—it may be an instantaneous intensifying of all-over dull pain, or it may come as a sharp stab or fiery sensation. It can summon someone out of a deep sleep or freeze him mid-motion like a vicious bolt out of the blue. Its unpredictability and severity make an immediate antidote imperative. Guarding against the possibility of breakthrough pain should be a part of any prescription for fighting end-of-life pain.

Speed is of the essence in devising a weapon for breakthrough pain. For decades, the fastest way to combat it has been through an intravenous tube that is in place and ready to deliver an opioid wallop, now usually in the form of PCA. Recently, drug manufacturers have devised an equally fast, noninvasive method of stopping breakthrough pain. The product is called Actiq, and it looks like an unappetizing lollipop—a sweetened lozenge on a stick that's laced with high-powered fentanyl that travels through mucosa tissue on the inner walls of the mouth, an exceptionally clever and speedy delivery system to the bloodstream. The Actiq unit has only to be rubbed on the inside of your cheek to rush opioids to the brain, traveling faster than any pill and just about as fast as an intravenous injection of morphine. Patients say that they can feel the relief from breakthrough pain within five minutes of putting the device in their mouth.

All routine pain-relieving delivery systems can cause side effects, and rarely they become intolerable. In such cases, I may advise implanting a pump that infuses tiny amounts of drug directly into the spinal fluid. This is an elaborate mechanical device, a small disk-shaped object a bit smaller than a hockey puck, that is embedded in a patient's abdomen. It is connected by a catheter line to a space in the spinal canal and delivers a steady drip of opioids or other pain relievers. If a patient's pain changes or gets worse, the dose can be increased and other drugs can be added to the mixture. And the mixture can be adjusted to deliver heavier doses at certain times, like during the night to help a patient sleep. The pump is loaded with drugs every one to three months, depending on the dosage, and needs to be removed only when the battery wears out, which usually takes many years.

When opioids are inserted right into the spinal fluid, the amount needed for pain relief is much less than when they travel via the blood and through organs. And since the drugs bypass the gastrointestinal system, they stir up much less constipation, vomiting, nausea, and other side effects. Pumps require a surgical procedure and are expensive, and not all patients get pain relief from them. Before implanting a pump, I may do a simple epidural or intrathecal injection of an opioid as a trial run to see if a pump might be effective.

The fentanyl patch helped curb Gabriella's pain, and for a while her spirit bounced back and she resumed the areas of her life with John and her children that she so much enjoyed. With opioids seeping into her around the clock instead of intermittently or only when she was actively uncomfortable, her pain subsided to mildly annoying background noise. But over a period of months, the achy, sometimes shooting pain inched back into her life. On a return visit to the cancer pain center, she wondered aloud whether her remission had run its course. Although she had put back some of the forty pounds she had lost, she looked washed out and exhausted. I examined her, feeling her stomach and pancreas, where I detected a new mass, and suggested she have another abdominal scan. In the meantime, I renewed my recommendation that she get a celiac plexus block. This nerve block, which is performed on the low back near the top of the lumbar spine, would intercept the pain signal for months. Gabriella still resisted, I think out of fatigue and discouragement as much as anything else, and only with John's insistence did the couple finally agree to the procedure.

I wish I could have offered them a brighter hope than the possibility that the disease had progressed, coupled with yet another palliative treatment. I was frustrated to be powerless against the cancer but determined to help them find personal comfort, closure, and a measure of peace. The celiac plexus block helped, as did several other interventions along the way. I moved from Boston to California several months before Gabriella passed away. We said good-bye during an emotional visit in my clinic. She died in comfort, with support from her family and friends. I learned that she had very little pain in her last weeks and died an easier death as a result.

These patient stories illustrate a few of the innumerable variations of profound experiences at the end of life. I hope they highlight the importance of effective and aggressive pain management for someone who is dying. There is no reason for pain and suffering to rob a dying person and his or her loved ones of one of the most meaningful times of life. Nowhere is effective pain management more important, because it is impossible to die well in pain.

12

TOWARD A WORLD WITHOUT PAIN

The Promise of the Future

Life begins on the other side of despair.
—JEAN-PAUL SARTRE

When I was in medical school, pain medicine was changing before my eyes: Acute pain was retreating in the face of potent analgesics and innovative delivery systems that we now take for granted, discoveries about brain chemistry were inspiring the creation of highly targeted drugs, and advances in computerized scanners were just beginning to produce images of the body in pain. Neuroscientists were discovering nerve pathways and receptors. Revelations about endorphins and the power of acupuncture were shining light on how the mind and body collude to create, and defeat, pain.

The pace and momentum of those discoveries are continuing to build, like a plane taxiing towards takeoff. Even within the relatively few years of its existence, pain medicine has made great strides in unraveling the mysteries of pain. Within the past couple of years, the underlying anatomy of pain has become clearer, and treatments for headaches, low back pain, arthritis, and neuropathic pain have become more effective, more direct, and safer. Huge breakthroughs are coming yearly, and I suspect that within the next ten years, pain medicine will advance dramatically. Pain medicine is to medical specialties as microprocessing is to computer science—every year, the technology is capable of doing more, and the people running it get smarter and more adept at applying it. The pain medicine of tomorrow is going to be an exciting time for patients and doctors. If you suffer from chronic pain, the near future offers tremendous hope as medical science brings to bear the latest in technology, biochemistry, psychology, and behavioral science.

As I was researching this book, I asked colleagues and leading pain specialists what they saw in their crystal ball. "Look ten years out," I said, "and tell me what you see ahead." These experts gave me snapshots of the future and intriguing theories about how the body and brain interact, as well as glimpses of revolutionary treatments to come. I want to share with you their predictions—and my own views—of a brighter future for pain sufferers.

INTEGRATING PAIN SPECIALTIES INTO COMPREHENSIVE, MIND-BODY CARE

Among doctors, treating patients in pain is widely viewed as one of health care's most challenging tasks because it calls on so many different areas of expertise. Most doctors today are not prepared to deal with this complexity, grounded as they are in single disciplines such as anesthesiology or neurology. However, medical schools are now training future pain doctors with much broader scope and wider knowledge bases.

A new generation of pain specialists is being trained in crossover fields that only a few years ago would have been overlooked but that are now becoming recognized as critical to halting the progression of pain's destruction: mind-body therapies, including psychology, behavioral science, and the basic physical therapies. Alternative treatments are becoming much more common; acupuncture's integration into the pain clinic at Massachusetts General Hospital is simply one sign of the changing times in pain medicine.

In the Pain Center at UC Davis, anyone coming in for chronic pain that has persisted for at least six months receives a psychological evaluation as part of their comprehensive care. This doesn't mean we think the pain isn't real or that it isn't physical. On the contrary, the new approach understands that the chronic pain is so real that it must be having negative effects on the patient's life. This type of comprehensive care, which looks at a person's entire life as well as at nerves and cells, blood tests, and CAT scans, requires physicians and psychologists to understand the complex relationship of the body and the mind. In the world of treating chronic pain, this has become much more commonplace.

As part of this meshing of specialties into a total mind-body approach to pain medicine, the future pain center will also look different. Instead of a free-standing facility or a clinic tucked into the corner of a large medical complex, pain centers will be better integrated into health-care facilities. Pain medicine will be a routine element of all health care, much in the same way that dispensing an antibiotic for an infection is today. Pain specialists are beginning to work with surgeons, family practitioners, and other doctors to anticipate every aspect of a patient's pain well before a crisis. At the same time, health-care professionals, be they physicians, nurses, physician therapists, or pharmacists, will learn the tools of effective pain control early in their training. As I write this, the California legislature is voting on a new bill to require medical schools to offer more training on pain control to medical students and to make training in pain management a compulsory prerequisite to getting a medical license.

Pain medicine is also working to make comfort and quality of life a priority of health care. Part of what is motivating this shift toward treating the person and not just the pain is the gradual realization by health-care officials that comprehensive care that improves patients' lives over the long haul—as opposed to simply applying a Band-Aid to a syndrome or condition—will ultimately reduce hospital costs. The medical center at UC Davis, for example, has built services that combat pain and suffering at every level. The hospice program, the department of anesthesiology, and the rest of the medical community have integrated treatments and resources for pain and suffering across a wide variety of specialties. This means that lines that typically separate medical disciplines, like the cordoning off of internal medicine or pediatrics from anesthesiology or psychiatry, no longer are in place. Until very recently, hospitals working in this way have been rare, proof positive that the revolution of comprehensive pain medicine has begun.

THE PROMISE OF TECHNOLOGY

Continued advances in technology are going to make pain medicine increasingly accurate and precise. Technology will transform the instruments, the drugs, and the very foundations of the science of pain management. The tools I use to silence nerve pathways will become so exact that I will be able to pinpoint single nerves—a microstrand smaller than a human hair—and deliver a drop of medication, a nanosecond of heat, or a blip of electricity to an individual nerve cell anywhere in the human anatomy. Medical instruments employing laser technology, microprocessors, and fiber optics may well be guided by the steady hand of robotics able to probe tangled webs of nerves or delicate layers of brain tissue.

One of the latest tools to come on the market employs a laser that is placed through a small hole in the skin and guided with a tiny video camera into a "slipped" or herniated disk in the back to surgically repair the problem. What is now an office procedure once required a large operation and an extended hospital stay. Although this treatment is still experimental and not yet widely used, it heralds an important advance in medical technology. It demonstrates that a laser attached to a tiny video camera can be sent to a space deep within the body, without major surgery or other risks. It shows that technology is limited only by our knowledge of what can be done with it—and that medical practitioners are well on their way to finding out exactly how these tools can best be deployed.

Enhancing the effectiveness of these tools will be improvements in imaging and scanning devices, enabling doctors to view processes and parts of the human body never seen before. Some of this equipment, like functional magnetic resonance imaging (fMRI), is already at work and is providing pictures that extend beyond medicine's current knowledge base. As often happens with scientific research, technological developments may be introduced before people understand all that the tool can do. Today, fMRI is generating pictures of the brain that scientists do not yet completely understand, and they are rushing to catch up with the technology. The same is true with the various scopes that are being used in pain medicine that enable scientists and physicians to peer into parts of the body previously hidden. In viewing the spinal cord through a highly sophisticated scope, I have seen what looks like fluffy white clouds. I am not yet sure of what it means, but soon I will.

Today's scopes and imaging instruments are like radar or night vision, enabling doctors to see where they never could before. When using the latest scope, I sometimes feel like an explorer going into a dark cave with a flashlight, shining light into corners and recesses I have never seen and trying to figure out what I'm looking at. I may have a rough idea of how the cave and its tunnels are laid out, but I still must orient myself and make sense of the small area illuminated by the flashlight. Every year, these scopes become smaller and more versatile, able to go further into the body and brain and capture images that are clearer and sharper. Their possible uses for treating pain are dazzling. Scientists already have pictures of what the brain looks like when a person is in pain and how morphine affects neurochemistry. I imagine in the near future that doctors will be able to watch on a video monitor a patient's brain as he ingests a drug, then adjust the drug or the dose based on how the brain responds.

DRUGS THAT WORK LIKE "SMART BOMBS"

Another facet of the advancing technological tide will be an array of new drugs. Already, three-dimensional computer imaging is helping scientists build designer drugs. Using this imaging, pharmaceutical manufacturers are now able to structure a drug molecule by molecule according to how the drug interacts with brain chemicals. Some of the new imaging technologies, like fMRI, produce live, moving pictures of brain activity and give scientists vivid, real-time pictures of how the brain reacts to drugs like morphine—potentially speeding up development of better drugs to combat pain. Using these devices, drug manufacturers will be able to engineer and modify chemicals to precisely target pain and tailor drugs according to how they affect brain activity. These can act like guided missiles, navigating through the body to impact only the targeted areas and leaving the rest unharmed by collateral side effects.

Big advances in drugs will come from finding new uses and combinations of existing drugs and developing entire new classes of drugs. New drugs will not only treat symptoms of pain but also block the destructive aftermath that can lead to chronic pain or produce intolerable side effects. Thus, pain medications are on the verge of advancing from controlling symptoms to promoting cures. As you know, opioids remain pain medicine's most potent drug, and so scientists are devising new formulas of opioids that have even stronger analgesic effects, but with many fewer side effects. Researchers are also beginning to understand the neurochemistry of addiction and drug tolerance, which will enable them to design better opioids.

Some of the new drugs most likely to revolutionize pain medicine may well come from psychiatry. A possible new category of antidepressant that blocks the pain-related neurochemical Substance P holds promise as a new pain medication. New classes of psychiatric drugs that combat thought disorders, such as schizophrenia, could also have a large impact on pain-related disorders. I am not implying that schizophrenia and chronic pain are the same thing, only that thought processing affects pain and that some of the safer new drugs may also combat the fear and agitation that so frequently coexist with, and magnify, pain.

New technology is also altering how drugs are inserted into the body. Needles and syringes may someday go the way of the typewriter. The current ways you take medicine, by pill or injection, have shortcomings. Anything you swallow naturally travels through the gastrointestinal tract and may irritate this system, as happens with many anti-inflammatories. A pill winding through the GI tract also sheds some of its active molecules and so loses potency. An injection bypasses the GI tract, but for someone already in pain, it introduces another level of discomfort, especially a series of injections. The new delivery technologies are using other routes into the body. Delivery of medication via nasal sprays, skin patches, and even lollipop-style applicators that send drugs directly through the walls of the mouth are already here, and coming soon are inhalers and needleless injectors that painlessly drive drug molecules into the skin at supersonic speeds. I've recently seen a prototype for a new way of introducing medication using electricity—the drug is pushed painlessly through the skin and into the bloodstream using an electric charge.

NEW SURGICAL FRONTIERS OF PAIN MEDICINE

At the far end of the technology rainbow are advances in brain surgery for pain. As you have read, defeating chronic pain by cutting nerves usually doesn't work for very long and can produce even worse pain. For this reason, most nerve surgery today that goes after pain is reserved for people who have a short time to live. But we've had previews of surgical procedures that, instead of severing nerves, target areas of the brain where the emotional side of pain resides. The brain surgery that dispelled Robert Evans's depression and crushing back pain, the cingulotomy, offers hope that someday doctors will discover exactly where in the brain pain and suffering lodge and be able to selectively excise it while keeping all other brain functions intact. Psychosurgery that erases physical pain and suffering is many years away, yet it is not a pipe dream. Someday doctors will understand the brain as thoroughly as they comprehend the heart today, and in the same way cardiac surgeons can operate on valves or insert pacemaking devices, the brain surgeons of tomorrow will use their instruments to dislodge pain at its source.

Low-Tech Weapons Against Pain

As technology speeds pain medicine toward a brighter future, another equally powerful force is helping steer the direction of treatment. This is the frontline, here-and-now side of pain medicine. Sometimes, doctors seem to believe that improving care requires developing new treatments. But the problem is often simply delivering the therapies that are already available to the patient. Doctors already have a very effective arsenal of drugs and other treatments for pain. But for treatment to work, it has to get to the patient. As simple as this may sound, a lot of manageable pain frequently goes untreated simply because the system doesn't recognize the problem or doesn't value the solution.

Today, nowhere is the application of our present treatments used more creatively and effectively than in the care of patients at the end of life. Palliative care and hospice programs are growing because they have harnessed a full spectrum of treatments and delivered them right to the patient and family in need. These programs use a grass-roots approach to treating patients who may be suffering and offer support to family as well as the dying in order to make the remaining time as positive and meaningful as possible. Discomfort and suffering are always addressed within the context of the patient's culture, family, and personal wishes. These programs bring commonsense solutions to situations that might otherwise become a tangle of frustration, or simply be ignored. The solutions are possible because a sector of health-care professionals ask about pain and are willing to consider all the variables that impact suffering. Hospice and palliative care programs have made a big difference for those at the end of life—and they have taught me a great deal about treating pain and suffering at every stage of life. As a model of comprehensive and human care, these programs are showing the rest of the medical community that treating discomfort with dignity and respect is possible for every patient in pain.

THE POTENTIAL OF COMPREHENSIVE CARE

Without a single new drug, injection, high-tech scan, or special laser, the future of pain medicine will advance by making present skills widely available. It will continue to push into other specialties, harnessing the experience and skills of physical therapy, psychiatry, behavioral medicine, and cognitive therapy. Concern about how a pain condition has affected a person's quality of life—from simple activities like walking to complex family relationships—will increasingly occupy the center of pain management programs. Symptoms that are usually part of pain but that are often dismissed as unimportant or overlooked by medical professionals will come under close scrutiny. In the same way that depression is becoming recognized as an unacceptable companion to pain, other symptoms of suffering, like fear and anxiety, will be tolerated less and less. Pain professionals—teams of medical doctors, psychologists, nurses, and physical therapists—will marshal their resources to defeat the emotional damage that usually accompanies pain. Their primary weapon will not be any single drug, procedure, or other intervention. It will be a collection of them all. Some of these therapies will be new, while others will be drawn from existing treatments that can be applied more effectively.

INTEGRATION OF ALTERNATIVE THERAPIES

It's difficult to predict exactly what role alternative therapies will play in the future of pain medicine, but the huge interest in such treatments—on the part of both patients and doctors—convince me that many will find a lasting place in the arsenal against pain. The popularity of many alternative therapies reflects the expansion of pain medicine into more humanistic realms. I think one reason people try alternative medicine is that they believe it's kinder and gentler than conventional medicine. Acupuncture has become widely accepted in pain management because of its safety, effectiveness, and lack of unpleasant side effects. Even though medical experts are uncertain why it seems to work for many people, they readily acknowledge that it's safe and seems to be effective. If you are in chronic pain, few pain specialists would quarrel with you if you wanted to try acupuncture.

The rise in alternative medicine is generating welcomed attention. As alternative medicine shoves its nose under the tent of conventional medicine, it is coming under increasing scrutiny, and this is going to benefit practitioners as well as patients. Scientists are starting to look critically at alternative remedies—herbs, supplements, unproven procedures, and unusual healing tools—subjecting them to rigorous testing and looking for results that can be replicated and verified. In coming years, you will be reading about these tests and studies. For instance, doctors at Massachusetts General Hospital are participating in one of the first double-blind studies of the effectiveness of acupuncture, and the results may help clear up the mystery about this ancient treatment. Another alternative treatment, a dietary supplement available as a pill in health-food stores that people say relieves the pain of osteoarthritis, is also under the microscope. The supplement, glucosamine combined with chondroitin sulfate, has receive lots of attention in the popular press and is now in controlled studies. So far, the results look very encouraging.

However, to me, stories about the curative powers of acupuncture and glucosamine highlight an ignored danger of alternative remedies. Advocates of alternative treatments seem to assume that they are both kinder and gentler—as well as highly potent. In the world of medicine, this is a flawed assumption. Potency is not a one-sided event; if a drug (and herbs *are* drugs) has enough muscle to knock out pain, then it will probably impact other systems in the body. Medical science has yet to find many drugs that are so selective in their chemical targets that they do not produce any side effects. Last week, I tried an over-the-counter herbal remedy to help me sleep. The next morning, I was so knocked out I had a hard time getting up. I don't know how it worked, but I do know that it was a strong drug. Had I also been taking other medications, there could have been serious interactions.

While alternative medicine cannot be dismissed as harmless placebos occupying the fringe of pain medicine, they do need to be subjected to laboratory and clinical tests that show if and how they work. If they are truly effective, I want to know that they work and are safe for my patients. If not, I want to be able to choose something else that does work. In a few years, I believe the safe treatments will be sorted from the dangerous, and they'll lose the adjective "alternative" as they become a part of my medicine bag. At that point, a new group of new "alternatives" will surely arise, and the cycle of experimentation and research will continue.

THE GROWING ROLE OF BEHAVIORAL THERAPIES

A vital part of a humanistic approach to pain medicine will be to harness the healing power within us all. Improved pain medicine will include more emphasis on behavioral therapies. The treatments used by some of the people I've written about, like Dr. Margaret Caudill and Dr. Daniel Rockers, will grow more widespread. Today, behavioral therapy is often viewed as a last resort. Chronic pain patients who are hurting despite months of medical attention and standard therapies give up looking for a cure and start to look for ways to manage their condition. They are often most frustrated by the loss of control in their lives. Behavioral therapy offers a treatment that demands a person's active participation in order to succeed, with increased control over pain as the reward. The patient becomes a full partner in the healing process by learning to control how his body reacts to pain, and how it mends itself. And, within a fairly short period of time, these treatments offer tangible tools that patients can use over a lifetime. I suspect that in the near future, the main goal of behavioral therapy—learning to control the body's response to pain—will be among the first steps for treatment, as basic to pain management as opioids are today.

CONQUERING PAIN: A CAVEAT

Pain medicine has a promising future for patients and doctors alike. It's not hard to envision a world in which chronic pain joins the ranks of other human plagues, like smallpox, that have faded into extinction. But before you celebrate the impending end of pain, recall the lessons of chapter 1: Pain is not only the enemy of our happiness, it is also our inborn defense system and evolutionary ally. There is a limit to how far pain medicine can and should travel toward complete eradication. Total and complete anesthesia, like that of Edward Gibson, the human pincushion, is not only impossible but undesirable. There are consequences to removing a natural defense system that is as integral a part of each of us as our brain and heart.

A world without pain is really a world without suffering. But pain and suffering are an inescapable and indispensable part of being human. Just as a cold rainy day makes warm sunny ones more special, physical hurt and psychic suffering add texture and depth to our lives. While everyone would like to diminish pain's impact, living completely without it would be a two-dimensional existence indeed.

Although medicine is a long way from manufacturing a drug that completely shields us from all pain, I wonder how far we want to go toward eliminating all unpleasant sensations and emotions. For example, as each generation of medication is better able to defeat depression, we need to ask ourselves where we're going. As a doctor, and as a person, do I want to witness the triumph of the ultimate mood drug that confines each of us to the same "normal" or even "happy" state of mind? In banishing physical pain, do I want to also vanquish any disquieting emotion that might make us suffer? I don't think so. Pain and suffering exist on a spectrum of human experience that includes pleasure and joy and as well as sadness and grief. These painful emotions are often telltale signs of important life issues that we may otherwise avoid dealing with. (Even "the blues" have an evolutionary purpose—to make us retreat temporarily from the fray and regroup after a setback.) The lives of each of us would be much poorer without this essential dimension of our humanity.

EPILOGUE
Making Peace with Pain

In war, diplomacy can be as powerful as brute force. We should never surrender to pain—but neither should we become too entrenched in combat to negotiate a truce. If you've been battling chronic pain, you may be locked in a struggle that's consumed precious months or years. Life is just too short to remain in a war zone any longer than absolutely necessary.

As a doctor, I negotiate with pain every day. So do my patients. We decide on a medication that may have side effects or procedures that have risks that are carefully weighed against possible benefits. We choose a therapy that limits rather than eradicates pain because it's noninvasive and reduces the pain to a manageable level. We recognize that each of us lives with pain, even if it's psychological suffering— career disappointments, romantic heartbreak, or the pain of watching a parent grow old and die. But we manage to find a balance between the inescapable suffering of life and the joys that make life worth living.

Total eradication of pain—even when it's possible—is not always the optimal result. For instance, a high dose of pain medication may totally subdue pain but might also dull your enjoyment of your relationships or your favorite pastimes. The difference hinges on recognizing what's most important to you in terms of your meaningful pleasures in life, and pursuing treatment strategies that keep those pleasures as accessible as possible. Complete pain relief may not always be a feasible goal, but having decent quality of life always is.

I hope you've come away from this book with a heightened understanding of how pain works and how many highly effective weapons we currently have that can combat it. Doctors no longer consider pain an inevitable and inescapable symptom of disease. Medicine has grown to respect the function and purpose of pain while increasingly taking action when its presence has no value. And as you look toward the future, you should be comforted by the accelerating pace of research and development of pain treatments that would have seemed impossible only a few years ago. I hope that by reading about how different doctors and patients have struck their own best deals with difficult situations, you can appreciate the importance of flexibility, creativity, and tenacity. In the end, we each fight our own war on pain. We don't make the rules, but the strategy and tactics are ours to decide.

We've made enormous strides in pain medicine over the past decade. But unless it remains a priority—and our society is currently embroiled in a fierce debate about our health-care priorities—we risk losing the benefits pain medicine has recently won for patients. Since pain is intrinsically subjective, its treatment will always remain vulnerable to neglect or apathy on the part of the bureaucracy that administers health care. So many of us will be afflicted by acute and chronic pain at some point in our lives that it would be terribly short-sighted not to maintain our awareness of suffering and invest in its comprehensive treatment.

The war on pain is being waged in many theaters: state and national legislatures, the researcher's laboratory, the surgeon's operating room, the clinician's office—and most of all, in the hearts, minds, and bodies of pain sufferers. While the future will be full of more weapons against pain, they will only be as valuable as our shared commitment to utilize them. The enemy in the war on pain is not just disease but also indifference. Making a difference for people in pain will require more attention to quality of life by all caregivers. Patients and doctors need to stand up and make it known that treating pain is important. Society must never lose sight of the inhumanity of allowing suffering to persist.

Major Pain Clinics in the United States

ARIZONA

The University of Arizona Health Science Center, Pain Management Services
1501 N. Campbell Avenue
P.O. Box 245114
Tucson, AZ 85724–5114
Phone: (520) 626–5119
Fax: (520) 626–3007
Email: bdavis@u.arizona.edu
Department Chairman: Steven J. Barker, Ph.D., M.D.
Director, Pain Fellowship Program: Bennet E. Davis, M.D.

CALIFORNIA

University of California, Davis Medical Center
2315 Stockton Blvd.
Sacramento, CA 95817
Phone: (916) 734–6824
Fax: (916) 734–6826
Email: dasyme@ucdavis.edu
Department Chair: Peter G. Moore, M.D., Ph.D. Professor, M.D.
Director, Pain Fellowship Program: Scott Fishman, M.D.

University of California at San Francisco, Pain Management Center
2255 Post Street
San Francisco, CA 94143–1654
Phone: (415) 885–7534
Fax: (415) 885–7575
Fellowship Information Email: randy-callahan@quickmail.ucsf.edu
Department Chairman: Ronald D. Miller, M.D.
Director, Pain Fellowship Program: Robert W. Allen, M.D.

Stanford University Pain Management Center
A–408 Boswell Building,
300 Pasteur Drive
Stanford, CA 94305
Phone: (650) 725–5852
Fax: (650) 725–7743
Email: gateta@leland.stanford.edu
Department Chairman: Frank Sarnquist, M.D.
Director, Pain Fellowship Program: Raymond R. Gaeta, M.D.

COLORADO

**University of Colorado Health
    Sciences Center**
Pain Management Center
4701 E. 9th Ave.
Denver, CO 80262
Phone: (303) 372–1650
Fax: (303) 372–1732
Department Chairman: Charles P.
    Gibbs, M.D.
Director, Pain Fellowship Program: Jose
    M. Angel, M.D.

CONNECTICUT

Yale Center for Pain Management
40 Temple St., Suite 3C
New Haven, CT 06520–8073
Phone: (203) 764–9170
Fax: (203) 764–9180
Department Chairman: Roberta Hines,
    M.D.
Director, Pain Fellowship Program:
    Lloyd Saberski, M.D.

FLORIDA

Mayo Clinic Jacksonville
4500 San Pablo Rd.
Jacksonville, FL 32224
Phone: (904) 296–5288
Fax: (904) 296–3877
Email: marshall.Kenneth@mayo.edu
Department Chairman: Tim J. Lamer,
    M.D.
Director, Pain Fellowship Program:
    Kenneth Marshall, M.D.

**University of Miami, Jackson
    Memorial Medical Center**
1611 NW 12th Avenue
Miami, FL 33136
Phone: (305) 585–6970
Fax: (305) 545–6753
Department Chairman: N.W. Brian
    Craythorne, M.D.
Director, Pain Fellowship Program:
    Vincent Pallares, M.D.

GEORGIA

Emory University Hospital
Allen H. Hord, M.D.
3B South
1364 Clifton Rd., NE
Atlanta, GA 30322
Phone: (404) 778–5582
Fax: (404) 778–5194
Email: allen_hord@emory.org
Department Chairman: John Waller,
    M.D.
Director, Pain Fellowship Program:
    Allen H. Hord, M.D.

ILLINOIS

**Northwestern Pain Management
    Clinic**
303 E. Superior, Rm. 360
Chicago, IL 60611
Phone: (312) 908–2500
Fax: (312) 908–3233
Department Chairman: Barry A.
    Shapiro, M.D.
Director, Pain Fellowship Program:
    Honorio T. Benzon, M.D.

IOWA

**University of Iowa, Department of
    Anesthesia**
200 Hawkins Drive
Iowa City, IA 52242–1079
Phone: (319) 356–2633
Fax: (319) 356–2940
Department Chairman: David L. Brown,
    M.D.
Medical Director: Richard W.
    Rosenquist, M.D.

MARYLAND

**Johns Hopkins University School of
    Medicine**
550 N. Broadway, #301
Baltimore, MD 21205
Phone: (410) 955–1818
Fax: (410) 502–6730
Email:slpancha@gwgate1.jhmi.jhu.edu

Department Chairman: Edward Miller, M.D.
Director, Pain Fellowship Program: Sunil J. Panchal, M.D.

MASSACHUSETTS

Beth Israel Deaconess Medical Center, Harvard Medical School
330 Brookline Avenue
Boston, MA 02215
Phone: (617) 754–2713
Fax: (617) 754–2677
Department Chairman: Leonard S. Bushnell, M.D.
Director, Pain Fellowship Program: Carol Warfield, M.D.
Director, Residency Education: Zahid Baiwa, M.D.

Brigham and Women's Hospital
75 Francis Street
Boston, MA 02115
Phone: (617) 732–6708
Fax: (617) 731–5953
Email: ross@zeus.bwh.harvard.edu
Department Chairman: Simon Gelman, M.D., Ph.D.
Director, Pain Management Center: Edgar L. Ross, M.D.

Massachusetts General Hospital Pain Management Fellowship, Department of Anesthesia
15 Parkman Street, WACC 324
Boston, MA 02114–3139
Phone: (617) 726–3332
Fax: (617) 724–2719
Department Chairman: Warren M. Zapol, M.D.
Director, Pain Center: David Borsook, M.D., Ph.D.

New England Medical Center, Tufts University, Department of Anesthesia
Box 298, 750 Washington Street
Boston, MA 02111
Phone: (617) 636–6208 or 6044
Fax: (617) 636–4674
Department Chairman: W. Heinrich Wurm, M.D.

Director, Pain Fellowship Program: Andrew W. Sukiennik, M.D.

MINNESOTA

Mayo Clinic
200 First Street, SW
Rochester, MN 55905
Phone: (507) 284–9694
Fax: (507) 284–0120
Email: wilson.jack@mayo.edu
Department Chairman: Duane K. Rorie, M.D.
Director, Pain Fellowship Program: Jack Wilson, M.D.

NEW HAMPSHIRE

Dartmouth Hitchcock Medical Center
Medical Center Drive
Lebanon, NH 03756
Phone: (603) 650–8391
Fax: (603) 650–8199
Email: leana.wiechnik@hitchcock.org
Department Chairman: D. David Glass, M.D.
Director, Pain Fellowship Program: Gilbert J. Fanciullo, M.D., M.S.

NEW MEXICO

University of New Mexico School of Medicine, Department of Anesthesia
Surge Bldg. 2701 Frontier St. NE
Albuquerque, NM 87131–5216
Phone: (505) 272–2610
Fax: (505) 272–1300
Email: sabram@salud.unm.edu
Department Chairman: Stephen E. Abram, M.D.

NEW YORK

Albany Medical Center, Anesthesia A–131
47 New Scotland Ave.
Albany, NY 12208
Phone: (518) 262–4302

Fax: (518) 262–4736
Department Chairman: Philip Lumb,
  M.B.B.S.
Director, Pain Fellowship Program:
  Howard Smith, M.D.

**Beth Israel Medical Center,
  Department of Pain Medicine &
  Palliative Care**
First Avenue at 16th Street
New York, NY 10003
Phone: (212) 844–1500
Fax: (212) 844–1503
Email: mglajchenethisraelny.org
Web: www.stoppain.org
Medical Director: Russell K. Portenoy,
  MD

**Cornell University Medical College,
  The New York Hospital
  (Tri-institutional Fellowship)**
525 East 68th St.
New York, NY 10021
Phone: (212) 746–2960
Fax: (212) 746–2023
Department Chairman: John Savarese,
  M.D.
Director, Pain Fellowship Program:
  Howard L. Rosner, M.D.

**Memorial Sloan-Kettering Cancer
  Center**
1275 York Avenue
New York, NY 10021
Phone: (212) 639–6848
Fax: (212) 717–3206
Department Chairman: Roger S.
  Wilson, M.D.
Director, Pain Fellowship Program:
  Richard Payne, M.D.

NORTH CAROLINA

Duke Pain Clinic
P.O. Box 3094
Duke University Medical Center
Durham, NC 27710
Phone: (919) 493–8829
Fax: (919) 439–7927
email: urban005

Department Chairman: J. G. Reves,
  M.D.
Director, Pain Fellowship Program:
  Bruno J. Urban, M.D.

OHIO

**Cleveland Clinic Foundation Pain
  Management Center**
9500 Euclid Avenue, U–21
Cleveland, OH 44195
Phone: (216) 444–2674
Fax: (216) 444–0797
Email: omabegb@cesmtp.ccf.org
Division Chair: F. George Estafanous, M.D.
Director, Pain Management Center and
  Director, Pain Fellowship Program:
  Nagy A. Mekhail, M.D., Ph.D.

OREGON

Oregon Health Sciences University
3181 SW Sam Jackson Park Road,
  UHS–2
Portland, OR 97201
Phone: (503) 494–3542
Fax: (503) 494–7635
Email: staceyb@ohsu.edu
Department Chairman: Harry Kingston,
  M.D.
Director, Pain Fellowship Program:
  Brett Stacey, M.D.

PENNSYLVANIA

**University of Pennsylvania Health
  System, Presbyterian Medical
  Center**
Suite 140, Medical Office Building
39th & Market Streets
Philadelphia, PA 19104–2699
Phone: (215) 662–8650
Fax: (215) 349–4616
Department Chairman: David E.
  Longnecker, M.D.
Director, Pain Fellowship Program: F.
  Michael Ferrante, M.D.

SOUTH CAROLINA

Medical University of South Carolina
171 Ashley Ave.
Charleston, SC 29425–2207
Phone: (803) 792–2322
Fax: (803) 792–2726
Department Chairman: Joanne M.
  Conroy, M.D.
Director, Pain Fellowship Program:
  Jeffrey W. Folk, M.D.

TENNESSEE

**Vanderbilt University Pain Control
  Center**
1211 21st Ave. South, Medical Arts
  Bldg., Suite 324
Nashville, TN 37232–4125
Phone: (615) 936–1206
Fax: (615) 936–1198
Department Chairman: Charles Beattie,
  M.D., Ph.D.
Director, Pain Fellowship Program:
  Benjamin W. Johnson, Jr., M.D.,
  M.B.A., DABPM, CIME

TEXAS

**University of Texas M.D. Anderson
  Cancer Center**
Box 42
1515 Holcombe Blvd.
Houston, TX 77030
Phone: (713) 745–0091
Fax: (713) 794–4590
Email: rpatt@earthlink.net
Department Chairman: Thomas Feeley,
  M.D.
Director, Pain Fellowship Program:
  Richard Patt, M.D.

**Texas Tech University, Health
  Sciences Center**
3601 4th Street–1C282
Lubbock, TX 79430
Phone: (806) 743–3112
Fax: (806)743–2984
Email: anepjb@ttubsc.edu or prithvi-
  raj@msn.com
Department Chairman: Gabor B. Racz,
  M.D.

UTAH

**University of Utah Health Sciences
  Center, Pain Management Center**
546 Chipeta Way, Suite 2000
Salt Lake City, UT 84108
Phone: (801) 585–7690
Fax: (801) 585–7694
Email: brobison@anesth.med.utah.edu
Interim Chairman: Dr. Michael A.
  Ashburn
Director, Pain Fellowship Program:
  Michael A. Asburn, M.D., MPH

VIRGINIA

**University of Virginia Health Science
  Center**
P.O. Box 10010, UVA HSC
Department of Anesthesiology
Charlottesville, VA 22906–0010
Phone: (804) 924–2283
Fax: (804) 982–0019
Email: jcr3t@virginia.edu
Department Chairman: Carl Lynch,
  M.D., Ph.D.
Director, Pain Fellowship Program:
  John C. Rowlingson, M.D.

APPENDIX B
Web Sites, Associations, Professional Organizations

GENERAL

American Chronic Pain Association
ACPA is a support and informational system for those suffering with chronic pain.
P.O. Box 850
Rocklin, CA 95677–0850
Phone: (916) 632–0922
Fax: (916) 632–3208
Email: ACPA@pacbell.net
Web: www.theacpa.org

American Pain Foundation
A consumer information, education and advocacy organization dedicated to helping people in pain.
111 South Calvert Street, Suite 2700
Baltimore, MD 21202
Email: ampainfoun@aol.com
Web: www.painfoundation.org

National Chronic Pain Outreach Association
Clearing house on chronic pain materials for physicians, sufferers, and family members.
P.O. Box 274
Millboro, VA 24460
Phone: (540) 862–9437
Email: ncpoa@cfw.com

The National Foundation for the Treatment of Pain
A not-for-profit organization dedicated to providing support for patients who are suffering from intractable pain, their families, and friends.
1330 Skyline Drive, #21
Monterey, CA 93940
Phone: (831) 655–8812
Fax: (831) 655–2823
Web: www.paincare.org

"Living in Pain Affliction: For Chronic Pain Sufferers, Even Hope Can Hurt," by Carl T. Hall.
Part One of a Two part series published by the San Francisco Chronicle, April 5, 1999
Web: www.sfgate.com/cgi-bin/article.cgi?file=/chronicle/archive/1999/04/05/MN37A1P.DTL

"Getting at the Molecular Roots of Pain," by Karen Hopkin. *The Scientist*, Volume 13, #1, January 4, 1999.
Researchers investigate how to eliminate difficult-to-control pain while leaving normal sensation intact.
Web: www.thescientist.library.upenn.edu/yr1999/jan/research_990104.html

SPECIFIC CONDITIONS

ARTHRITIS

Arthritis Foundation
Has written material; support groups; will provide list of arthritis specialists in patient's area.
1330 W. Peachtree Street
Atlanta, GA 30309
Phone: (404) 872–7100 or 1-800-283–7800
Email: help@arthritis.org
Web: www.arthritis.org

BACK PAIN

Back Pain Association of America
Has written materials; quarterly newsletters; six support groups in Northeastern U.S.; will refer to specialists/spine centers nationwide.
P.O. Box 135
Pasadena, MD 21122–0135
Phone: (410) 255–3633
Fax: (410) 255–7338
Email: backpainassoc@Fmsn.com

CANCER PAIN

Cancer Care, Inc.
Has written material; telephone support groups and counseling; will locate other community services in patient area.
275 Seventh Avenue, 22nd flr
New York, NY 10001
Phone: (212) 221–3300 or 1-800–813-HOPE (4673)
Email: info@cancercare.org
Web: www.cancercareinc.org

OncoLink
OncoLink is the first multimedia oncology information resource placed on the Internet. OncoLink was founded in 1994 by Penn cancer specialists with a mission to help cancer patients, families, health care professionals and the general public get accurate cancer-related information at no charge.
Web: www.oncolink.org

Resource Center for the American Alliance of Cancer Pain Initiatives
Has written material; videos/books for sale/loan; provides an advocacy network for cancer pain.
Univ. of Wisconsin-Madison, Medical Sciences Center
1300 University Avenue, Room 4720
Madison, WI 53706
Phone: (608) 265–4013
Fax: (608) 265–4014
Email: aacpi@aacpi.org
Web: www.aacpi.org

CHRONIC FATIGUE SYNDROME

American Association for Chronic Fatigue Syndrome (AACFS)
Promotes the stimulation, coordination, and exchange of ideas for CFS research.
c/o Harborview Medical Center
325 Ninth Avenue
Seattle, WA 98104
phone: 206–521–1932
fax: 206–521–1930
Email: info@aacfs.org
Web: www.aacfs.org

The CFIDS Association of America
Charitable organization dedicated to conquering chronic fatigue and immune dysfunction syndrome (CFIDS), also known as chronic fatigue syndrome (CFS), myalgic encephalomyelitis (M.E.) and many other names.
P.O. Box 220398
Charlotte, NC 28222–0398
phone: 800–442–3437
fax: 704–365–9755
Email: info@cfids.org
Web: www.cfids.org

HEADACHE PAIN

American Council for Headache Education
Publishes quarterly newsletter; other printed material available; books and videos for sale; 50 support groups nationwide; will provide list of physicians who specialize in headache.

19 Mantua Road
Mount Royal, NJ 08061
Phone: (856) 423–0258 or 1-800-255-
    ACHE (255–2243)
Fax: (856) 423–0082
Email: achehq@talley.com
Web: www.achenet.org

JAMA Migraine Information Center, The Journal of the American Medical Association

The JAMA Migraine Information Center is designed as a resource for physicians and other health professionals. The site is produced and maintained by JAMA editors and staff under the direction of an editorial review board of leading migraine authorities.
Web: www.ama-assn.org/special/
    migraine/newsline/newsline.htm

National Headache Foundation

Has written material; about 25 support groups nationwide; will mail list of physicians in patient area.
428 W. St. James Place, 2nd Floor
Chicago, IL 60614
Phone: (773) 388–6399 or
    1–888–NHF–5552
Fax: (773) 525–7357
Web: www.headaches.org

INTERSTITIAL CYSTITIS

Interstitial Cystitis Association

Founded in 1984, the Interstitial Cystitis Association (ICA) is a not-for-profit health organization dedicated to providing patient and physician educational information and programs, patient support, public awareness and, most importantly, research funding. The ICA has 100 support groups nationwide; will do physician referrals.
51 Monroe Street
Suite 1402
Rockville , MD 20850
Phone: (301) 610–5300 or
    1-800-HELP ICA

Fax: (301) 610–5308
Email: ICAmail@ichelp.org
Web: www.ichelp.com

MULTIPLE SCLEROSIS

National Multiple Sclerosis Society

Has written material; support groups and physician referrals through local chapters.
733 3rd Avenue
New York, NY 10017–3288
phone: 800–344–4867
fax: 212–986–7981
Email: info@nmss.org
Web: www.nmss.org

OROFACIAL PAIN

American Academy of Head, Neck and Facial Pain

Focus is on the diagnosis and treatment of TMJ.
520 West Pipeline Road
Hurst, Texas 76053
Phone: (800) 322–8651
Web: www.aahnfp.org

American Academy of Orofacial Pain (AAOP)

Offers a TMJ brochure for patients on-line.
19 Mantua Road
Mount Royal, NJ 08061
Phone: (609) 423–3629
Fax: (609) 423–3420
Email: aaophq@talley.com
Web: www.aaop.org

TMJ Association, Ltd.

Has written material; 29 support affiliates; hotline will refer to other patients; no physician referrals.
5418 W. Washington Boulevard
Milwaukee, WI 53213
Phone: (414) 259–3223
Fax: (414) 259–8112
Email: info@tmj.org
Web: www.tmj.org

Trigeminal Neuralgia Association
*Has written materials; 23 support groups
nationwide; telephone contact network of
patients: limited specialist referral.*
Claire W. Patterson, President
P.O. Box 340
Barnegat Light, NJ 08006
Phone: (609) 361–1014
Fax: (609) 361–0982
Web: www.neurosurgery.mgh.harvard.
edu/tna/

**"A Lifetime of Motion:
Temporomandibular Joints" by
Harold C. Slavkin, DDS, Director,
National Institute for Dental
Research, NIH**
Web: www.nidr.nih.gov/slavkin/
joint.htm

PERIPHERAL NEUROPATHY

Neuropathy Association
*A nonprofit organization established by peo-
ple with neuropathy and their families or
friends to help those who suffer from disor-
ders that affect the peripheral nerves.*
60 E. 42nd Street
Suite 942
New York, NY 10165
Phone: (212) 692–0662
Fax: (212) 692–0068
Web: www.neuropathy.org

RSD/CRPS
**Reflex Sympathetic Dystrophy
Syndrome Association**
*Has written material; about 100 support
groups nationwide; will send list of physi-
cians in patient area.*
P.O. Box 821
Haddonfield, NJ 08033
Phone: (609) 795–8845
Fax: 856–795–8845
Web: www.rsds.org

SHINGLES

VZV Research Foundation
*Has written material on Zoster/Shingles pain;
no support groups; no physician referrals.*
40 E. 72nd Street, 4B
New York, NY 10021
Phone: (212) 472–3181 OR (800)
472–8478
Web: vzvfoundation.org/index.cfm

SICKLE CELL DISEASE

**Sickle Cell Disease Association of
America, Inc.**
*Has written materials; will provide list of
physicians in patient area.*
200 Corporate Pointe, Suite 495
Culver City, CA 90230–7633
Phone: (310) 216–6363 or 1-800-
421–8453
Fax: (310) 215–3722

VULVAR PAIN

National Vulvodynia Association
*A nonprofit organization created in 1994 to
improve the lives of individuals affected by
vulvodynia, a spectrum of chronic vulvar
pain disorders.*
Executive Director: Phyllis Mate
P. O. Box 4491
Silver Spring, MD 20914–4491
Phone: (301) 299–0775
Fax: (301) 299–3999
Web: www.nva.org

The Vulvar Pain Foundation
*The Vulvar Pain Foundation was estab-
lished in 1992 as a non-profit organiza-
tion to end the isolation of women
suffering from vulvar pain and related
disorders.*
Prefer written requests for information
and $2 for S/H.
P.O. Drawer 177
Graham, NC 27253
Phone: (910) 226–0704
Fax: (910) 226–8518
Web: www.vulvarpainfoundation.org

CHILDREN IN PAIN

Cancer Pain Relief and Palliative Care in Children, 1998

New publication available from the World Health Organization

Web: www.who.int/dsa/justpub/just-pub.htm#Cancer

The Candlelighters Childhood Cancer

CCCF is an international, nonprofit, tax-exempt organization whose mission is to educate, support, serve, and advocate for families of children of cancer, survivors of childhood cancer, and the professionals who care for them.

7910 Woodmont Ave., Suite 460
Bethesda, MD 20814–3015
Toll-free information line: 1-800–366–2223
Or: (301) 657–8401
Fax: (301) 718–2686
Email: info@candlelighters.org
Web: www.candlelights.org

The Pediatric Pain Research Lab Web Site

Located in the IWK Grace Health Centre and the Psychology Department of Dalhousie University in Halifax, Nova Scotia, Canada.

Offers professional resources for health care workers caring for children in pain, resources for researchers, and self help resources for children in pain and their parents. Available in a booklet called Pain, Pain, Go Away: Helping Children With Pain, *by Patrick J. McGrath, Ph.D., G. Allen Finley, M.D., FRCPC, and Judith Ritchie, R.N., Ph.D.*

Web: is.dal.ca/~pedpain/pedpain.html

PAIN AT THE END OF LIFE

Last Acts Web Site

An online community dedicated to improving end-of-life care.

Web: www.lastacts.org

Last Acts Email Discussion Group

Health care professionals, educators, authors, clergy, and consumers discuss strategies on the national, state and local level to improve care at the end of life. To join the discussion, send an e-mail to join-lastacts-discussion@lists.lyris.net.

"In Search of a Good Death, Sometimes when Pain Holds On, the Greatest Challenge is Letting Go," by Carl T. Hall

Part Two of a two-part series published by the San Francisco Chronicle, *April 6, 1999.*

Web: www.sfgate.com/cgi-bin/article.cgi?file=/chronicle/archive/1999/04/06/MN55PAI.DTL&type=health

PROFESSIONAL ORGANIZATIONS/ RESOURCES

American Academy of Pain Management

13947 Mono Way #A
Sonora, CA 95370
Phone: (209) 533–9744
Fax: (209) 533–9750
Email: aapm@aapainmanage.org
Web: www.aapainmanage.org

American Academy of Pain Medicine

4700 West Lake Avenue
Glenview, IL 60025–1485
Phone: (847) 375–4731
Fax: (847) 375–4777
Email: aapm@amctec.com
Web: www.painmed.org

American Association for the Study of Headache

AASH is a professional society of health care providers dedicated to the study and treatment of headache.

19 Mantua Road
Mount Royal, NJ 08061
Phone: (856) 423–0043
Fax: (856) 423–0082
Email: aashhq@talley.com
Web: www.aash.org

American Pain Society

4700 West Lake Avenue
Glenville, IL 60025–1485
Phone: (847) 375–4715
Fax: (847) 375–4777
Email: info@ampainsoc.org
Web: www.ampainsoc.org

American Society of Addiction Medicine

A medical specialty society dedicated to educating physicians and improving the treatment of individuals suffering from alcoholism or other addictions.
4601 North Park Ave, Arcade Suite 101
Chevy Chase, MD 20815
Phone: (301) 656–3920
Fax: (301) 656–3815 Email@asam.org
Web: www.asam.org

American Society of Pain Management Nurses

7794 Grow Drive
Pensacola, FL 32514
Phone: (850) 473–0233 or 1-888-34-
ASPMN (342–7766)
Fax: (850) 484–8762
Email: aspmn@aol.com
Web: www.nursingcenter.com/
people/nrsorgs/aspmn

American Society of Regional Anesthesia

P.O. Box 11086
Richmond, VA 23230–1086
Phone: (804) 282–0010
Fax: (804) 282-0090
Email Asra@SocietyHQ.com
Web: www.asra.com/welcome.htm

Mayday Pain Resource Center

The purpose of the Mayday Pain Resource Center is to serve as a clearinghouse to disseminate information and resources that will enable other individuals and institutions to improve the quality of pain management. The MPRC is a central source for collecting a variety of materials related to pain including pain assessment tools, patient education materials, quality assurance materials related to pain,

research instruments used in pain research and other resources. The MPRC is a compilation of materials in use and disseminated by the City of Hope National Medical Center and Beckman Research Institute professionals and materials contributed by other individuals and organizations.
Web: mayday.coh.org

PainLink

A virtual community of health professionals working in institutions that are committed to alleviating pain.
Web: www.edc.org/PainLink

Society for Neuroscience

11 Dupont Circle, NW
Suite 500
Washington, DC 20036
Phone: (202) 462–6688
Email: info@sfn.org
Web: www.sfn.org

Talaria: The Hypermedia Assistant for Cancer Pain Management

Talaria provides interactive tools for healthcare providers to assist with managing pain in cancer patients.
Web: www.statsci.com/talaria/talaria-home.html

ADVOCACY GROUPS, PUBLIC POLICY

American Society for Action on Pain

Skip Baker
P. O. Box 3046
Williamsburg, VA 23187
Email: skipb@widomaker.com

American Society of Law, Medicine & Ethics

This is the Web Site of the American Society of Law, Medicine & Ethics. Presently, the Society is carrying out research on pain management.
Phone: (617) 262–4990
Fax: (617) 437–7596
Web: www.aslme.org

International Association for the Study of Pain
Louisa E. Jones, Executive Officer
909 NE 43rd Street
Suite 306
Seattle, WA 98105–6020
Phone: 206–547–6409
Fax: 206–547–1703
Web: www.halcyon.com/iasp

University of Wisconsin Pain and Policy Studies Group
The purpose of this Web site is to facilitate public access to information about pain relief and public policy.
Web: www.medsch.wisc.edu/painpolicy

MEDICAL RESOURCES ON THE INTERNET/WEB SITES

Medical Matrix Guide to Internet Clinical Medicine Resources
Web: www.medmatrix.org/index.asp

National Network of Libraries of Medicine
Dedicated to making the world's biomedical information available throughout the U.S.
Web: www.nnlm.nlm.nih.gov

Neurosciences on the Internet
A searchable and browsable index of neuroscience resources available on the Internet: Neurobiology, neurology, neurosurgery, psychiatry, psychology, cognitive science sites and information on human neurological diseases.
Web: www.lm.com/~nab

Online version of the journal *Pain*
The official publication of the International Association for the Study of Pain, publishing original research on the nature, mechanisms and treatment of pain.
Web: www.elsevier.nl/homepage /sah/pain

Systematic reviews on pain topics
Known meta-analyses/systematic reviews around the pain area.
Web: www.jr2.ox.ac.uk/bandolier/ painres/MApain.html

NEWS GROUPS

News groups are discussion groups about a certain topic. To access them, you need an internet browser with a News Reader (like Netscape or Internet Explorer) and your Internet access provider must carry access to these groups.

ARTHRITIS

alt.support.arthritis

CANCER

alt.support.cancer
alt.support.cancer.prostate
sci.med.diseases.cancer

ENDOMETRIOSIS

alt.support.endometriosis

HEADACHES

alt.support.headaches
alt.support.headaches.migraine

MULTIPLE SCLEROSIS

alt.support.mult-sclerosis

PAIN

alt.support.chronic-pain

RECOMMENDED READING

Back Pain: How to Relieve Low Back Pain and Sciatica, by Loren Fishman and Carol Ardman, 1999, W.W. Norton.

The Body in Pain: The Making and Unmaking of the World, by Elaine Scarry, 1987, Oxford University Press.

Care of the Soul: A Guide for Cultivating Depth and Sacredness in Everyday Life, by Thomas Moore, 1994, HarperPerennial.

The Culture of Pain, by David B. Morris, 1993, University of California Press.

Dying Well: Peace and Possibilities at the End of Life, by Ira Byock, M.D., 1998, Riverhead Books.

Freedom from Headaches, by Dr. J. Saper, Dr. K. Magee, and Kenneth R. Maggee, 1986, Simon & Schuster.

Full Catastrophe Living: Using the Wisdom of Your Body and Mind to Face Stress, Pain, and Illness, by John Kabat-Zinn, Thich Nhat Hanh (Preface), and Joan Borysenko, 1990, Delta.

Headache Relief: A Comprehensive, Up-To-Date, Medically Proven Program That Can Control and Ease Headache Pain, by Alan M. Rapaport, M.D. and Fred D. Sheftell, M.D., 1991, Fireside.

Headache Relief for Women : How You Can Manage and Prevent Pain, by Alan M. Rapaport, M.D. and Fred D. Sheftell, M.D., 1996, Little Brown & Company.

Healing Back Pain: The Mind-Body Connection, by John E. Sarno, 1991, Warner Books.

How We Die: Reflections on Life's Final Chapter, by Sherwin B. Nuland, 1995, Vintage Books.

Learning to Master Your Chronic Pain, by Robert N. Jamison, 1991, Professional Resource Exchange.

Making Peace With Chronic Pain: A Whole-Life Strategy, by Marlene E. Hunter and Marlene E. Hunter, M.D., 1996, Brunner/Mazel.

Managing Pain Before It Manages You, by Margaret A. Caudill, M.D., Ph.D., 1999, Guilford Press.

Mastering Pain: A Twelve-Step Program for Coping With Chronic Pain, by Dr. Richard A. Sternbach, 1995, Ballantine Books.

Natural Pain Relief: A Practical Handbook for Self-Help, by Jan Sadler with Patrick Wall, 1997, Element.

On Death and Dying, by Elisabeth Kubler-Ross, M.D., 1997, Collier Books.

Pain and Suffering, by William K. Livingston and Howard L. Fields, 1998, International Association for the Study of Pain.

Phantoms in the Brain: Probing the Mysteries of the Human Mind, by V. S. Ramachandran and Sandra Blakeslee, 1999, Quill.

Suffering, by Betty Rolling Ferrell (editor), 1996, Jones & Barlett Publishers.

When Bad Things Happen to Good People, by Harold S. Kushner, 1992, Avon Books.

Wherever You Go, There You Are: Mindfulness Meditation in Everyday Life, by Jon Kabat-Zinn, 1995, Hyperion.

You Don't Have to Suffer: A Complete Guide to Relieving Cancer Pain for Patients and Their Families, by Susan S. Lang and Richard B. Patt, M.D., 1995, Oxford University Press.

acetaminophen: a pain-relieving drug and the main ingredient in Tylenol.

acupuncture: a Chinese healing art in which thin needles are inserted in specific spots around the body to produce a healing effect, like reducing pain.

acute pain: an unpleasant sensation that results from recent injury, such as from surgery or trauma, and is short-lived.

allodynia: pain arising from something that normally doesn't produce pain, like a breeze of air or the touch of a feather.

analgesia: a drug or substance that eliminates pain.

anesthesia: a drug or condition that produces the general loss of sensation.

anticonvulsants: a family of drugs that prevents seizures in nerves and muscles and helpful in relieving some kinds of pain.

autoimmune disease: a disease that causes the body's immune system to attack its own tissue. Rheumatoid arthritis is an autoimmune disease.

Bier block: a procedure where pain numbing medications are injected intravenously into a limb (are or leg) with a tourniquet above the limb to keep the medication from flowing out of the limb.

biofeedback: a technique for controling certain body functions, like skin temperature and muscle tension.

barbiturate: a drug that depresses the central nervous system.

benzodiazepines: a family of drugs that are minor tranquilizers (includes Valium and Klonopin).

bupivicaine: a local anesthetic drug used for peripheral nerve blocks, epidurals and spinal anesthesia.

block: injecting a chemical to halt the transmission of pain signals almost anywhere in the body.

calcium-channel blockers: a family of drugs that block small channels on the walls of cells that are responsible for movement of calcium—an ion that can have profound effects throughout the body. Most are used to lower blood pressure but are also possibly pain relievers.

CAT scan (computerized axial tomography): x-rays from various angles that produce a three-dimensional picture.

casualgia: a kind of pain that feels like severe burning which is typically due to nerve injury.

caudal space: referring to the tail-end of the spine.

celiac: relating to the abdominal cavity.

celiac plexus: confluence of nerves that are responsible for many organs within the abdomen such as the pancreas.

central pain: pain that stems from the central nervous system, as opposed to the peripheral nervous system.

cingulotomy: a brain surgery used to treat unusual kinds of psychiatric conditions such as severe depression or obsessive compulsive disorder and which rarely may help reduce some kinds of pain.

cluster headache: fierce head pain that usually strikes middle-aged men and often occur at night. The headaches frequently come in groups, hence the name.

complex regional pain syndrome (CRPS): a type of chronic pain, also called reflex sympathetic dystrophy, marked by intermittently bluish/reddish skin tone, burning sensations, and loss of muscle tone.

dermatome: area of skin or part of the body connected to a particular nerve root and named according to its position on the spine. For example, the C1 dermatome emanates from the first cervical joint.

endorphin (beta-endorphin): a hormone the body generates which is similar in its action to morphine or opiates that can eliminate pain and produce euphoria. It is a member of a larger group called endogenous opioids; meaning opioids that are made within the body.

enkephalin: a kind of endogenous opioid.

epidural: refers to the space between the layer of tissue just outside the spinal cord.

epinephrine: a hormone of the sympathetic nervous system also known as adrenalin. It is a member of a larger group called catecholamines.

facet: one of a series of joints running down the spine which connect each vertebrae to the one above and below.

failed back syndrome: back pain that persists after surgery has tried to correct the problem.

fascia: a layer of connective tissue.

fibromyalagia: a pain syndrome that is diffuse throughout the body and distinguished by tender areas within muslces.

fluoroscopy: an X-Ray machine in the shape of a C-arm that wraps above and below the treatment table and enables a doctor to see precisely where a needle or injection is being placed.

Gate control theory: a theory about why some sensations are felt as pain and others are not. It suggests that a chemical "gate" into the brain regulates which sensations a person feels. This theory is now challenged by newer models of pain transmission.

herpes zoster: a virus that causes Chicken Pox afterwhich also lives quietly within us throughout our lives and sometimes reactivates to causeshingles.

ibuprophen: the generic name for a pain-relieving drug that is classified as a non-steroidal anti-inflammatory.

idiopathic: of unknown origin.

intercostal: referring to space between the ribs.

intrathecal: referring to of the fluid space within the spinal cord and brain.

intravenous: introduced into or situated within a vein.

ischemia: reduced flow of blood to a part of the body.

lidocaine: the most commonly used local anesthesic drug.

lumbar: refers to an area of the spine below the lowest rib and above the pelvis.

median nerve: one of the three major nerves in the hand.

MRI (magnetic resonance imaging): a kind of imaging technique that uses magnetic energy to create three dimensional images without x-ray exposure.

migraine: a severe headache frequently distinguished by sensitivity to light and nausea.

morphine: derived from the opium plant and one of the strongest pain killers.

musculoskeletal: referring to both muscles and skeleton.

myelin: an insulating fatty sheath surrounding nerve fibers.

myofascial pain: muscle pain stemming from muscles.

neuron: a nerve cell including all of its branches.

neuralgia: nerve pain along a nerve pathway.

neuritis: inflammation of a nerve.

neuropathy: a disease or condition involving individual or groups of nerves.

neurotransmitter: any chemical that carries messages between nerve cells.

nociceptor: a nerve that is receptive to painful sensations.

nocebo effect: a negative effect, like increased pain, produced by thoughts and emotions. The opposite of a placebo effect.

nonsteroidal anti-inflammatory drugs (NSAIDs): a family of drugs that block inflammation and also are potent pain relievers. These drugs include aspirin, ibuprofen, ketoprofen, noproxen and other similar over the counter and prescription medications (but not Tylenol).

norepinephrine: a hormone of the sympathetic nervous system associated with function of heart rate and blood pressure. It is a member of a larger group called catecholamines.

opiate: any drug made from opium.

opioid: any drug that acts like an opiate.

opium: extract from the opium plant.

PCA (patient-controlled analgesia): a device that allows a patient to regulate the amount and timing for receiving pain-relieving medication.

phantom limb pain: pain that feels like it's coming from a part of the body that's been amputated or otherwise removed.

peripheral nerves: nerves that connect sensory or motor organs to the central nervous system.

placebo: an effect attributed to a drug that is related to the idea of having taken a drug rather than the intrinsic pharmacological effect of the drug.

post-herpetic neuralgia: The chronic form of shingles caused by nerve irritation resulting from expression of the same herpes virus that causes chicken pox.

radiculopathy: pain that is caused by irritation of a nerve root as it exits the spinal cord. Such pain occurs in the area of the involved nerve called a dermatome.

reflex symympathic dystrophy: a type of chronic pain, also called complex regional pain syndrome, marked by intermittently bluish/reddish skin tone, burning sensations, and loss of muscle tone.

steroid: a family of chemicals that usually act as hormones in the body, meaning that they travel in the body to produce change in organs and tissue distant from where they are produced. These chemicals are also used as medications, each one with different properties that range from potent anti-inflammatory and pain relieving effects to birth control and muscle growth.

sympathetic nervous system: a part of the unconscious autonomic nervous system that carries signals to internal organs, blood vessels and glands and controls basic functions such as heart rate and blood pressure.

TENS (transcutaneous electrical nerve stimulation): a small electric device that diminishes pain by emitting a mild, electric current to the skin.

threshold: the lowest intensity of sensation that feels like pain.

tic douloureaux: a condition that produces sharp pain in the face due to abnormal firing of the trigeminal nerve. Also known as trigeminal neuralgia.

tolerance: the greatest intensity of sensation that a person is able or willing to endure.

trigeminal nerve: the largest nerve in the face and head.

trigeminal neuralgia: a condition that produces sharp pain in the face due to abnormal firing of the trigeminal nerve. Also known as **tic douloureaux.**

trigger point: an area within a muscle or connective tissue that transmits pain to a distant area called referred pain.

visceral pain: pain in an internal organ which is usually experienced as distant from the affected organ.

ACKNOWLEDGMENTS

I have been blessed with wonderful mentors, colleagues, friends and family, without whom I would have been unable to develop my career or produce this book. I would not have become a pain specialist, and possibly not a physician, without early guidance and kindness from Dr. Daniel Carr, a genuine authority on treating pain and a role model physician, scientist, scholar, mentor and friend. There are so many others who have influenced the approaches and types of treatments presented in this book and, unfortunately I can only mention a small minority of those who deserve my thanks. I must thank my former teachers and colleagues at Massachusetts General Hospital where I was privileged to train and work. These include Sal Abdi, Joseph Audette, Zahid Bajwa, Jane Ballantyne, Andy Billings, Onassis Caneris, Ned Cassem, Jeanette Cohan, Annabel Edwards, Donna Greenberg, James Groves, Steve Hyman, Alyssa LeBel, Jerrold Rosenbaum, Mei Sang, Milan Stojanovic, Donald Todd, Jeff Uppington, Warren Zapol, and so many others. David Borsook played a special role in my development as a pain specialist — he directed the pain program at Mass General for the later years that I was there and gave me opportunities for which I am grateful. Penny Herbert is an extraordinary clinician and kindred spirit who has convinced me, by her shining example, of the intrinsic healing power of special people.

Many others have been significant parts of my life and career, to whom I must thank for their support and inspiration. These include Tony Melchionda, Martin Roseman, Anne Hutchins, Raul Navarro,

Janet Bookey, Wanessa Risko, Ginger Wright, Rey Cordero, Vicki Reider, David Morris, Ana Collins, William Berg, Leon Specthrie, JoEllen Habas, Irene DeFelice, Jim Snyder, Anna Holmgren, Susan Cooney, and so many others.

I am now indebted to my present pain management family at The University of California, Davis. Dr. Peter Moore, Chairman of the Department of Anesthesiology and Pain Medicine in which I serve, has a remarkable vision of pain medicine and without his foresight, support and mentoring, I would not have been able to take this most recent advance in my career. I am privileged to work with a talented and committed group of clinicians who make my work easier and more enjoyable. In particular, I must thank Eugene Becker, Betsey Benkin, Joseph Condon, Dianna Copas, Martha Daschbach, Paul Duran, Marcia Figaroa, Aretha Gillis, Chris Harkin, Kay Harse, Jay Hendrickson, Paul Klein, Paul Kries, Kathey Lammers, Brian Mack, Steve Macres, Laura Mansouri, Sharon Melberg, Fred Meyers, Patty Morrow, Blythe Myers, Karen Pantazis, Aida Phelen, Claudette Prevots, Steven Richeimer, David Robinson, Daniel Rockers, Diane Siegal, Brian Smith, Debbie Syme, David Teichera, Kalle Verav, Barth Wilsey, and many others.

I also have to thank my new colleagues who have been instrumental in producing this book. Even prior to my involvement, Johua Horwitz took the original idea of a unique book about pain and suffering from its conception and has nurtured it to its completion and beyond. He has been a constant source of energy in this project. Gail Ross has been instrumental in fostering this book and allowing it to proceed smoothly. I was blessed with a remarkable editor in Gail Winston, who was able to see the potential in this project, and skillfully navigate through rough construction to a polished product. And this book could not have been the product it is without the critical collaboration with Lisa Berger. She added form to my perspective, translated endless amounts of medical technobabble and unfortunate metaphors, and made it possible for she and I to sculpt a formless block of knowledge and experience into a polished image that will hopefully be recognizable to anyone who suffers. Lastly, many thanks to Bridget Sweeney at HarperCollins.

My dear family continues to enrich and balance my life, without which I would be ill prepared to go to work. They are what make my life most worthwhile. In particular, I must thank my parents for their constant love and encouragement. There aren't words to fully describe how they, as well as Jodi, Jeff, Keith, Sarah, Darren, Jillian, Graham, Jarryd, Hannah, Gabriel, and Eliza mean to me. My rich immigrant heritage is personified by my great aunt Goldie, who fought for workers' rights in the 1920s and 1930s, and continues to teach me about the urgency of making the best of our lot in life. My grandmothers Annette and Ann were loving, strong-minded matriarchs. As a small boy, my grandfather Herman blew into my socks to warm them before he put them on me. He was a gentle soul from whom I learned about simple kindness. Without loud displays or declarations of affection, each of his grandchildren was convinced that they were his favorite. Through his kind gestures, I first knew unconditional love. I can only hope that some of his qualities are within me and find their way to my patients.

I must offer special thanks to the patients that have allowed me to tell their stories. While their specific identities have been disguised, they will recognize themselves by the essence of their experiences, which have been preserved. I have been most fortunate to be allowed into the lives of so many patients who have offered profound dimension to my life. I am indebted to all of my patients who have enhanced my life by sharing theirs with me and who never cease to convince me of the power of the human spirit.

INDEX